Community as Partner

Theory and Practice in Nursing

Community as Partner

Theory and Practice in Nursing

Second Edition

Elizabeth T. Anderson, R.N., Dr. PH., F.A.A.N.
Professor
University of Texas
School of Nursing at Galveston
Galveston, Texas

Judith McFarlane, R.N., Dr. PH., F.A.A.N.
Parry Chair in Health Promotion and Disease Prevention
College of Nursing
Texas Woman's University
Houston, Texas

With 17 Contributors

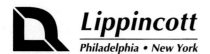

Lippincott
Philadelphia • New York

Sponsoring Editor: Jennifer E. Brogan
Coordinating Editorial Assistant: Danielle J. DiPalma
Production Editor: Virginia Barishek
Indexer: Impressions, a division of Edwards Brothers, Inc.
Interior Designer: Tenenbaum Design
Cover Designer: Anne R. Bullen
Production and composition: Impressions, a division of Edwards Brothers, Inc.
Printer/Binder: R. R. Donnelley & Sons Company/Crawfordsville

Second Edition

Library of Congress Cataloging-in-Publication Data
Anderson, Elizabeth T.
      Community as partner : theory and practice in nursing / Elizabeth
   T. Anderson, Judith McFarlane, with 17 contributors.
         p.   cm.
      Includes bibliographical references and index.
      ISBN 0-397-55088-X (pbk.)
      1. Community health nursing. 2. Community health nursing--Case
   studies. I. McFarlane, Judith M. II. Title.
   RT98.A533 1995
   610.73′43--dc20   95-14909
                                                            CIP

   The material contained in this volume was submitted as previously unpublished material, except in the instances in which credit has been given to the source from which some of the illustrative material was derived.

   Any procedure or practice described in this book should be applied by the health-care practitioner under appropriate supervision in accordance with professional standards of care used with regard to the unique circumstances that apply in each practice situation. Care has been taked to confirm the accuracy of information presented and to describe generally accepted practices. However, the authors, editors, and publisher cannot accept any responsibility for errors or omissions or for any consequences from application of the information in this book and make no warranty, express or implied, with respect to the contents of the book.

   The authors and publishers have exerted every effort to ensure that drug selection and dosage set forth in this text are in accordance with current recommendations and practice at the time of publication. However, in view of ongoing research, changes in government regulations, and the constant flow of information relating to drug therapy and drug reactions, the reader is urged to check the package insert for each drug for any change in indications and dosage and for added warnings and precautions. This is particularly important when the recommended agent is a new or infrequently employed drug.

   Materials appearing in this book prepared by individuals as part of their official duties as U.S. Government employees are not covered by the above-mentioned copyright.

9 8 7 6 5 4 3 2 1

For inspiriting Community as Partner, *we wish to acknowledge communities everywhere* . . .

> *public health service areas;*
> *rural villages;*
> *shelters for battered women, the homeless, refugees,*
> *and migrants;*
> *factories;*
> *urban neighborhoods;*
> *schools* . . .

and the nurses who work in partnership with them.

Community as Partner: Theory and Practice in Nursing
is dedicated to you.

Contributors

Doris F. Campbell, M.S., R.N.C.S.
Assistant Professor
University of Texas
School of Nursing at Galveston
Galveston, Texas

Judith C. Drew, R.N., Ph.D.
Assistant Professor
University of Texas
School of Nursing at Galveston
Galveston, Texas

John Fehir, Ph.D.
Program Evaluator
Houston, Texas

Sally Gadow, R.N., Ph.D.
Professor
University of Colorado,
School of Nursing
Denver, Colorado

Janet Gottschalk, R.N., Dr. PH., F.A.A.N.
Kate Hanna Harvey, Visiting Professor
of Community Health Nursing
Co-Director, WHO Collaborating
Center for Nursing
Bolton School, Case Western Reserve
University
Cleveland, Ohio

Charles Kemp, R.N., C.R.N.H.
Clinical Instructor
Baylor University School of Nursing
Dallas, Texas

John McDonough, M.A.
Manager, Aboriginal Health
Alberta Health
Edmonton, Alberta, Canada

Robert McFarlane, Ph.D.
Consulting Ecologist
University of Texas

Jean F. Mouch, M.D., Msc. in M.C.H.
Primary Care Health Services Research
Fellow
Department of Family Health
UMDNJ, Robert Wood Johnson Medical
School
New Brunswick, New Jersey

Rachel Rodriguez, R.N., Ph.D.
Assistant Professor
University of Colorado Health Science
Center
School of Nursing
Denver, Colorado

Carole A. Schroeder, R.N., Ph.D.
Assistant Professor
University of Washington, School of
Nursing
Department of Community Health Care
Systems
Seattle, Washington

Maija Selby-Harrington, R.N., Dr. PH.
Professor and Director of Research
School of Nursing
University of North Carolina at
Greensboro
Greensboro, North Carolina

Sharon Snell, R.N., B.S.N.
Manager Health Outcomes
Area Services—Calgary
Alberta Health
Edmonton, Alberta, Canada

Anita Tesh, B.S.N., M.S.N., Ed.D.
Assistant Professor, School of Nursing
University of North Carolina at
Greensboro
Greensboro, North Carolina

Karen Titanich, R.N., M.Sc.N., M.P.H.
Workforce Planning Branch
Alberta Health
Edmonton, Alberta, Canada

Mary Wainwright, R.N., M.S.
Program Coordinator
East Texas Area Health Education
Center
The University of Texas at Galveston,
School of Nursing
Galveston, Texas

Sandra Woodhead-Lyons, B.Sc.
Manager of Physician Manpower
Alberta Health
Edmonton, Alberta, Canada

Foreword

More than 20 years ago, Dr. Doris E. Roberts* had a dream. She envisioned a contemporary nursing role in which the skills of the professional nurse were combined with those of the community "detective," the epidemiologist. This role was to focus entirely on the community, the population, and it was to complement the individual-focused role of the nurse as caregiver. Critical elements of the role were identified, taught, and tested at the University of Texas School of Public Health in Houston through contract with the U.S. Department of Health and Human Services (at that time the Department of Health, Education, and Welfare) Division of Nursing. This pioneering work has been recognized as having contributed to nursing programs throughout the United States and other parts of the world; it truly blazed a trail for those teaching the community-focused role in graduate programs in nursing today.

Based firmly in the roots of public health nursing and the practice of public health nurses such as Lillian Wald and consistent with the tenets of the World Health Organization, this book continues the spirit of innovation seen in the authors' earlier work, *Community as Client: Application of the Nursing Process*. In *Community as Partner: Theory and Practice in Nursing*, they have captured not only the structure and process but also the "heart" of community health nursing as well. The authors provide the reader (nursing student, practitioner, teacher, or interested observer from another discipline) with the theoretical underpinnings of community work, in particular the concepts of primary health care, environmental health/ecology, ethics, epidemiology, and culture—all of which are surely critical for working in and with any community in the world today. One hallmark of the earlier edition, application of the community model to an actual community, has been

*Doris E. Roberts, R.N., Ph.D., F.A.A.N., Chief, Nursing Practice Branch, Division of Nursing, U.S. Department of Health and Human Services.

expanded to include a number of outstanding exemplars from places as diverse as rural Arkansas and the West African country of Ghana.

With its global focus, including WHO concepts of primary health care (and a look into the future provided by one WHO publication), and its incorporation of nursing and "detecting," I believe that Dr. Roberts's vision has come to realization in this book. As one of the people who assumed Dr. Roberts' mantle when she retired from the Division of Nursing, I can say with candor that the role she conceived is portrayed in *Community as Partner.* The authors have performed a real service to public health nurses everywhere by providing this "reader friendly" guide to the nurse's community-focused role.

O. Marie Henry, R.N., D.N.Sc.
Deputy Surgeon General, ret.
U.S. Public Health Service
Potomac, Maryland

Preface

Building on an earlier edition in which the community was characterized as "the client," we have expanded our thinking and elaborated the community-as-*partner* concept as the basis for nursing practice in and for the community. Key theoretical underpinnings of nurse/community partnership are delineated and illustrated throughout this edition. The nursing process provides the framework for a real-life, step-by-step, community partnership.

Part I: Foundations of Community as Partner

This section describes content areas basic to the practice of community health nursing. The areas encompassed include primary health care; epidemiology, demography, and research; environment and ecology; cultural competence; and ethics, an advocacy approach. Emphasis is on theory-based practice, with those theories critical to community health described and explicated.

Part II: The Process of Community as Partner

This section begins with a model for practice in the community. The model and one sample community are used to apply each step of the nursing process to the practice of community health nursing. The student is guided through the processes of community assessment; data analysis; formulation of a community nursing diagnosis; and the planning, implementation, and evaluation of a community health program. The emphasis is on understanding the community as a dynamic system that is both more than the sum of its parts and in continual interaction with its environment.

Part III: Exemplars of Community as Partner

This section provides a number of community "stories" in which nurses played a major role as partners in the promotion of health. Communities included are Ghana, West Africa; rural Arkansas; a refugee center in Dallas, Texas; Houston, Texas; migrants in Colorado; and Back Lakes in rural Alberta, Canada. Each narrative includes a description of the process of working in partnership with the community as well as a description of the outcomes of working together.

Part IV: The Future: Nursing Beyond the Year 2000

This section includes the outcome of an iterative project sponsored by the World Health Organization wherein nursing experts exchanged views on the future of nursing. Current global health issues are discussed, as are trends in nursing and midwifery. Concluding recommendations provide guidelines for community health nurses everywhere.

Elizabeth T. Anderson, R.N., Dr. PH., F.A.A.N.
Judith McFarlane, R.N., Dr. PH., F.A.A.N.

Acknowledgments

Community as Partner: Theory and Practice in Nursing could not have been written without the thoughts, critiques, and examples of our students. We thank each of you. Special thanks go to those whose work directly contributed to "Rosemont": Kathy Falkenhagen, Anne Stewart Helton, Mary Luckett, Carol Pyles, and Marianne Zotti.

For editing and editorial assistance, thanks for exceptional help go to Danielle DiPalma and Jennifer Brogan at J. B. Lippincott Company and Nicole Brogdon at The University of Texas School of Nursing at Galveston. One last note: Greg Everitt, the copyeditor at Impressions, made the often tedious work of proofing and checking references a joy at times: thanks.

Contents

Part I

Foundations of Community as Partner

1

Primary Health Care
The Foundation

Janet Gottschalk

Objectives

This chapter initiates the conceptual underpinning of the community as partner. As such, it introduces the major concepts underlying primary health care, which are the foundation for our work in the community,

> After studying this chapter, you should be able to
> - Describe primary health care
> - Understand the basic elements necessary for health in the community
> - Explain the need for a multisectoral approach in improving the community's health

Today, community health nurses, and their colleagues who work in communities throughout the world, are increasingly basing their practice on concepts such as partnership, collaboration, empowerment, human rights (especially for women and the most vulnerable populations), and above all, a commitment to social justice and equity. In addition, it has also become more evident to community health nurses that they must view their health-promotion efforts as being part of broader socioeconomic contexts and in terms of their relationships to global issues and concerns.

Introduction

In a time when national borders in their traditional sense continue to disappear and other barriers are being lifted, the interconnected nature of our world—and its problems—can be readily seen in the multiplicity of international, regional, and local efforts to solve these problems. At the same time, our world is much more politically unstable than it was during the Cold War, when identifying our "friends" and "enemies" was relatively easy. In addition, new forms of nationalism, ethnic identity, religious fundamentalism, and even fascism appear to be gaining ground and threatening people's earlier hopes for a "new" world based on peace and justice for all.

These same forces that are affecting political structures and their functioning around the world are also reshaping health issues, gradually transforming them from national and international concerns to *global* ones (Morgan & Mutalik, 1992). In addition, our understanding of what comprises "health"—whether local, national, or global—has itself changed.

Factors Affecting Health

Speaking in Geneva, Switzerland, at a recent World Health Assembly in which all of the sovereign nations of the world participated, Dr. Hiroshi Nakajima, the director general of the World Health Organization (WHO), identified the changes occurring in our understanding of health and its component parts as a "paradigm shift" (World Health Organization [hereafter referred to as WHO], 1991). As recently as 20 to 30 years ago, *health* was defined biologically and quantified in negative terms such as the "absence of death, disease, and disability." However, during the past two decades, it has become evident that social, economic, and political issues are additional essential determinants of a society's health. An especially strong link between a society's health and its economic development has been identified.

Also on a global scale, a phenomenon known as *epidemiologic transition* is occurring. This means that the poorest countries of the world, those already heavily burdened by communicable diseases like AIDS, cholera, malaria, and tuberculosis, are now also suffering from epidemics of diseases formerly regarded as primarily restricted to the industrialized nations, such as cancer, heart disease, stroke, and diabetes (WHO, 1993).

Another health-related global phenomenon is that many of those countries in which this transition is occurring are also being confronted with growing numbers of "displaced persons" (refugees) who are "escaping from persecution, environmental deterioration and economic collapse" (Blewett, 1993). In our Western industrialized society, these same displaced persons can daily be seen on our streets and in our bus and train stations. We usually call them "the homeless" and are often equally challenged to deal with these and other vulnerable groups who are experiencing "unnecessary pain and suffering from preventable diseases, economic deprivation, social isolation, violence, abuse, and war" (WHO, 1992).

Because of a deepening awareness of the multiple factors relating to a community's or society's health, persons concerned about the health of people throughout the world are today developing a new pragmatism. This pragmatism, based on traditional public health principles, is directed toward making the basic principles of democracy ("governments in which the people hold the ruling power either directly or through elected representatives" [Neufeldt, 1991]) and development the ground upon which communities can build healthy societies for themselves and their families.

Development, understood in economic terms, is usually considered to be a process of improving the quality of life, increasing economic productivity, raising standards of living, achieving greater political participation, and broadening access to basic goods and services (Rodriguez-Garcia, 1993). However, the *Human Development Report,* published annually by the United Nations Development Program, speaks of development as the "process of enlarging the range of people's choices" (1992). It is this broader understanding of development that is guiding the community health practitioners of today (and tomorrow) to work collaboratively and in a spirit of solidarity with communities as they seek better health.

Acknowledging people's and communities' needs for economic and human development that is sustainable, health practitioners everywhere are beginning to join forces in new ways that reinforce the dignity, self-reliance, and independence of all concerned (Blewett, 1993). They realize, of course, that in order to achieve the sustainable development that our fragile planet requires, the often exploitative relationships many people and societies currently have with the earth must change to mutually enhancing relationships. Such new forms of partnership will not only be more sustainable but will also become more equitable and participatory. Consequently, at the same time that the larger human community learns to care more for its environment, individual communities will—with these collaborative experiences—become more empowered to meet their basic needs.

If current trends are any indication, the peoples and nations of the 21st century will continue to face many of the same health-related problems that we struggle with today: poverty, hunger, unemployment, homelessness, illiteracy, racism, sexism, ageism, environmental deterioration, militarism, and human rights violations of all kinds from torture and death in conflict situations to the lack of basic necessities such as food, housing, and health care.

If one looks at recent history, many of these same problems, or their seeds, were evident in some form during the 1970s. At that time, many were hopeful (quite unrealistically, as it turned out) that the marvels of modern science, technology, and economics would usher in an era of continued improvements in health and human development to a world weary of war. However, by the mid-1970s, it became clear that only *some* of the world's peoples were benefiting from these new marvels. Just as is still happening today in much of the world, the gap between rich and poor continued to widen. And while the number of unmet human needs (and humans) was growing, the degree of social inequality in the world was increasing even more rapidly. In addition, health and development workers were becoming disenchanted with purely technological approaches to the problems faced by struggling communities. Reports of the failure of many development efforts based on purely economic principles were also beginning to make these workers seek alternative theories and methods of development that could assist peoples and communities in their struggles for a better life.

Primary Health Care

In their annual assessment of the world's health, delegates to the 28th World Health Assembly, meeting in Geneva, judged the current global situation to be both unhealthy and unjust (WHO, 1975). Numerous examples from different parts of the world convinced them that the use of an approach called *primary health care (PHC)* could contribute greatly to freeing all people from *avoidable* suffering, pain, disability, and death. They predicted that if sufficient political will and commitment on the part of the global community could be guaranteed, much of the massive burden of unnecessary illness and death borne by millions throughout the world could be prevented through the use of PHC (Bryant, 1969; Newell, 1975). These predictions led them to make the historic determination in a spirit of social justice to set in motion a new global revolution in health care.

Because of the global nature of the problem, a worldwide mobilization of personnel and resources was considered necessary. Two of the United Nations' specialized agencies, the World Health Organization and the United Nations Children's Fund (UNICEF), began immediately to coordinate the world's effort to study and implement PHC on a global scale.

As with all U.N. conferences, especially those of such magnitude, initial preparatory meetings were held in many parts of the world to gather additional experiences and to further refine the principles and basic elements of PHC. Although the majority of these meetings were held in what were then called the "developing," or poorer, nations of Asia, Africa, and Latin America, one meeting for the nations of the Western, or "industrialized," world was held in New York. At this conference, efforts were made to counter the belief that PHC was appropriate *only* for poor countries and not for the richer, more industrialized ones. A final preparatory meeting was held in Halifax, Nova Scotia, where nongovernmental organizations (NGOS)—ranging from large, internationally active humanitarian organizations to small religious groups active in only one country—were able to review the final draft of the actual conference document.

After such extensive preparation, delegates from 134 nations of the world, plus representatives from those NGOs officially accredited to the World Health Organization, met during September 1978 in what was then known as Alma Ata, USSR (now Almatay, Kazakhstan). In that historic meeting, the nations of the world committed themselves and their resources to the achievement of health for all by the year 2000 through PHC.

The *health for all* (HFA) era was from its very beginning based on the defining principles of social justice and equity. In Alma Ata, the original WHO definition of health, "a state of complete physical, mental and social well-being and not merely the absence of disease," (WHO, 1975) was revised on the basis of the newer understanding of health and its many component parts. According to WHO, health was now to be defined as "a state of enough physical, mental and social well-being to enable people to work productively and participate actively in the social and economic life of the community in which they live" (WHO, 1978). A major consequence of this new definition is that every nation is now challenged to provide a basic level of health for *all* its citizens so that they are able to lead socially and economically productive lives.

As determined at Alma Ata, the principal means by which this level of health can be realized is primary health care, which was defined as follows:

PRIMARY HEALTH CARE
- Is essential health care
- Based on practical, scientifically sound, and socially acceptable methods and technology
- Universally accessible to all in the community through their full participation
- At an affordable cost
- Geared towards self-reliance and self-determination

(WHO, 1978)

Although PHC was conceived as a global view, the issues addressed and the solutions adopted should be country-specific. This means that HFA visions should be both conceptualized and utilized within national and local contexts. As explained in the original *Alma Ata Declaration,* PHC

- Forms an integral part of both the health system and . . . the overall social and economic development of the community
- Is the main focus and central function of the health system
- Is the first level contact of people with the health system
- Is health care as close as possible to where people live and work
- Constitutes the first element of a continuing health process

(WHO, 1978)

Many of the concepts basic to PHC would be familiar to community health practitioners: prevention, universal coverage and accessibility, affordability, teamwork, priority setting to address the main local problems, effective management, community participation, and cultural sensitivity. However, building on the delegates' new knowledge and understanding, four additional concepts were identified in Alma Ata as *essential* to the achievement of health for all:

- Maximum involvement of people in their own health care and the development of their self-reliance
- Involvement and cooperation of persons and agencies from many sectors (housing, employment, environment, education, safety and transportation, communications, and so forth)
- Use of scientifically sound technologies that are appropriate, acceptable, and affordable
- Availability of essential medicines

As should be evident, PHC shifts the emphasis to the people themselves and their needs, thus reinforcing and strengthening their capacity to shape their own lives. Although hospitals and health centers will always be extremely important to people in their search for healthier lives, PHC is based on the principle that health begins where people live and work—that is, in their homes, schools, communities, and places of employment. Understood in its totality, PHC becomes not only a level of care but a philosophy and a strategy as well.

As a philosophy, PHC is based on the tenets of social justice, equity, and self-reliance. As a strategy, PHC bases itself upon individual community needs; maximizes the involvement of the community; includes all relevant sectors and agencies; and uses only health technologies that are accessible, acceptable, affordable, and appropriate. As a level of care, PHC is the one closest to the people; it relies on the maximum use of both lay and professional workers and includes a minimum of eight essential components, which will be discussed later in this chapter.

This shifting of emphasis away from dependence on health professionals and toward personal involvement, as well as the need for more than just improved health and medical services, was echoed again in 1986 at another international conference in Ottawa, Canada. The *Ottawa Charter for Health Promotion* defined health promotion as "enabling people to increase control over and improve their health." Repeating many of the same concepts identified at Alma Ata, the Ottawa Charter stresses that the prerequisites to health promotion include "peace, shelter, education, food, income, a stable ecosystem, social justice, and equity" (WHO, 1986).

Although representatives from 134 nations signed the original Alma Ata document, thus affirming their commitment to the goals of PHC, differences continue to arise over how the basic concepts of PHC should be put into practice in specific countries. In the United States, a relatively affluent country, many policymakers believed until quite recently that they could afford to emphasize optimum functioning and a "high level of wellness." More recently, it has become evident that the technologies required for such high-level functioning may be excessively expensive and more than the present system can afford. In addition, because so many millions of people have no access to health care or even health insurance, serious ethical questions are being raised regarding the maldistribution of health resources in the country. Others are beginning to question the appropriateness of U.S. health care priorities and the possible need to revise them. On the other hand, in areas where the burden of disease, poverty, and death continues while the resources for health care remain very limited, many nations are beginning to see the wisdom of adopting a PHC approach (Ulin, 1989).

The Eight Elements of Primary Health Care

The eight elements essential to the PHC approach should be seen in the light of the priorities identified at Alma Ata. Although applied differently around the world, they remain valid for all countries, whatever their level of socioeconomic development.

As envisioned at Alma Ata, the priorities in PHC should be

1. **Education for the identification and prevention/control of prevailing health problems.**
    This means that in countries such as the United States, emphasis should be placed on such health-related problems as violence (homicide, suicide, domestic violence), substance abuse, AIDS, tuberculosis, sexual exploitation, and high infant morbidity and mortality rates. Although these problems are found throughout the United States, they are often more prevalent in poor communities as well as among ethnic and racial minorities.

    In countries with much more limited resources than the United States, emphasis still needs to be placed on malnutrition, diarrhea, acute respiratory infections, and of course, the killer diseases of poverty:

measles, malaria, tuberculosis, and cholera. More recently, AIDS, sexually transmitted diseases (STDs), and childhood disabilities have also become major health problems in many of these same countries, often overwhelming their already limited health care systems.

In all countries, the education required to identify and prevent the prevailing health problems should also extend to health professionals, who may be more knowledgeable about the diseases treated in secondary and tertiary health care facilities.

2. Proper food supplies and nutrition.

First of all, because of the direct relationship between nutrition and illness, attention to the "food security" of communities is essential. This has become especially critical in many parts of the world where civil disturbances continue to exacerbate problems of drought and underdevelopment. Access to food, unfortunately, is now frequently used in many of the world's war-torn areas as a weapon specifically directed at civilian populations. However, lack of food or of the appropriate kind of food is not a problem only of the poor in Asia, Africa, and Latin America. Hidden (and not-so-hidden) forms of malnutrition, with often disastrous health consequences, can also be found in almost every country in the world today.

3. Adequate supply of safe water and basic sanitation.

A safe water supply and clean disposal of wastes are also essential to the health and well-being of any community. UNICEF reported that for more than 1.6 billion people, water "is a rare and precious resource" (1993a). Ian Steele (1993) also reported that 43% of the world's people, a great percentage of whom live in marginal urban and rural communities, are still without adequate sanitary disposal systems.

Once again, problems related to water and sanitation are also becoming more prominent in countries such as the United States where this had been thought to be a thing of the past. News of the inadequate disposal of toxic wastes, hospital syringes, blood products, and nuclear by-products has been routinely reported in the Western media. Unable safely and locally to dispose of the mountains of waste generated by their consumer societies, some countries are even attempting to dump these wastes in poorer countries that have less-stringent environmental regulations. Where this occurs, additional health hazards are being added to already overburdened economic and ecological systems.

4. Maternal and child care, including family planning.

UNICEF has played a major role in alerting the Western world to the enormous burden of disease and death that is borne by the world's children. However, in spite of decades of concentrated efforts to ameliorate this problem, it is estimated that throughout the world *35,000 children under the age of five still die in the developing world each day* (UNICEF, 1993b). What is even sadder is that the majority of these deaths could be prevented.

What is less well known is that the burdensome level of disease and death borne by the women of the world, especially during their child-bearing years, is also extremely high (Women's Environment and Development Organization, 1991). At the same time that women are demanding increased respect for their rights as women (including their reproductive rights), they are also calling attention to the needs of their entire families for PHC. Although no one questions that improved maternal and child health (MCH) care is essential for healthier families, it is important to realize that education, employment opportunities, an end to gender discrimination and the general empowerment of women may ultimately have more impact on women's and children's health status than specific MCH efforts. Women's groups and networks became an integral part of international deliberations at the U.N.-sponsored Earth Summit held in Rio de Janeiro in 1992 and at the 1994 International Conference on Population and Development in Egypt; they will no doubt continue to press for reform at the 1995 Women's Conference.

5. Immunization against the major infectious diseases; prevention and control of locally endemic diseases.

Great strides have been made in immunizing the world's children against the six major vaccine-preventable diseases. UNICEF and WHO report that their campaign for universal immunization against these killers is now reaching more than 80% of the world's children before their first birthday (1993b). However, the same immunization levels are rarely found among the poorer populations of the United States. In fact, some sections of U.S. cities have immunization levels similar to or lower than those of many of the poorest countries in the world (UNICEF, 1993a). Wherever they live in the world, children have the right to protection from the preventable suffering and death caused by the major childhood diseases. When their lack of immunization is compounded by poverty, malnutrition, abuse, and locally endemic diseases—what

UNICEF calls the "silent" emergencies—children have little hope of living "socially and economically productive lives" as adults. These silent emergencies are in addition to the "loud" emergencies we see reflected in the faces of suffering children from Somalia, Sudan, and the former Yugoslavia each night on our television screens (UNICEF, 1993c).

In addressing the main health problems not just of the community's children but of the community as a whole, a PHC approach requires the provision of appropriate "promotive, preventive, curative, and rehabilitative services." Where and when this cannot be done locally, referral should be made to "integrated, functional and mutually-supportive referral systems, leading to the progressive improvement of comprehensive care for all . . . giving priority to those most in need" (WHO, 1978). Hospitals and health professionals who work in tertiary care facilities have, unfortunately, often misunderstood their role in the provision of PHC. Secondary and tertiary care facilities, as well as more complex rehabilitative and long-term care facilities, *do* have a critical role to play in the provision of PHC. Without adequate backup and referral systems, PHC—at the local level—will ultimately fail (Aga Khan Foundation, 1982). Likewise, effective management practices are also critically important for the development of successful PHC systems. Without such management systems, valuable human and financial resources are used poorly.

6. Appropriate treatment of common diseases using appropriate technology.

Over and over again, community workers of all kinds have found that simple, affordable technologies, often produced locally, can be extremely effective in easing common health problems. "Technologies" can be as simple, yet scientifically sound, as oral rehydration solutions for diarrhea or orthopedic aids built of local materials to give mobility and independence to a community's disabled members. Other health workers and communities have found the use of herbal medicines and alternative healing methods—ranging from acupuncture/acupressure to Ayurvedic and "New Age" practices—as effective in the treatment of common illnesses as their more expensive counterparts (Health Action Information Network, 1992). There is an extreme need for additional research in this area. Although such research is not currently viewed as equal in status to more sophisticated biomedical studies and therefore receives less funding, it is gradually (and fortunately) receiving more support and acceptance.

At all levels, the appropriate treatment of common diseases relies on the appropriate mix of health workers. This means that the PHC health team may include not only physicians, nurses, midwives, and auxiliaries but also community health workers (agents, promotoras de salud, and so on) and traditional practitioners (herbalists, curanderos, shamans). When such nontraditional members are added to the health team, care should be exercised in their selection, training, and ongoing supervision. Whatever the makeup of the local health team, the goal should be to concentrate on the expressed needs of the community and to work with it in achieving its health-related goals.

7. Promotion of mental health.

Although not included as an essential element of PHC in all countries, the promotion of mental health is extremely important for the well-being of any community. Working together with the community from a proactive stance, the PHC team should concentrate on those mental health problems that are preventable and can lead to more serious mental and emotional concerns. Assistance from and collaboration with many other disciplines and civic groups active in the broader community are usually crucial in such efforts. In communities where persons and groups have often been treated more like "objects than subjects" (Freire, 1982) and have become dependent on welfare systems, the involvement and mobilization of the community in meeting its needs may contribute positively to the mental health of many of its members.

8. Provision of essential drugs.

WHO has long been convinced that the adequate provision of essential drugs at a cost that the community can afford is critical to the success of PHC. Efforts to identify and permit the sale of *only* those drugs that are essential for a nation's PHC system have, however, met with great opposition from many in the pharmaceutical industry as well as from many health professionals. Appropriate treatment requires the provision of essential drugs that are safe and effective; of high quality; capable of being adequately supplied, stored, and distributed; and of course, affordable. To achieve this, the pharmaceutical industry, health professionals, community, schools, universities, and governments must all collaborate and cooperate. An effective drug marketing and distribution policy has, fortunately, become reality in countries such as Kenya, Uganda, and Bangladesh (not the United States). However, attaining this goal, like other goals of PHC, will require political will and commitment.

In addition to the provision of essential drugs, many countries are studying the use of herbal and other traditional medicines and treatments in PHC (le Grand & Wondergem, n.d.).

It should be obvious that although PHC builds on traditional public health practice, its emphasis on community participation, a multisectoral approach, the use of appropriate technologies, and the availability of essential drugs adds new dimensions to community health efforts, bringing additional challenges to all those who are involved.

Primary Care or Primary Health Care?

In the United States, the terms *primary care* and *primary health care* are often used interchangeably, but they do not always mean the same thing. In reality, the latter term, as used in the United States, frequently does not include all of the elements deemed essential at Alma Ata. One example of this difference of understanding can be found in *Report of a Study: A Manpower Policy for Primary Health Care* (Institute of Medicine, 1978). The report identified four factors considered absolutely necessary for the practice of good primary care: accessibility, comprehensiveness, coordination, and continuity. It emphasized comprehensive health care, professional attention by accountable providers, and the provision of personal health services at the primary level (Franks, Nutting, & Clancy, 1993). This form of primary health care, although it includes fundamental components of PHC as defined at Alma Ata, unfortunately excludes public health services as well as environmental and occupational health services and makes no mention of community participation. When PHC is discussed outside the United States, the Alma Ata definition of PHC is more frequently used. Given the commitment of the majority of nations to this version of PHC, U.S. nurses and other health personnel who wish to work in the changing health scene in the United States as well as in other countries must thoroughly understand the dimensions of PHC as identified at Alma Ata. It is especially critical that U.S. nurse educators include them in nursing curricula at all levels (Pew Health Professions Commission, 1993).

Health for All Through Primary Health Care

Ten years after Alma Ata, a meeting of international health experts was held in Riga, Latvia, to evaluate the progress made toward achieving the goal of health for all by the year 2000. Although it was clearly evident that efforts toward this goal would have to be ongoing, the ethical precepts, political imperatives, and technical directions identified at Alma Ata were reaffirmed. Health for all was confirmed as a permanent goal for the nations of the world. Some of the specific goals set at Riga relate to the need for intensified social and political action, the renewal and strengthening of PHC strategies, the development and mobilization of leadership, increased participation of people, and sustained intersectoral collaboration (Bryant, 1988).

Since the Riga conference, the world has continued to change at a rapid pace. Political and economic realignments, social and demographic changes, and the continuation of armed conflicts—with their disastrous health and environmental consequences—have added a new urgency to the world's need for more justice and equity.

At the U.N. Conference on the Environment and Development (UNCED) held in June 1992, delegates, aware of the critical issues facing our communities and the planet, urgently affirmed that

> Humanity is at a defining moment in history.
>   We are confronted with a perpetuation of disparities
>   between and within nations,
>   A worsening of poverty, hunger, ill health and illiteracy,
>   and the continuing deterioration of the
>   Ecosystems on which we depend for our well-being.
>
> *(UNCED, 1992)*

Building on the principles expressed in WHO's goal of making it possible for all to "lead socially and economically productive lives," UNCED emphasized that human beings are the center of concern for sustainable development and are entitled to healthy and productive lives in harmony with nature.

The need for partnerships has never been more critical. As Dr. Nakajima stated at the 46th World Health Assembly (1993), "Together we can herald a world in which health is an unquestionable human right." Because it is evident that no single entity can do the job alone, he proposed a new partnership that "implies a new social covenant, a new international bargain. It means mutual responsibility, respect and sharing."

Communities that are empowered to choose health strategies based on appropriate information and that have access to local resources and support as well as the needed institutional, organizational, and social approval will be integral elements in such a partnership, in which the range of people's choices will be widened (McMurray, 1991; American Public Health Association, 1993; Morgan & Mutalik, 1992; International Council of Nurses, 1988). One of the many ways in which U.S. communities are formalizing these new relationships is through the Healthy Cities movement (Flynn, 1992), which "brings together politicians, scientists, health professionals, educators, business people, and community people to be a unified force for health" (Asvall, 1992).

The Nurse and Primary Health Care

Where is nursing's role in the creation and strengthening of these new partnerships? Nurses, especially in the United States, have also been undergoing a paradigm shift in their practices, moving from a medical/curative orientation to one of prevention and health promotion. Increasingly active in policy arenas, nurses are also forming new broad-based partnerships with communities and organizations at local, regional, and national levels. Community health nurses have always been active in these arenas, but today their role is even more important (Mason, Talbott, & Leavitt, 1993).

In speaking of PHC as one of the social phenomena of our times with a powerful potential for improving the quality of human life, Dr. Halfdan Mahler, the former director general of WHO, identified nurses as leading the way in PHC: "Millions of nurses throughout the world hold the key to an acceptance and expansion of primary health care because they work closely with people, whether they are community health nurses in the Amazon rainforests or intensive care nurses in a heart transplant unit." During the same WHO executive board meeting, Dr. Mahler predicted that the role of nurses would change, moving more from the hospital to the community; become more innovative; entail greater responsibility; and become more involved in program planning and legislation (Mahler, 1985).

His prediction that nurses would increase their community involvement has now become a reality. The process of "enabling people to increase control over and to improve their health" is now an integral part of nursing's role. This new partnership, involving nurses, communities, and their environments, is a common search, based on personal choice and social responsibility, for a healthier future (Maglacas, 1988).

REFERENCES

Aga Khan Foundation. (1982). World health organization: The role of hospitals in primary health care. Report of a conference held in Karachi, Pakistan, November 1981. Geneva, Switzerland: Author.

American Public Health Association. (1993, July). APHA's vision: Public health and a reformed health care system [Editorial]. *The Nation's Health, 23,* p. 9.

Asvall, J. (1992, June). Copenhagen Healthy Cities symposium focuses on healthy public policy. In *Copenhagen healthy cities conference.* Conference conducted in Copenhagen, Denmark.

Blewett, J. (1993). In G. Barney (Ed.), *Global 2000 revisited.* Arlington, Virginia: Public Interest Publications.

Bryant, J. (1969). *Health and the developing world.* Ithaca, New York: Cornell University Press.

————. (1988, August–September). Ten years after Alma Ata. *World Health.*

Flynn, B. (1992, April). Healthy Cities: A model of community change. *Family and Community Health.*

Franks, P., Nutting, P., & Clancy, C. (1993). Health care reform, primary care, and the need for research. *JAMA, 270*(12), 449–453.

Freire, P. (1982). *Pedagogy of the oppressed.* New York: Continuum Press.

Health Action Information Network (HAIN). (1992, October). Traditional medical practitioners in the Philippines. *Health Alert* #134. Manila.

Institute of Medicine, Division of Health, Manpower, and Resources Development. (1978). *Report of a study: A manpower policy for primary health care.* Washington, DC: National Academy of Sciences.

International Council of Nurses. (1988). *Nursing and primary health care: A unified force.* Geneva, Switzerland: Author.

leGrand, A., & Wondergem, P. (n.d.). Herbal Medicine and health promotion: A comparative study of herbal drugs in primary health care. Amsterdam: Royal Tropical Institute.

Maglacas, A.M. (1988). Health for all: Nursing's role. *Nursing Outlook, 36*(2), 66–71.

Mahler, H. (1985, October). Nurses lead the way. *The New Zealand Nursing Journal.*

Mason, D.J., Talbott, S.W. & Leavitt, J.K. (1993). *Policy and politics for nurses.* Philadelphia: W.B. Saunders Company.

McMurray, A. (1991). Advocacy for community self-improvement. *International Nursing Review, 38*(1), 19–21.

Morgan, R.E., & Mutalik, G. (1992). Bringing international health back home. A policy paper for the 19th annual conference of the National Council for International Health, Washington, DC.

Neufeldt, V. (Ed.) (1992). *Webster's New World dictionary of American English.* Englewood Cliffs, NJ: Prentice-Hall.

Newell, K.W. (Ed.) (1975). Health by the people. Geneva, Switzerland: World Health Organization.

Pew Health Professions Commission. (1993). Health professions education for the future: Schools in service to the nation. San Francisco: UCSF Center for Health Professions.

Rodriguez-Garcia, R. (1992, August). Health and development: Revitalizing the link. *Health Link (NCIH).* Washington, DC.

Steele, Ian. (1993, August–September). Water and sanitation: Governments and donors must change priorities. *First Call for Children, 3.*

Ulin, P.R. (1989). Global collaboration in primary health care. *Nursing Outlook, 37*(3).

United Nations Children's Fund (UNICEF). (1993a, July–September). Setting the water standard. *First Call for Children, 3.*

———. (1993b). The state of the world's children 1993. Oxford: Oxford University Press.

———. (1993c). UNICEF annual report 1993. New York: Author.

United Nations Conference on Environment and Development (UNCED). (1992). Proceedings of "Earth Summit." Rio de Janeiro, Brazil, 1992.

United Nations Development Program (UNDP). (1992). Human development report 1992. Oxford: Oxford University Press.

Women's Environment and Development Organization (WEDO). (1991). *Women's Action Agenda 21.* New York, NY.

World Health Organization. (1975). Official records, Twenty-Eighth World Health Assembly. Geneva, Switzerland: Author.

———. (1978, September). Report of the International Conference on Primary Health Care, held in Alma Ata, USSR. Geneva, Switzerland: Author.

———. (1986). Ottawa charter for health promotion. Developed at an International Conference on Health Promotion. Ottawa, Ontario, Canada: Author.

———. (1991). Report of the 44th World Health Assembly. 1991. Geneva, Switzerland, 1991.

———. (1992). Forty-Fifth World Health Assembly, agenda item 30.1. Collaboration within the United Nations system: General matters: Health and development. Geneva, Switzerland: Author.

———. (1993). WHO director general calls for a new partnership on health. Press Release WHA/4. Geneva, Switzerland: Author.

2

Epidemiology, Demography, and Research

Maija Selby-Harrington
Anita S. Tesh

Objectives

To assess community health needs and to plan, implement, and evaluate programs to meet those needs, the community health professional must understand basic concepts in epidemiology, demography, and research. This chapter will help you to

- Interpret and use basic epidemiologic, demographic, and statistical measures of community health
- Apply principles of epidemiology, demography, and research to your practice in community health

The EPSDT study described in this chapter was supported by grants from the Agency for Health Care Policy and Research of the U.S. Public Health Service (Grant Number RO1 HS 06507); the United Way of North Carolina; the Gamma Zeta Chapter of Sigma Theta Tau; the University of North Carolina at Greensboro; and the University of North Carolina at Chapel Hill. The study received the Region 7 (Southeastern United States) Research Utilization Award for Sigma Theta Tau, the international honor society for nursing.

Introduction

Epidemiology and *demography* are sciences for studying population health; *research* is a structured process for acquiring new knowledge. To restore, maintain, and promote the health of populations, the community health professional integrates and applies concepts from these fields. In this chapter, we will explore the meaning and usefulness of these concepts and apply them to an actual community health investigation.

Research

Research is a systematic process for obtaining new knowledge through examination of data and empirical testing of hypotheses. The term *research* may conjure images of the laboratory scientist applying treatments to test tubes. In community health, research is more likely to deal with populations as they exist in natural settings. This chapter explains why research is essential to community health practice.

Demography

Demography (literally, "writing about the people," from the Greek *demos* [people] and *graphos* [writing]) is the science of human populations and is concerned with population size, characteristics, and change. Examples of demographic studies—that is, *demographic research*—are descriptions and comparisons of populations according to such characteristics as age; race; sex; socioeconomic status; geographic distribution; and birth, death, marriage, and divorce patterns. Demographic studies often have health implications that may or may not be addressed by the investigators. The census of the United States population is an example of a comprehensive descriptive demographic study that is conducted every 10 years.

Epidemiology

Epidemiology ("the study of what is upon the people," from the Greek *logos* [study], *demos* [people], and *epi* [upon]) is the science of population health. Epidemiology incorporates concepts from demography and research as they relate to health and illness and investigates the characteristics, distribution, and determinants of health conditions. Epidemiology overlaps with demography, and epidemiologic methods are special research methods. Epidemiologic studies sometimes take on the intrigue of detective stories as the investigators track the factors associated with illness and death. In fact, a number of novels concerning epidemiologic studies have become popular classics. (Try *The Black Death* [Cravens & Mair, 1977], *The Andromeda Strain* [Crichton, 1969], and *The Scourge* [Dunne, 1978].)

Early epidemiologic studies were concerned chiefly with the control of epidemics. (An *epidemic* is an outbreak of an illness beyond the levels expected in a population.) John Snow's study of a cholera epidemic in London in 1853 is a classic in epidemiologic history. At that time, the mode of transmission of cholera was unknown. Snow suspected it was spread by contaminated water. Applying epidemiologic principles, Snow determined that death rates from cholera were highest in areas served by two specific water pumping systems. He learned that the water from these systems came from portions of the Thames River in which London sewage was discharged. Thus, this early epidemiologist was able to identify a waterborne mode of transmission of cholera and determine measures to control its spread (Snow, 1936).

Contemporary Community Health Research and Practice

Today, advanced epidemiologic and demographic measures and research methods are used not only to study disorders such as food poisoning and acquired immune deficiency syndrome (AIDS) but also to investigate environmental conditions, lifestyles, health-promotion strategies, and other factors that influence health. This chapter provides an introduction to epidemiologic, demographic, and research concepts that are useful for the practice of community health. If you need more in-depth study, numerous textbooks are available (for example, Lilienfeld & Stolley, 1994; Mausner & Kramer, 1985; Polit & Hungler, 1991; Singleton, Straits, & Straits, 1993).

Levels of Prevention in Community Health Practice

The concept of *prevention* is a key component of modern community health practice. In popular terminology, prevention means warding off an event before it occurs. In community health practice, we consider three levels of prevention: primary, secondary, and tertiary.

Primary prevention involves true avoidance of an illness or adverse health condition through health-promotion activities and protective actions. Primary prevention encompasses a vast array of areas, including nutrition, hygiene, sanitation, immunization, environmental protection, and general health education, to name but a few. Research into the causes of health problems provides the basis for primary prevention. For example, just as Snow's 1853 investigation of cholera paved the way for provision of pure water to the residents of London, modern research into motor vehicle accidents has led to seat belts and air bags.

Secondary prevention is the early detection and treatment of adverse health conditions. Secondary prevention may result in the cure of illnesses that would be incurable at later stages, the prevention of complications and disability, and confinement of the spread of communicable diseases. An important component of secondary prevention is *screening,* the examination of asymptomatic individuals for disorders such as tuberculosis, diabetes, and hypertension. Screening methods are developed through research.

Tertiary prevention is employed after diseases or events have already resulted in damage to individuals. The purpose of tertiary prevention is to limit disability and to rehabilitate or restore the affected individuals to their maximum possible capacities. Examples of tertiary prevention include provision of "meals on wheels" for the homebound, physical therapy services for stroke victims, and mental health counseling for rape victims.

To plan appropriate methods of primary, secondary, and tertiary prevention, the community health professional must first assess the health of the community. The following section covers some basic measures used in community health assessment.

Descriptive Measures of Health

Demographic Measures

Certain human characteristics, or *demographics,* may be associated with wellness or illness. Age, race, sex, ethnicity, income, and educational level are important demographics that may affect health outcomes. For example, men are more likely than women to develop certain heart diseases, and blacks are more likely than whites to have low-birth-weight infants. To plan for the health of a community, a health professional must be familiar with the demographic characteristics of the community and with the health problems associated with those characteristics.

Morbidity and Mortality

Although epidemiology encompasses wellness as well as illness, wellness is difficult to measure. Therefore, many measures of "health" are expressed in terms of *morbidity* (illness) and *mortality* (death).

Incidence

The *incidence* of a disease or health condition refers to the number of persons in a population who develop the condition during a specified period of time. The calculation of incidence, therefore, generally requires that a population be followed over a period of time in what is called a *prospective* (forward-looking) study.

Prevalence

The *prevalence* of a disease or condition refers to the total number of persons in the population who have the condition at a particular time. Thus, prevalence may be calculated in a "one-shot" *cross-sectional* ("slice of time") or *retrospective* (backward-looking) study.

Interpretation of Incidence and Prevalence

Measures of incidence and prevalence provide different information and have different implications. For example, an increase in the prevalence of cancer means that there are more persons with cancer in the population. This may be because there are more new cases (in other words, increased incidence) or because persons with cancer are living longer. In either case, the community may need to direct resources toward cancer. However, if knowledge of incidence is lacking, it will be difficult to decide whether to target the resources toward primary prevention or toward secondary and tertiary treatment services.

Rates

Incidence and prevalence usually are expressed as mathematical measures called *rates*. Because epidemiology is the study of *population* health, these measures must relate the occurrence of a health condition to the population base. Rates do exactly this. They express a mathematical relationship in which the *numerator* is the number of persons experiencing the condition and the *denominator* is the *population at risk,* or the total number of persons who have the possibility of experiencing the condition.

Rates must not be confused with other proportions that do not use the population at risk as the denominator. For example, the death rate from cancer is not the same as the proportion of deaths from cancer. In each, the numerator is the number of deaths from cancer. However, the denominators differ. In the death rate, the denominator is all persons at risk of dying from cancer. Therefore, the cancer death rate is an expression of the risk of dying from cancer. In the proportion of deaths, also called *proportionate mortality,* the denominator is the total number of deaths from all causes. Therefore, the proportionate cancer mortality simply describes the proportion of deaths attributable to cancer.

Calculation of Rates

Rates are calculated in this general format:

$$\text{rate} = \frac{\text{number of persons experiencing condition}}{\text{population at risk for experiencing condition}} \times \text{K}$$

K is a constant (usually 1,000 or 100,000) that allows the ratio, which may be a very small number, to be expressed in a meaningful way. Let us apply this formula to the calculation of the infant mortality rate, which estimates an infant's risk of dying during the first year of life.

Example of a Rate: The Infant Mortality Rate

The infant mortality rate (IMR) usually is calculated on a calendar-year basis. The number of infant deaths (deaths before the age of one year) during the year is divided by the number of live births (infants born alive) during the year. The numerator represents the number of infants experiencing the "condition" of dying in the first year of life, and the denominator represents the population of infants at risk for dying in the year.

Preliminary totals of 4,084,000 live births and 34,400 infant deaths were reported for the United States for 1992 (National Center for Health Statistics, 1993). Applying the formula for a rate, we divide 34,400 by 4,084,000 and find that 0.0084 of the infants died during the first year of life. Because it is difficult to relate to 0.0084 of an infant, we multiply by a constant, in this case 1,000, and find that 8.4 infants per 1,000 live births died during the first year of life; that is, the infant mortality rate was 8.4 infant deaths per 1,000 live births.

Interpretation of Rates

Rates enable researchers to compare different populations in terms of health problems or conditions. To assess whether the population in a specific community is at greater or lesser risk for the problems or conditions, the rates for the community should be compared with rates from similar communities, from the state, or from the United States as a whole.

Some cautions must be taken in interpreting rates. Like most statistical measures, rates are less reliable when based on small numbers. This must be kept in mind when assessing relatively infrequent events or conditions, or communities with small populations.

Many rates are based on data from a calendar year, which may also present some difficulties. In the example of the infant mortality rate, some of the infants who died during calendar year 1992 were actually born in 1991 and thus were not part of the 1992 population at risk, and some of the infants who were born in 1992 might die in 1993 and not be reflected in the 1992 infant mortality rate. Also, populations may increase or decrease during a calendar year. In such cases, the midyear population estimate is generally used because the population at risk cannot be determined exactly. A study that follows a *cohort,* or specified group, forward into time can help overcome the limitations of the conventionally calculated calendar-year rate.

Commonly Used Rates

Table 2-1 summarizes a number of important rates. Note that the measures of natality and mortality are, in essence, measures of incidence of the conditions of "being born" and "dying." Note also the various ways in which the denominator, or population at risk, is determined in different rates.

Crude, Specific, and Adjusted Rates

Rates that are computed for a population as a whole are called *crude rates.* Subgroups of a population may have differences that are not revealed by the crude rates. Rates that are calculated for subgroups are referred to as *specific rates.* Specific rates help identify groups at increased risk within the population and also facilitate comparisons

TABLE 2-1 Commonly Used Rates

Measures of Natality

$$\text{Crude birth rate} = \frac{\text{Number of live births during time interval}}{\text{Estimated midinterval population}} \times 1000$$

$$\text{Fertility rate} = \frac{\text{Number of live births during time interval}}{\text{Number of women aged 15–44 at midinterval}} \times 1000$$

Measures of Morbidity and Mortality

$$\text{Incidence rate} = \frac{\text{Number of new cases of specified health condition during time interval}}{\text{Estimated midinterval population at risk}} \times 1000$$

$$\text{Prevalence rate} = \frac{\text{Number of current cases of specified health condition at a given point in time}}{\text{Estimated population at risk at same point in time}} \times 1000$$

$$\text{Crude death rate} = \frac{\text{Number of deaths during time interval}}{\text{Estimated midinterval population}} \times 1000$$

$$\text{Specific death rate} = \frac{\text{Number of deaths in subgroup during time interval}}{\text{Estimated midinterval population of subgroup}} \times 1000$$

$$\text{Cause-specific death rate} = \frac{\text{Number of deaths from specified cause during time interval}}{\text{Estimated midinterval population}} \times 1000$$

$$\text{Infant mortality rate} = \frac{\text{Number of deaths of infants aged} < 1 \text{ year during time interval}}{\text{Total live births during time interval}} \times 1000$$

$$\text{Neonatal mortality rate} = \frac{\text{Number of deaths of infants aged} < 28 \text{ days during time interval}}{\text{Total live births during time interval}} \times 1000$$

$$\text{Postneonatal mortality rate} = \frac{\text{Number of deaths of infants aged} \geq 28 \text{ days but} < 1 \text{ year during time interval}}{\text{Total live births during time interval}} \times 1000$$

between populations that have different demographic compositions. Most frequently, specific rates are computed according to demographic factors such as age, race, or sex.

In comparing populations with different distributions of a factor that is known to affect the health condition being studied, the use of *adjusted rates* may be advisable. An adjusted rate is a summary measure that statistically removes the effect of the difference in the distributions of that characteristic. In essence, adjustment produces an estimate of what the crude rate would be if the populations were identical in respect to the factor for which adjustment is made. A rate can be adjusted for age, race, sex, or any factor or combination of factors suspected of affecting the rate. Adjusted rates are helpful in making community comparisons, but they are *imaginary rates* and so must be interpreted with care.

Analytic Measures of Health

As you have learned, rates are used to describe and compare the risks of dying, becoming ill, or developing other health conditions. It is also desirable to determine if health conditions are associated with, or related to, other factors. The related factors may point the way to preventive actions, as, for example, the linking of air pollution to health problems has led to environmental controls. To investigate potential relationships between health conditions and other factors, analytic measures of community health are required. In this section, three analytic measures will be discussed: relative risk, odds ratio, and attributable risk.

Relative Risk

To determine if a relationship or association exists between a health condition and a suspected factor, it is necessary to compare the risk of developing the health condition for the population exposed to the factor with the risk for the population not exposed to the factor. The *relative risk* (RR) does exactly this by expressing the ratio of the incidence rate of those exposed and those not exposed to the suspected factor:

$$RR = \frac{\text{incidence rate among those exposed}}{\text{incidence rate among those not exposed}}$$

The relative risk tells us whether the rate in the exposed population is higher than the rate in the nonexposed population and, if so, how many times higher it is. A high relative risk in the exposed population suggests that the factor is a *risk factor* in the development of the health condition.

Internal and External Risk Factors

The concept of relative risk is understood readily when one group of people clearly is exposed and another is not exposed to an external agent such as a virus, cigarette smoke, or an industrial pollutant. However, it may be confusing to see relative risks applied to internal factors such as age, race, or sex. Nevertheless, as can be seen in the next example, persons are also "exposed" to intrinsic factors that may carry as much risk as extrinsic ones.

Example of Relative Risk: Homicide

Hammett, Powell, O'Carroll, & Clanton (1992) found that the 1988 U.S. homicide rate (incidence rate) was 9 per 100,000 persons. Among blacks (those "exposed" to the intrinsic condition of being black), the rate was 34.4 per 100,000, and among whites (those "not exposed" to the condition of being black), the rate was 5.9 per 100,000. Thus, the relative risk of homicide for blacks can be calculated as follows:

$$RR = \frac{34.4 \text{ per } 100,000}{5.9 \text{ per } 100,000} = 5.83.$$

In other words, the risk of dying from homicide was nearly six times greater for blacks than for whites. Clearly, race is a risk factor. The risk factor itself cannot be altered, but the information provided by this analysis can be used to plan protective services for the population at greatest risk.

Odds Ratio

Calculation of the relative risk is straightforward when incidence rates are available. Unfortunately, not all studies can be carried out prospectively as is required for the computation of incidence rates. In a retrospective study, the relative risk must be approximated by the *odds ratio*.

As shown in Table 2-2, the odds ratio is a simple mathematical ratio of the odds in favor of having a specific health condition when the suspected factor is present and the odds in favor of having the condition

TABLE 2-2   Crosstabulation for Calculation of Odds Ratio

	Health Condition		
	PRESENT	*ABSENT*	*TOTAL*
Exposed to factor	*a*	*b*	*a + b*
Not exposed to factor	*c*	*d*	*c + d*
Total	*a + c*	*b + d*	*a + b + c + d*

when the factor is absent. The odds of having the condition when the suspected factor is present is represented by a/b in the table. The odds of having the condition when the factor is absent is c/d. The odds ratio is thus

$$\frac{a/b}{c/d} = \frac{ad}{bc}$$

An example may help. When toxic shock syndrome (TSS), a severe illness involving high fever, vomiting, diarrhea, rash, and hypotension or shock, was first reported, it was neither practical nor ethical to consider cases only on a prospective basis. Therefore, existing cases were compared retrospectively with noncases, or *controls*. Early studies noted an association between TSS and tampon use and suggested that users of a specific brand of superabsorbent tampon might be at especially high risk. To clarify the issue, researchers analyzed data from TSS cases and controls, all of whom used tampons. Let's use the TSS data in Table 2-3 to calculate the odds ratio for users of the specific brand of tampons.

$$\text{odds ratio} = \frac{ad = 30 \ (84)}{bc = 30 \ (12)} = 7$$

Users of the specific brand were seven times more likely to develop TSS than were users of other brands. Based on this and other studies, the brand was voluntarily withdrawn from the market.

TABLE 2-3	*Toxic Shock Syndrome Cases Among 146 Tampon Users*		
	Toxic Shock Syndrome		
BRAND OF TAMPON USED	*PRESENT*	*ABSENT*	*TOTAL*
Suspected brand	30	30	60
Other brands	12	84	96
Total	42	114	146

(Data from Centers for Disease Control (1980). Follow-up on toxic shock syndrome. MMWR, 29(37), 441–444.)

Relative Risk and Odds Ratio: Caution in Interpretation

A word of caution: Regard a high odds ratio or relative risk with appropriate concern, but do not allow the finding to obscure the potential involvement of other factors. Refer to Table 2-3 again and note that 12 persons in the sample had TSS even though they did not use the specific brand of tampons. In other words, this product was not the sole cause of TSS. Subsequent research showed that certain superabsorbent materials in tampons or certain aspects of tampon use foster growth of *Staphylococcus aureus,* the probable causal organism in TSS (Centers for Disease Control [CDC], 1981, 1983; Davis, Chesney, Ward, LaVenture, & the Investigation and Laboratory Team, 1980).

Attributable Risk and Attributable Risk Percent

Another measure of risk is *attributable risk* (AR), or the difference between the incidence rates for those exposed and those not exposed to the risk factor. This measure estimates the excess risk attributable to the factor being studied. It shows the potential reduction in the overall incidence rate if the factor could be eliminated:

$$AR = \text{incidence rate in exposed group } \textit{minus} \text{ incidence rate in nonexposed group}$$

AR usually is further quantified into attributable risk percent:

$$\frac{\text{attributable risk}}{\text{incidence rate in exposed group}} \times 100$$

This provides an estimate of the percent of occurrences of the health condition that could be prevented if the risk factor were eliminated. For example, studies of the relation between physical inactivity and mortality from coronary heart disease (CHD) showed that the attributable risk associated with physical inactivity was 35% (CDC, 1993). Thus, improved physical activity has the potential to greatly reduce CHD mortality.

Cause and Association

Ultimately, community health professionals hope to determine causes of health conditions so that steps can be taken to improve health. In view of the complexity of the human body and human behavior, establishing causality is very difficult. Therefore, investigations of population health generally examine relationships or *associations* between variables. The *variables* are the characteristics or phenomena (such as age, occupation, or physical exercise) and the health conditions (such as heart disease) being studied.

Variables and Constants

An important requirement in any study is that the factors studied must have the potential to vary from person to person. If a factor cannot vary, it is not a variable but a *constant*. It is impossible to establish an association between a constant and a variable because the constant, by definition, cannot change when the variable changes. Thus, a study that looks only at men cannot establish an association between gender and, for example, heart disease; the study has made gender a constant. A study that looks only at persons with heart disease cannot establish an association between heart disease and any other variable; heart disease has become a constant in the study.

Control or Comparison Groups

To ensure that associations between variables can be examined, *control groups* or *comparison groups* may be needed. A study of heart disease might compare persons with the disease with a control group of persons without the disease. An investigation of a new treatment would study persons who receive the treatment and a control group of persons who do not receive the treatment.

Independent and Dependent Variables

Frequently variables are referred to as *dependent* or *independent*. The dependent variable is the outcome or result that the investigator is studying. It is a characteristic that conceivably could be altered, for example, health status, knowledge, or behavior. The independent variable is the presumed "cause" of or contributor to variation in the dependent variable. For example, in the heart disease study cited earlier (CDC, 1993), physical inactivity, the independent variable, is seen to contribute to heart disease, the dependent variable. An independent variable may be a naturally occurring event or phenomenon such as level of usual physical activity, exposure to ultraviolet radiation, or type of employment, or it might be a planned intervention such as an exercise regimen, a medical treatment, or an educational program. An independent variable might also be an intrinsic quality such as age, race, or sex. (Note that these intrinsic qualities, though they cannot vary *within* an individual, can vary from person to person; thus, they can be studied as independent variables.)

Confounding Variables

When an association is identified between variables, it is tempting—but incorrect—to assume that one variable causes the other. If, for example, a study found that communities with lower salaries for public health workers had higher crime rates, we could not conclude that low public health salaries lead to high crime. Common sense suggests that economic conditions might influence both salaries and crime, that is, economic conditions intervene in the study and confound the results. Any factor that may influence a study's results is referred to as an extraneous, intervening, or *confounding variable.*

Criteria for Determining Causation

If an association is found between variables, it means the variables tend to occur or change together, but it does not prove that one variable causes the other. Because of the possibility of confounded results, very strict criteria for determining causation have been established. An association must be evaluated against all of these criteria; the more criteria that are met, the more likely it is that the association is causal. However, an association may meet all the criteria for causation and later be shown to be spurious because of factors that were not known at the time the study was done. For this reason, investigators must interpret their results with great caution; they rarely consider a cause "proven." Six widely used criteria for evaluating causation are listed below.

1. The association is strong.

The strength of the relationship may be evaluated statistically by a variety of measures. For example, the higher the relative risk or odds ratio, the stronger the association.

2. The association is consistent.

The same association must be found repeatedly in other studies, in other settings, and with other methods.

3. The association is temporally correct.

The hypothesized cause of the health condition must occur *before* the onset of the condition.

4. The association is specific.

The hypothesized cause should be associated with relatively few health conditions. For example, speaking English may be associated with many health conditions, but it is a cause for none. This criterion must be tempered by the knowledge that certain factors, such as cigarette smoking, have been shown to have multiple effects.

5. The association cannot be explained as being the result of a confounding variable.

Not all potential intervening variables can be explored, of course, but alternate explanations for the association must be examined carefully before considering an association to be causal.

6. The association is plausible and consistent with current knowledge.

An association that contradicts current scientific views must be evaluated very carefully. However, associations may be inconsistent with current knowledge simply because current knowledge is not as advanced as a new discovery.

Sources of Community Health Data

To be an effective community health professional, you will also need to interpret and use data from various sources. In this section we will review the use of several important sources of data.

Census

The census is probably the most comprehensive source of health-related data for the United States. Every 10 years, the Bureau of the Census enumerates the U.S. population and surveys it for basic demographics such as age, race, and sex as well as numerous other factors such as employment, income, migration, and education. Only a limited number of questions are asked of the entire population. More detailed surveys are taken of selected samples of the population.

Census data are available in many public libraries. The *Census of the Population* addresses the entire census. Special *Subject Reports* (for example, on Hispanic populations) also are published. In noncensus years, segments of the population are surveyed to monitor ongoing demographic trends. These are published as *Current Population Reports.*

Even though census data are comprehensive, bias does occur. For example, people may answer personal questions dishonestly. Perhaps more significantly, the census is believed to underrepresent low-income residents, minorities, and transients. These people are more difficult to locate and enumerate and tend to be less likely to respond to census surveys.

Vital Statistics

Vital statistics are the data on legally registered events (such as births, deaths, marriages, and divorces) collected on an ongoing basis by government agencies. State health departments usually publish vital statistics annually. The U.S. Public Health Service also gathers data from the states and publishes annual volumes as well as periodic reports on specific topics.

Beginning researchers tend to consider vital statistics "hallowed" because they are, after all, legal data. However, legality does not guarantee validity. For example, an individual's race sometimes differs on birth and death certificates, and the manner in which cause of death is recorded on death certificates is inconsistent. The numbers of unmarried but cohabiting couples—and the occasional news reports of newly discovered bigamists—also demonstrate that marriage and divorce records are also not completely valid measures of reality. Despite their limitations, vital statistics are often the best available data, and much useful information can be gained from them.

Notifiable Disease Reports

The Centers for Disease Control and Prevention of the U.S. Public Health Service reports data collected by state and local health departments on legally reportable diseases and also periodically requests voluntary reporting of nonnotifiable health conditions of special interest. The CDC weekly publication, *Morbidity and Mortality Weekly Report* (*MMWR*), is valuable for community health practice.

Even legally mandated disease reports may not be representative of all cases of the disease. Thus, they may not provide valid descriptions of the disease as it exists in the community. In practice, health care providers may fail to report diseases that should be reported.

Medical and Hospital Records

Medical and hospital records are used extensively in community health research. These records, however, do not provide a completely representative or valid picture of community health. In the first place, not all clients with health problems receive medical attention, so medical records are obviously biased. Second, medical documentation is not always complete. Finally, hospitalized patients are also more likely to have another illness along with the one being studied. This phenomenon, called *Berkson's bias,* creates the likelihood of finding a false association between the two illnesses.

Autopsy Records

Autopsy records have a very severe inherent bias: The patients were so sick that they died. Autopsies are not performed for all deaths. Autopsy records include a disproportionate number of cases of violent death and persons for whom the cause of death was unknown until after autopsy; for example, the manifestation of the illness was unusual. Religious groups that do not sanction autopsy are underrepresented. These factors influence the validity and representativeness of the findings of any study using autopsy records.

Screening for Health Conditions

Thus far we have focused on methods for studying community health problems and assessing health risks for populations. In this section, we will discuss *screening,* a method of secondary prevention. Screening is an effort to detect unrecognized or preclinical illness among individuals. Screening tests are not intended to be diagnostic. Their purpose is to rapidly and economically identify persons who have a high probability of having (or developing) a particular illness so that they can be referred for definitive diagnosis and treatment.

Considerations in Deciding to Screen

Screening goes further than identifying groups at risk for illness; it identifies *individuals* who may actually have an illness. Screening carries an ethical commitment to continue working with these individuals and provide them access to diagnostic and treatment services. In general, screening should be conducted only if

- Early diagnosis and treatment can favorably alter the course of the illness
- Definitive diagnosis and treatment facilities are available, either through the screening agency or through referral
- The group being screened is at risk for the illness (in other words, the group is likely to have a high prevalence of the illness)
- The screening procedures are reliable and valid

Screening Test Reliability and Validity

Reliability refers to the consistency or repeatability of test results; *validity* refers to the ability of the test to measure what it is supposed to measure. Reliability and validity of assessment instruments, including screening tests, are discussed extensively later in this chapter. A few considerations specific to screening tests are discussed below.

Screening Test Reliability

A reliable screening test yields the same result even when administered by different screeners. Training for all screening personnel in use of the test is essential. Lack of reliability may suggest that the screeners are administering the test in an inconsistent manner.

Screening Test Validity: Sensitivity and Specificity

To be valid, a screening test must distinguish correctly between those individuals who have the condition and those who do not. This is measured by the test's sensitivity and specificity, as shown in Table 2-4.

Sensitivity is the ability to correctly identify individuals who have the disease; that is, to call a *true positive* "positive." A test with high sensitivity will have few *false negatives*.

TABLE 2-4   *Sensitivity and Specificity of a Screening Test*

		Reality
SCREENING TEST RESULTS	**DISEASED**	**NOT DISEASED**
Positive	True positive	False positive
Negative	False negative	True negative
Total	Total diseased	Total not diseased

$$\text{Sensitivity (true positive rate)} = \frac{\text{True positives}}{\text{Total diseased}}$$

$$\text{Specificity (true negative rate)} = \frac{\text{True negatives}}{\text{Total not diseased}}$$

$$\text{False negative rate} = \frac{\text{False negatives}}{\text{Total diseased}} \; or \; 1 - \text{Sensitivity}$$

$$\text{False positive rate} = \frac{\text{False positives}}{\text{Total not diseased}} \; or \; 1 - \text{Sensitivity}$$

Specificity is the ability to correctly identify individuals who do not have the disease, or to call a *true negative* "negative." A test with high specificity has few *false positives.*

Relationship Between Sensitivity and Specificity

Ideally, a screening test's sensitivity and specificity should be 100%; in practice, however, screening tests vary in this regard. As shown in Table 2-4, sensitivity, or the *true positive rate,* is the complement of the *false negative rate,* and specificity, or the *true negative rate,* is the complement of the *false positive rate.* Thus, as sensitivity increases, specificity decreases. Therefore, decisions regarding screening test validity may require uncomfortable compromises, as you will see from the following examples.

Decision Making in Screening: Practical and Ethical Considerations

Suppose you are screening for a deadly disease that is curable only if detected early and you have a choice between a test with high sensitivity and low specificity or one with high specificity and low sensitivity. To save the most lives, you need high sensitivity, that is, a low rate of false negatives (people who have the disease but are not detected by the screening test). However, if you select the test with high sensitivity, its low specificity means that you will have a high rate of false positives (people who do not have the disease but whom the test identifies as having it). That is, you will alarm many people needlessly and will cause unnecessary expenses by overreferring them for nonexistent disease. Which test would you choose?

Now suppose you are screening for the same disease, but the diagnostic and treatment facilities in the community are already overloaded, and further budget cuts are projected. To minimize unnecessary referrals of false positives, you'd want the test with high specificity. However, because of the low sensitivity of this test, you will have to weigh the benefits of a low false positive rate against the ethics of a high false negative rate. Is it justifiable to lull the undetected diseased persons into a false—and potentially fatal—sense of security? Which test would you choose now?

Decisions regarding screening involve seeking the most favorable balance of sensitivity and specificity. Sometimes sensitivity and specificity can be improved by adjusting the screening process (for example, adding another test or changing the level at which the test is considered positive). At other times, evaluating sensitivity and specificity may result in a decision not to conduct a screening program because the economic costs of overreferral or the ethical considerations of underreferral outweigh the usefulness of screening. An understanding of the principles discussed in this section will help you make informed decisions regarding community screening. You also are encouraged to pursue further study regarding screening (see, for instance, Morrison, 1992).

Epidemiologic Approaches to Community Health Research

In studying the determinants of population health, investigators may be guided by epidemiologic models. This section describes three models and explains how each might guide the approach to the same problem.

The problem to be considered is an increase in the infant mortality rate in a hypothetical community. The infant mortality rate is a particularly important health index that should be understood even by health professionals whose main concern is not maternal or child health. Because infant mortality is influenced by a variety of biological and environmental factors affecting the infant and mother, the infant mortality rate is both a direct measure of infant health and an indirect measure of community health as a whole.

The Epidemiologic Triangle

The *epidemiologic triangle* or *agent-host-environment model* is a traditional view of health and disease, developed when epidemiology was concerned chiefly with communicable disease. As you will see, however, the model is applicable to other health conditions as well. In the model, the *agent* is an organism capable of causing disease. The *host* is the population at risk for developing the disease. The *environment* is a combination of physical, biological, and social factors that surround and influence both the agent and the host. According to this model, health and illness can be understood by examining characteristics of, changes in, and interactions among the agent, host, and environment.

Figure 2-1 shows the triangle in its normal state of equilibrium. Equilibrium does not signify optimum health but simply the usual pattern of illness and health in a population. Any change in one of the sides

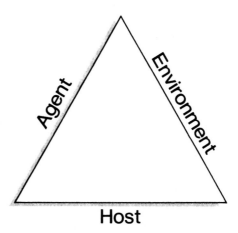

FIGURE 2-1
The epidemiologic triangle is the traditional view, showing health and disease as a composite state of three variables.

(agent, host, or environment) will result in disequilibrium, in other words, a change in the usual pattern.

How would this model guide the investigation of increased infant mortality? To understand this, let us consider the three facets of the model.

Agent

At first glance, it might be concluded that the investigation should focus on types of infections as agents that cause infant deaths. However, major causes of infant mortality in the United States include prematurity and low birth weight, birth injuries, congenital malformations, sudden infant death syndrome (SIDS), accidents, and homicides. Therefore, the investigation will try to determine whether there has been a change in any of these other agents.

Host

The investigators also will want to know the characteristics of the host, that is, the infant population. This involves examining infant birth and death patterns in terms of age, ethnicity, sex, and birth weight. These characteristics have been shown to be important risk factors for infant mortality. By studying these factors, it may be possible to identify groups of infants who are at particularly increased risk of dying.

Environment

Finally, the environment must be assessed. The mother is a significant part of the infant's prenatal and postnatal environment. Therefore, the investigators will analyze birth and infant mortality patterns according to factors such as maternal age, ethnicity, parity (number of previous live births), prenatal care, and education or socioeconomic status. Analysis of these factors, which have also been shown to be related to infant mortality, will help provide further identification of at-risk groups. Other conditions in the environment also need to be considered. For instance, has migration into the community from other areas increased? Has adult morbidity or mortality, particularly among pregnant women, increased? Have there been changes in health services, policies, personnel, funding, or other factors that could affect infant health?

Practical Application

The analysis of these three areas—the agent, host, and environment—should provide information regarding groups at risk for increased infant mortality and may point the way toward a program aimed at reducing that risk. Thus, the epidemiologic triangle, although it was designed with a communicable disease orientation, can provide a useful guide for studying the multifaceted problem of infant mortality, as well as other health problems.

The Person-Place-Time Model

An approach similar to the epidemiologic triangle is one that guides the investigators to consider the health problem in terms of person, place, and time (Mausner & Kramer, 1985; Roht, Selwyn, Holguin, & Christensen, 1982). The investigators examine characteristics of the persons affected (the host in the triangle model), the place (environment) or location, and the time period involved (which could relate to the agent, host, or environment). In studying infant mortality according to the person-place-time model, infant and maternal factors are considered traits of "person." Aspects of "place" are such factors as whether the community is rural or urban, affluent or poor. Aspects of "time" include seasonal or age-specific patterns or trends in mortality.

The Web of Causation

The *web of causation* (MacMahon & Pugh, 1970) views a health condition not as the result of individual factors but of complex interactions among multiple factors. One factor may lead to others, which in turn lead to others, all of which may interact with one another to produce the health condition.

Central to this model is the concept of *synergism,* wherein the whole is more than the sum of its separate parts. For example, the effects of a *Shigella* infection of the infant, combined with the effects of poverty, youth, and low educational level of the mother, are more deleterious to infant health than the sum of the effects of the individual risk factors.

Use of the web of causation may result in a more expansive study of infant mortality than one guided by other models. Ideally, investigators using this model first identify all factors related to infant mortality. Next, they identify factors that are related to each of these factors. These two comprehensive steps provide the outline for the web of causation for infant mortality. Finally, the investigators examine the relationships among all the identified components of the web and attempt to determine the most feasible point of intervention to improve infant mortality in the community. Figure 2-2 depicts a web of causation for infant mortality.

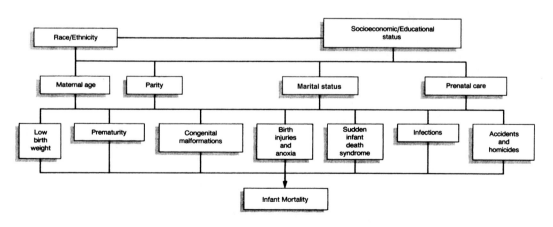

FIGURE 2-2
A web of causation for infant mortality, based on information available from birth and death certificates.

Practical Application

This multifaceted approach addresses the concept of causation in a manner consistent with current knowledge of human health. However, it may be overwhelming to carry out in everyday practice. In fact, it is more usual to examine only a portion of the web, acknowledging that other relationships exist. Thorough examination of one portion of the web may provide sufficient information for initiation of useful actions to improve community health.

Models: Guides to Investigation and Practice

In this section, we showed how three models each provide a slightly different approach to a community health problem. As you continue to study community health, you will find other models that can guide your practice and investigation. There is no one "right" model; as you gain experience, you will be able to choose or adapt those that are most appropriate for your work.

Community Health Research

The community health professional often acts as a researcher as well as a health care provider. In this section, we will review basic concepts of research as applied to community health practice.

Community health research is traditionally considered to have two major purposes: to describe and to explain the health conditions of populations. The authors of this chapter believe that the following four categories more completely describe the purposes and scope of research in community health.

1. *To describe* the health conditions of populations
2. *To identify* groups at risk for certain health conditions
3. *To explain* the health conditions of populations by exploring association and potential causation
4. *To evaluate* interventions for improving the health of populations

Focus of Community Health Research

The emphasis in community health research is the health of populations. The research is practical; it is used to identify and solve real, everyday problems in community health practice. Inherent in community health practice is the consideration of "the greatest good for the greatest number." For this reason, community health research usually does not focus on extremely rare health conditions, unless these conditions are expected to affect the health of the population as a whole. Thus, research priorities are likely to be related to the major causes of morbidity and mortality in a community rather than to such relatively unknown conditions as myositis ossificans progressiva or relapsing nodular nonsuppurative panniculitis. However, in certain areas, it might be very important to study a relatively uncommon condition such as dengue fever because of its potential for becoming epidemic in a community.

Community health research also focuses on the levels of prevention considered in community health practice. That is, the emphasis is on promoting health at primary, secondary, and tertiary levels of prevention but rarely on high-technology techniques for prolonging life such as organ transplantation. However, community health researchers might examine such techniques in the context of the overall impact of these programs on the health of the community or nation, for example, regarding allocation of scarce resources.

The Research Process

The research process, outlined in the accompanying display, is similar whether the research is in community health, high-technology medical intervention, or basic science. In this section, we will explain each step in the research process and demonstrate how the steps were applied in a specific community health study (Selby, Riportella-Muller, Sorenson, Quade, Stearns, & Farel, 1992). We will trace the study from its inception through its planning, implementation, and dissemination.

Step 1: Identify an Area of Interest

In community health practice, you will encounter many unanswered questions and unsolved problems. In the first step of the research process, identify a problem area that you haven't been able to solve satisfactorily or simply an area about which you would like to learn more. Be sure that the area is one in which you have a strong interest. It's very difficult to do research—or any other work—in an area that has little meaning for you.

In choosing an area of interest, be aware that research involves empirically demonstrable findings, not value judgments. For example,

Steps in the Research Process

1. Identify an area of interest.
2. Review the literature to formulate a problem statement based on theory and research.
3. State the assumptions.
4. Formulate the research questions or hypotheses.
5. Operationalize the variables.
6. Plan the methodology.
   A. Select the research design.
   B. Select the population, setting, and sample.
   C. Select or design the data collection instruments and procedures.
   D. Plan the data analysis.
7. Ensure the protection of human subjects.
8. State the limitations of the study.
9. Conduct a pilot study.
10. Implement the methodology.
11. Interpret the results.
12. Communicate the results.

research cannot determine whether abortion is morally or ethically good or bad. Research can be done on the social, economic, and health effects of abortion, but value judgments about the morality or ethics of abortion must be made outside the realm of research.

APPLICATION

How was the area of interest identified in our example? First, nurses in a number of rural North Carolina county health departments noted that use of the Early and Periodic Screening, Diagnosis and Treatment (EPSDT) program was declining in their clinics; they learned this from observing their clinics and reviewing clinic utilization statistics. The nurses were concerned because the EPSDT program is the major source of preventive health care for children from low-income families on Medicaid; thus, needy children were going without preventive health care. The nurses wanted to learn how to increase utilization of the program. They approached a senior nurse with research experience and asked her to help investigate their concerns; the nurse agreed.

Step 2: Review the Literature and Formulate a
Problem Statement Based on Theory and Research

This step is carried out chiefly at the library. Sometimes a preliminary *literature review* satisfies the need for knowledge on a topic, and further research is unnecessary. At other times, the literature raises as many questions as it answers, and a more comprehensive search is needed.

As you review the literature for *theory* and *research* regarding the problem of interest, it will become clear if the health condition is of sufficient importance to warrant research and if there is a need for such research, that is, if there are gaps in the literature that further research would fill. The literature will guide you to identify a preliminary *problem statement* or *purpose of the study*. As you learn more about the topic, the study purpose may undergo many revisions.

The literature also provides a *theoretical framework* or *scientific rationale* for a study. A framework or rationale helps a study stay grounded in theory and research. That is, it helps keep an investigator from going off on a tangent without justification. A framework or rationale also helps the investigator synthesize the findings of previous research into a meaningful pattern, and it guides the development of research questions, methods, and interventions that will yield meaningful and useful results.

The literature helps the investigator formulate a tentative methodology for the needed research and provides information for assessing whether the research is feasible to undertake. In community health practice, it is usual to find that a topic is too complex for one investigator to handle. Frequently community health research is conducted by a team of investigators who, as a whole, have the needed expertise to address the research problem.

APPLICATION

In the EPSDT example, the literature suggested that the EPSDT program could improve the health of children through early detection and treatment. The literature also documented that EPSDT underuse was a problem statewide and nationwide, especially in rural areas; in other words, the scope of the problem extended beyond the nurses' clinics. The literature had few clues about ways to improve EPSDT use, which showed that further study was needed.

From the literature it also became clear that an approach to EPSDT use would need to involve interdisciplinary collaboration. For example, in North

Carolina, application for and education about EPSDT services occurs at social services offices; eligibility for services is regulated by the state Medicaid office; and health services are provided by physicians and nurses, who are reimbursed by the Medicaid office. In addition, the literature showed that it was important to assess the economic costs associated with community health interventions; such analyses could be complex. Therefore, the senior nurse, who became the principal investigator (PI) of the study, assembled an investigative team that included expertise in social services, Medicaid, health education, nursing, medicine, health economics, and statistics.

The literature also described the PRECEDE model for planning health education programs (Green, Kreuter, Deeds, & Partridge, 1980), as well as theories of health education and behavior (e.g., Becker et al., 1977; Morley, Messick, & Aguillera, 1967; Pender, 1987; Rogers, 1969). The PRECEDE model, adapted to consider these theories, provided the conceptual framework for further study of EPSDT use. The adapted model indicated that interventions to improve EPSDT use would need to consider factors that (1) *predispose* families to use or not use EPSDT, (2) *enable* them to use EPSDT or deter them from using it, and (3) *reinforce* the likelihood of their continuing to use EPSDT (Selby, Riportella-Muller, Sorenson, & Walters, 1989).

The adapted model guided the investigators to develop interventions for this study. The usual process for informing parents about EPSDT was during the Medicaid eligibility interview, a stressful time. Based on the model, the team developed three enhanced educational interventions, to be compared with the usual, or *control*, procedure. The interventions were a home visit by a nurse, a phone call by a nurse, and a pamphlet mailed to the parent's home. The major purpose of the study was to determine whether there were differences in the effectiveness of the various interventions in terms of producing EPSDT use. The study also examined the cost-effectiveness of these interventions.

Step 3: State the Assumptions

Assumptions are ideas that form the basis or reason for the study, but for which there is no definitive proof. If the assumption were untrue, there might not be a reason to do the study. Assumptions should be derived from theory or research, and they should be stated explicitly.

APPLICATION

The major *assumption* for the proposed study was that EPSDT, if used, can improve the health of needy children. This assumption was based on past research as well as on theories of the levels of prevention in community health. However, the past studies were not conclusive, so there was no definitive "proof" that the assumption was true. Do you see how this assumption was basic to a study aimed at increasing EPSDT use?

Step 4: Formulate the Research Questions or Hypotheses

The *research questions* specify which questions must be answered in order to address the problem statement and carry out the purpose of the study. If a research question asks about relationships between variables or differences between groups, a *hypothesis,* or projected answer to the research question, may be formulated. A hypothesis is a statement that can be tested statistically. In general, a hypothesis is formulated only for studies that test for statistical significance, not for descriptive studies.

If a hypothesis is formulated, it generally will have an *independent variable* and a *dependent variable* (in complex studies, there may be multiple independent and dependent variables). When researchers are simply exploring relationships between variables rather than seeking potential causal relationships, a hypothesis may have two variables, neither of which is specified as independent or dependent.

APPLICATION

The EPSDT study involved a number of hypotheses, but the main purpose was to learn which of the interventions was the most effective in producing EPSDT use by children in the families targeted, that is, to test this hypothesis: There are differences in the effectiveness of the intervention and control procedures. Here, the independent variable is the *type of intervention or control procedure.* The dependent variable is the *effectiveness* of the procedure.

Step 5: Operationalize the Variables

It is necessary to specify the variables that must be measured to answer the research questions or test the hypotheses. The variables must be *operationalized,* or defined explicitly to ensure consistency in data collection and to enable other researchers to replicate a study.

The *operational definitions* must take into account the desired *level of measurement* for each variable. The levels of measurement are reviewed below.

- *Nominal:* The lowest (weakest) level, in which data are categorized into mutually exclusive groups (for example, based on sex or ethnicity)
- *Ordinal:* A higher level, in which data are categorized into mutually exclusive groups and placed in rank order (for example, based on "satisfaction," rated on a scale from very satisfied to very dissatisfied)
- *Interval* or *ratio:* The highest levels, in which data are categorized into mutually exclusive groups and placed in order on a continuum with equally spaced units that include zero as a possible value (for example, based on age in years or blood pressure in millimeters of mercury)

APPLICATION

In the EPSDT study, the investigators *operationalized* the key variables for the hypothesis as follows:

- Type of intervention or control procedure, the independent variable, was set up to accommodate two different studies of interventions for families with telephones and for families without telephones; this was necessary because phone call interventions could not be made to families without phones. In the study of families with phones, the independent variable had four nominal-level categories: control, mailed pamphlet, phone call, and home visit. In the study of families without phones, the variable had three nominal-level categories: control, mailed pamphlet, and home visit. Detailed protocols ensured that families received the proper interventions.
- Effectiveness, the dependent variable, was defined as the use of EPSDT by at least one previously nonusing child in the family, no later than four months after the intervention or control procedure. This was measured by presence of at least one health care provider's claim, on state Medicaid files, for an EPSDT visit for the child in the specified time interval. This measure also was at the nominal level; there either was or was not an EPSDT claim, and an intervention or control procedure either was or was not effective.
- Potential confounding variables also were measured. These included, for example, child's race (nominal level), number of children in the family (interval level), and child's age (ratio level). Data on these vari-

ables were obtained from the state Medicaid files; the operational definitions used by the state were used.

Step 6: Plan the Methodology

To plan the methodology, you must choose the research design, select the sample, select or design the data collection instruments and procedures, and plan the data analysis. You will do all of this before you collect any data. First we will consider the research design.

Step 6A: Select the Research Design

Research designs can be categorized as experimental, quasi-experimental, or nonexperimental. The choice of design is determined by the purposes of the research and by real-life resources and constraints. The discussion in this section will help you choose the appropriate research design for your needs.

Experimental Design.   Experimental design requires adherence to all of the following conditions:

1. *Manipulation* of the *independent variable* through intervention or treatment.
2. *Control* for confounding variables through use of a control group to which the intervention or treatment is not applied and through careful monitoring of the study.
3. *Randomization* or *random assignment* of subjects to the treatment or control groups; this means that a specific scientific procedure such as a table of random numbers or a computer-generated random list, rather than human judgment or choice, is used to decide which subjects will receive which treatment or control procedure.

The true experiment is the hallmark of excellence in research design. However, in community health, experimental research sometimes is impossible, unfeasible, unethical, or simply unnecessary. It is valuable to compare the requirements for experimental research to the four purposes of community health research: description, identification, explanation, and evaluation.

If the purpose of the research is to *describe* a human population or *identify* a population at risk, that is, to learn the relationship of a certain characteristic to a health condition, manipulation of the independent variable is usually impossible or unwarranted. For instance, it is impossible to manipulate a person's heredity, age, or race, and it is unwarranted to manipulate a person's lifestyle if there is no prior research that identifies the lifestyle as a risk factor. Therefore, experimental design is inappropriate for this type of research.

If the research purpose is to *explain* the cause of a health condition in humans, then even if it is possible to manipulate the independent variable, it may be unethical to do so; or it may be unethical to use random assignment. For example, it is unethical to randomly (or otherwise) assign children to consume varying quantities of lead in order to determine the dose at which lead becomes toxic. For such reasons, experimental research is rarely used for determining causal relationships in community health.

However, if the purpose of the research is to *evaluate* an intervention or treatment for a health condition, experimental research is highly desirable. The intervention or treatment constitutes the manipulation. The intervention, of course, must be justified by earlier research. Adhering to the other requirements for experimental research, namely, use of randomization and a control group, will help ensure that the intervention rather than a confounding variable leads to improvement—or lack of improvement—in health.

As you develop programs to address needs in your community, you must plan how to evaluate their impact. The principles of experimental research are excellent for this purpose. For further study, consult a research text (for example, Polit & Hungler, 1991; Singleton, Straits, & Straits, 1993).

Quasi-Experimental Design. Although experimental research is the preferred method for evaluating interventions, the constraints of real life may make it unfeasible to conduct a true experiment. If so, the best choice may be *quasi-experimental* research. This research design is used when

1. Experimental research is desirable
2. Manipulation of the independent variable (the treatment or intervention) is feasible
3. Either randomization or use of a control group, or both, is not feasible

In essence, quasi-experimentation is faulty experimental research and thus is considerably less reliable than a true experiment. However, careful attention to other methodological aspects can make quasi-experimental design a viable option. If you are responsible for program planning, you may wish to pursue further reading in quasi experimentation (such as Cook & Campbell, 1979; Fitz-Gibbon & Morris, 1987).

Nonexperimental Design.   Most community health research does not involve manipulation of variables; it is *nonexperimental.* If your practice involves *describing* populations, *identifying* populations at risk, or *explaining* possible causes of health conditions, you will be using nonexperimental research. Nonexperimental research is used whenever manipulation of variables is impossible, unethical, unfeasible, or unnecessary. Nonexperimental research can produce excellent results when sound epidemiologic principles are applied.

Nonexperimental research is usually categorized according to its time perspective: *retrospective,* in which data for a particular health condition are examined in relation to past events, or *prospective,* in which data are collected on an ongoing basis to be examined in relation to a possible future health condition. Nonexperimental research also may be categorized as *cross-sectional,* meaning that data are collected for a "slice of time" from the present or the past. Cross-sectional studies are often considered retrospective because even when they involve surveying a present population, they generally consider past as well as present events.

Prospective research design.   A well-designed nonexperimental prospective study approximates an experiment as closely as can be done without actual manipulation of variables. A prospective study begins with a group of people, or *cohort,* exposed to a particular event (the independent variable). The event may be as dramatic as the radiation leak at the Chernobyl nuclear reactor in the 1980s or as mundane as being born in a particular year. This event may be seen as the naturally occurring equivalent of manipulation of the independent variable. The study then follows the cohort forward in time to see whether the independent variable results in the health condition under study. Ideally, the study also follows a similar group of people who were not exposed to the event (a type of control group) in order to make comparisons. A nonexperimental prospective study cannot use randomization of subjects to groups; the change in the independent variable occurs naturally before the groups are identified. Incidence and relative risk can be deter-mined from a prospective study.

Despite the many advantages of prospective research, it has limita-tions. Prospective research is usually not practical for studying rare health conditions or those with a long latency period. Prospective stud-ies tend to be time-consuming and expensive and may suffer from loss or dropout of subjects over time.

Retrospective research design: The case-control study. Because of the difficulties in prospective research, retrospective studies are used fre-quently in community health. In the earlier example of the study of TSS, you were introduced to the *case-control* study, a special type of retro-spective study in which persons with a particular health condition (*cases*) and persons without the health condition (*controls*) are com-pared. An attempt is made to look backward in time to determine risk factors and potential causes of the health condition. The case-control study tries to approximate a prospective study by estimating relative risk using the odds ratio. At the same time, the case-control study has the advantage of being less costly in terms of time and money than a prospective study.

Guidance for Choosing a Research Design.   Now that you understand the basic types of research design, you may find Figure 2-3 useful in your practice. The figure provides a guide for choosing the research design appropriate for various types of community health studies.

APPLICATION

Refer to Figure 2-3 as we return to the EPSDT study and observe how the inves-tigators determined the research design for it. As you may recall, the purpose of the study was to test the effectiveness of various interventions in terms of increas-ing use of EPSDT. Thus, it is clear that the investigators intended to *evaluate* interventions.

In this case, it was possible to *manipulate* the independent variable (type of intervention). Some families would receive a specific enhanced educational intervention about EPSDT, and others would receive only the usual (*control*) educational information when they applied for Medicaid. In the setting being studied, it was feasible and ethical to *randomly assign* families to receive the intervention or control procedures. There was no indication that the interven-tions would be harmful and, although intervention group families would receive

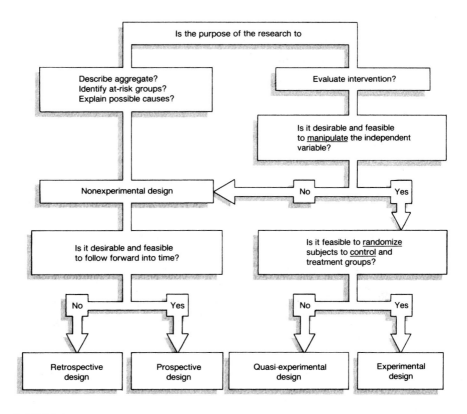

FIGURE 2-3
Selection of research designs for community health practice.

enhanced education, no one would be deprived of usual education. Thus, the investigators were able to choose an *experimental* design.

Step 6B: Select the Population, Setting, and Sample

The *population* is the group of people to whom the results are intended to apply; this population may be referred to as the *target population.* From the population, the investigator usually selects a *sample* or subset of the population. The *subjects* are the individual members of the sample. To select subjects for the sample, it is necessary to obtain a *sampling frame,* or list of members of the population; the sample is selected from this list. Sometimes the entire population, or *census,* is studied, but this usually is too costly.

The *setting* refers to the geographic or physical location of the population being studied. The characteristics of the setting affect the generalizability of the study. Clearly, the findings of a study in an affluent suburb may not apply to a rural, poor area.

A *probability sample* is one in which each member of the population has a probability, or chance, of being included in the sample. This is achieved by *random selection,* using a table of random numbers or some other probability selection device. Probability sampling helps ensure that the sample is *representative* of the population. Provided the sample size is sufficiently large and the study procedures are valid, this form of sampling allows *generalization* of the results from the sample to the population. Therefore, probability sampling is the preferred method.

A *nonprobability* sample is one for which random selection is not used. Thus, there is no assurance that each member of the population has a chance of being in the sample. Many studies report use of a *convenience sample,* a type of nonprobability sample. A nonprobability sample is unlikely to be representative of the population, so the results cannot be generalized to the population. In research that seeks to make inferences about the health of the population, the lack of ability to generalize is an important limitation.

Sampling Bias.   The possibility of making random and systematic errors that may affect data adversely is always a concern. In sampling, the most important error to avoid is systematic error, or bias. *Sampling bias* is the systematic over- or underrepresentation, in the sample, of a specific part of the population. The results from a biased sample cannot be generalized to the population. Sampling bias is most likely to occur in nonprobability sampling but may also occur in probability sampling by chance, because of a small sample, or because of inherent biases in the sampling frame or data source.

Sample Size.   Regardless of the sampling method, a sample that is too small may cause an investigator to make the wrong conclusion about the hypothesis. That is, the data from the sample may seem to indicate that there is no relationship between the variables being tested or no difference between the treatment and control groups, when there really is a relationship or a difference. Unfortunately, there is no magic number for adequate sample size. Sample size must be calculated for each study. It will vary according to a number of factors including the level of measurement of the variables, the statistical test and strength desired for the test, the number of groups in the study, and what already is known about the population.

Other Sampling Issues.   We have discussed only very basic issues of sampling. Because sampling issues are critical, we urge you to include a statistician on your community health investigative team. Should you desire further reading on sampling, try the article by Selby, Gentry, Riportella-Muller, Quade, Legault, & Monahan (1990) and the references therein or the research texts already cited.

APPLICATION

In the EPSDT study, the results would ideally apply to the population of families with children eligible for EPSDT. However, a study of this magnitude was impossible. Officials in six rural North Carolina counties, all having low rates of EPSDT use and all within reasonable distance of the investigators, were eager to collaborate in the study. The investigators chose these counties as their *setting*. The county officials were most concerned about children who were overdue for EPSDT checkups. Therefore, the *target population* consisted of families in these counties that had at least one child eligible for EPSDT who had not used EPSDT in the past one or two years (depending on the age of the child). The members of the population were identified from a computerized database of Medicaid recipients, provided by the state Medicaid office. From the database, the investigators listed all families with children meeting the study's age and EPSDT nonuse criteria; the list formed the *sampling frame* for the study. Sampling frames were created periodically over a two-year period (1990–1992), in accordance with the intervention schedule for the study. Over the two-year period, the investigators periodically chose *probability* or random samples of families from the current sampling frame. The families that were chosen were the *subjects* for the study. A total *sample size* of 2541 families was calculated to meet the statistical specifications of the study.

Step 6C: Select or Design the Data Collection Instruments and Procedures

Now that the research design and sample have been determined, it is time to plan the methods for obtaining data from the sample. At this point the information desired has already been outlined in the form of operational definitions for the variables of interest. Now, data collection procedures and *instruments,* or devices for gathering data, must be selected or designed to collect data in accordance with the operational definitions.

Valid and reliable instruments and procedures help prevent systematic and random error. The concepts of reliability and validity were introduced in the discussion of screening programs. We will now relate these concepts to data collection instruments and procedures. Readers who desire further study are encouraged to refer to the *Standards for Educational and Psychological Testing,* which provides reliability and validity criteria for users and developers of instruments (American Educational Research Association, American Psychological Association, & National Council on Measurement in Education, 1985). Further discussion of validity and reliability also is provided by Selby-Harrington, Mehta, Jutsum, Riportella-Muller, & Quade (1994).

Validity.   Validity refers to the ability of a test or instrument to measure what it should measure. Strictly speaking, it is not the instruments themselves that are valid; it is the use that the researcher makes of the results. An instrument that is valid for one purpose might not be valid for another.

In research, if the instruments consist of screening tests, their validity is assessed through evaluation of sensitivity and specificity. Most often, however, research involves the use of instruments other than screening tests. For these other instruments, evidence of validity may be categorized according to face, content, criterion-related, and construct validity.

Face validity.   Some researchers contend that face validity is a legitimate form of validity. In epidemiologic circles, however, face validity is referred to, tongue in cheek, as "faith validity." Essentially, *face validity* means that the instrument appears valid to the researcher. In your research, you are urged not to consider this a true form of validity. It is presented here so you will evaluate skeptically any study that reports only face validity for its instruments.

Content validity.   The presence of content validity in an instrument indicates that the individual items in the instrument are representative of the concept(s) to be measured. This type of validity, generally considered the weakest true form of validity, is easily achieved and should be documented for any data abstracting form, questionnaire, attitude scale, or knowledge test. To obtain content validity, the proposed instrument is submitted to a number of experts in the field, referred to as a *panel of experts.* These experts critique the instrument and may suggest revisions before they agree that the items are representative of the concept(s) being measured.

Criterion-related validity. This type of validity is more difficult to achieve. Essentially, *criterion-related validity* measures the correlation between the proposed instrument and another, supposedly valid, measure of the same concept. The other measure, or criterion, may be a more-established instrument or any other valid method of measuring the concept. For example, in designing an instrument to assess the seriousness of a particular disease, a researcher might correlate the results obtained by the proposed instrument with those obtained when a medical expert does the assessment personally.

A difficulty with criterion-related validity comes in deciding upon the criterion against which the proposed instrument is to be measured. If the criterion itself is not valid, the validity of the proposed instrument cannot be determined. In the example above, the medical expert conceivably could make mistakes in the assessments.

Construct validity. Construct validity is intended to ensure that the instrument measures the concept it is supposed to measure and not something else. This is the highest form of validity; essentially, it states that the instrument truly is valid. Construct validity is difficult to establish; it can rarely be done on the basis of one study. Discussion of the various techniques for determining this type of validity is beyond the scope of this text. These techniques include the *known-groups method,* the *multi-trait multi-method matrix,* and *factor analysis.* As you grow in research experience and expertise, you may wish to consider these methods.

Choosing a method for determining validity. Table 2-5 presents a summary of key issues to consider in choosing methods to determine instrument validity. The methods are hierarchical. That is, each succeeding level is a higher form of validity. Therefore, you will want to begin with the easiest method and advance to the highest level possible for your instrument, given your real-life resources and constraints. In no case should you settle for less than content validity.

Reliability.   Reliability refers to the consistency of results. Reliability may be expressed as a *correlation coefficient* (r), usually ranging from zero to 1, or as a *percentage of agreement,* from 0% to 100%. Reliability of 1 or 100% is ideal but rare. Reliability of under 0.8 or 80% is questionable.

In assessing reliability, you should be aware that the correlation coefficient or percent of agreement is influenced by the sample from which

TABLE 2-5	*Guide to Techniques for Determining Instrument Validity*		
Type	**Key Question**	**Technique**	**Comments**
Face	Does the instrument appear to be logical?	Researcher decision	Alone, this is *not* a legitimate form of validity
Content	Are the individual items representative of the concept?	Panel of experts	Weakest form of true validity Relatively simple to achieve
Criterion related	Is there a high correlation between this measure and another measure of the same concept?	Correlation coefficient (between the 2 measures)	Difficult to decide on appropriate criterion If another valid measure is already available, is there a legitimate reason for not using the other measure?
Construct*	Does the instrument truly measure the concept and not something else?	Known groups	Assumption is made about characteristics of the known groups Least difficult of 3 construct validity techniques
		Multi-trait multi-method matrix	Requires 2 or more methods and concepts Requires some statistical sophistication
		Factor analysis	Requires some statistical sophistication

Construct validity is the highest form of validity.

reliability is calculated; in other words, reliability is *sample-specific*. For example, an instrument that has high reliability in a sample of military recruits may be very unreliable in a sample of pregnant teenagers.

For screening tests and procedures, reliability is measured by *intraobserver* and *interobserver agreement*. For other types of instruments and procedures, reliability usually is measured according to three key aspects: *equivalence, stability,* and *internal consistency*. The aspect of reliability to be measured depends on the type and purpose of the instrument or procedure. In this section, we will discuss the major methods for measuring validity.

Intraobserver and interobserver agreement. In intraobserver agreement, a screening test must yield the same results when it is repeated on the same individual, under the same conditions, by the *same* investigator or observer. In interobserver agreement, the test must yield consistent results when it is repeated on the same individual, under the same conditions, by separate investigators or observers.

Lack of intra- or interobserver agreement may suggest that the criteria for the instrument are inadequately formulated. If so, the criteria may need to be clarified or revised. Another common cause of poor reliability is insufficient training of screening personnel. Adequate training will help ensure reliability of the screening program and may also prevent embarrassment and diplomatic difficulties among staff members.

Equivalence.   Equivalence examines whether different researchers using the same instrument on the same subjects under the same conditions will measure the same characteristic (*interrater reliability*) or if different instruments used on the same subjects under the same conditions will measure the same characteristic (*parallel forms reliability*).

Interrater reliability is identical to the concept of interobserver agreement in screening tests, discussed above. It is also expressed as a correlation or percentage of agreement between the observers or raters. Interrater reliability is necessary if more than one person will collect data.

Parallel forms reliability is necessary if two different instruments are used to measure the same characteristic. This sometimes is the case in pretest-posttest studies for program evaluation. Although most often the pretest and posttest are identical, in some cases the researcher wants the tests to be different but to measure the same concept. If so, parallel forms reliability first must be established. The two tests are administered simultaneously to one sample, and a correlation or percentage of agreement is calculated between the subjects' responses on the two tests.

Stability.   Stability refers to the ability of the instrument or procedure to give the same results on repeated use. Stability is measured by intrarater or test-retest reliability, depending on whether the instrument is intended to be completed by the researcher or by the subject.

For a data collection form that will be completed by a researcher, stability may be measured by *intrarater reliability,* the equivalent of intraobserver agreement for a screening test. For example, in assessing the stability of a form for abstracting data from medical records, the researcher will use the form on a sample of records; a week to 10 days later, the researcher will repeat the process and determine a correlation or percentage of agreement between the two sets of results. This method will also help identify particular items on the form that are unclear.

For a data collection form that is to be completed by the subjects, stability may be measured by *test-retest reliability*. The questionnaire or scale is administered to a sample of subjects; a week to 10 days later, it is readministered to the same group, and a correlation or percentage of agreement of responses is calculated. This method, like the intrarater method, also helps identify individual items in need of revision.

Stability is not an appropriate aspect of reliability to measure in cases in which the measured characteristic or concept is expected to change over time. If the trait itself is not stable, the data collection device is not expected to yield stable results on readministration. An example is the concept of state anxiety, a psychological condition that may vary from moment to moment, depending on the situation (Spielberger, Gorsuch, & Lushene, 1968).

Internal Consistency.   Internal consistency refers to the ability of the various subparts of an instrument to measure the same characteristic or concept. This type of reliability is important in scales or tests in which the purpose is to provide an overall estimate of a single characteristic, such as attitude or knowledge.

Various techniques are used to calculate reliability for such scales and tests. These include the *coefficient alpha* (Cronbach's alpha), *split-half* or *odd-even* method with correction by the *Spearman-Brown prophecy formula,* and the *Kuder-Richardson 20* (KR-20). These calculations produce coefficients that are interpreted in the same manner as other reliability coefficients.

Choosing a method for determining reliability. Table 2-6 lists key issues for choosing methods to establish reliability. The methods for reliability, unlike those for validity, are not hierarchical; they simply are different. You will need to choose the method or methods appropriate for your particular instrument and purpose.

Documentation of Procedures.   A final aspect of quality assurance in data collection is the need for explicit *documentation* of procedures or protocols. Protocols must be written in sufficient detail to ensure consistency in the study. Clear protocols help guarantee that even if there are changes in personnel, the research can continue without a compromise in reliability or validity. The documentation also enables other researchers to replicate the study in different settings and populations, and it helps practitioners evaluate whether they might be able to apply the procedures to real-life practice.

TABLE 2-6   Guide to Techniques for Determining Instrument Reliability

Type	Key Questions	Technique	Comments
Equivalence	Do different researchers using the same instrument measure the same characteristic?	Interrater reliability	Used when more than one researcher using an instrument that requires subjective judgment
	Do different instruments measure the same characteristic?	Parallel forms reliability	Used when it is advisable to have different items for the pretest and posttest
Stability	Will instrument give the same results on repeat administration?		
	Instrument to be completed by researcher	Interrater reliability	Not appropriate if data being measured are not stable over time
	Instrument to be completed by subjects	Test-retest reliability	Short period of time between first and second administration may give falsely high reliability because person completing instrument may simply remember earlier responses
Internal consistency	Do the subparts measure the same characteristic?	For Likert-type scale: Coefficient alpha Split-half or odd-even with correction by Spearman-Brown prophecy For right/wrong questions: Kuder-Richardson 20 (KR-20) Split-half or odd-even with correction by Spearman-Brown prophecy	This type of reliability is not appropriate unless the various items are intended to measure the *same* concept
	Are individuals responding consistently?	Agreement of responses between two items that ask for the same information	Used when researcher is concerned about possibility that a particular item will not be measured accurately

APPLICATION

In the EPSDT study, a panel of experts reviewed the instruments to establish content validity. Public health nurses who were to conduct the interventions and use the instruments received reliability training and had to achieve at least 80% *interrater agreement* before they were allowed to use the instruments in the study. They followed detailed protocols developed by the investigators.

Step 6D: Plan the Data Analysis

Data analysis should be planned before the data are collected. In essence, all the previous steps in the research process—formulation of the research questions and hypotheses, operational definitions, and research design; selection of the sample; and design of the instruments and procedures—are directed toward data analysis. If these steps are planned properly, data analysis should proceed relatively smoothly. However, many a study has bitten the dust after months of data collection because it was discovered, too late, that the data collected could not be analyzed to produce valid results. You can see, then, that it is imperative to plan the data analysis while you still have an opportunity to make revisions in the plan for data collection.

Data analysis involves two types of statistics: *descriptive statistics,* which describe and summarize data, and *inferential statistics,* which test for the significance of relationships in the data. All studies require descriptive statistics. Only those that test hypotheses use inferential statistics. An overview of the use of descriptive and inferential statistics is provided below. For an in-depth explanation of statistics, you should consult a statistics textbook (for example, Munro & Page, 1993; Remington & Schork, 1985).

Descriptive Statistics.   Descriptive statistics should be used to describe the sample in terms of each important variable. These will include the key outcome variable, that is, the dependent variable, and important confounding variables in the study, such as age, education, and the like. If the study compares different groups of subjects, descriptive statistics should be presented separately for each group.

Selection of the appropriate statistics for a variable depends partly on the level of measurement, as shown in Table 2-7, and on the study

TABLE 2-7 *Guide to Selected Descriptive Statistics*

	Minimum Level of Measurement Required		
	NOMINAL	*ORDINAL*	*INTERVAL/RATIO*
Central tendency	Mode	Median	Mean
Variability	Percent	Range	Standard deviation
Association (both variables must be at least the level specified)	Contingency coefficient Lambda Phi coefficient	Spearman rho Kendall tau	Pearson product moment

design. The variables can be summarized by *measures of central tendency* such as the *mean, median,* and *mode,* and *measures of variability* such as the *standard deviation, range,* and *proportions or percentages.* Analysis of the levels or categories of a variable in terms of numbers and percentages is referred to as describing the *distribution* of the variable. In epidemiologic studies, it also is helpful to compute rates or odds ratios, whichever is justified by the study design.

APPLICATION

The EPSDT researchers planned to use descriptive statistics to describe the entire sample of families, as well as the different intervention and control groups, according to a number of variables. For example, they planned to compute the mean, standard deviation, and median age of children and number of children in the families, and the distribution of families in each county. For the dependent variable, effectiveness in producing EPSDT use, they planned to calculate rates of EPSDT use for each intervention and control group.

Inferential Statistics. *Inferential statistics* are used in studies in which a hypothesis is tested. The hypothesis may be about an *association between variables* such as tampon-brand use and the occurrence of toxic shock syndrome or about a *difference between groups* such as the difference in pulse rates between persons who participate in an exercise program and those who do not. The inferential statistic tests if the association or difference is *statistically significant,* or divergent from that expected by chance alone.

Considerations in choosing inferential statistics. Essentially, inferential statistics test for the statistical significance of differences or relationships between descriptive statistics. In the study of tampon-brand use and TSS, an inferential statistic was used to test for significance of the odds ratio. In the case of exercisers and nonexercisers, an inferential statistic could be used to test for differences between the mean pulse rates of the exercisers and nonexercisers.

It should come as no surprise that selection of inferential statistics, like descriptive statistics, must consider the level of measurement of the variables and the design of the study. Table 2-8 is a guide for selecting inferential statistics in some common community health research situations. The table considers basic requirements for the level of measurement, study design, and sample. However, each statistical test may have additional specifications regarding the nature of the data. Therefore, it is advisable to consult a statistics text and a statistician when planning a study.

APPLICATION

In the EPSDT study, the dependent variable, EPSDT use, was measured at the nominal level. The hypothesis tested for differences in EPSDT use among three groups in one study (control, mailed pamphlet, home visit) and among four groups in the other study (control, mailed pamphlet, phone call, home visit). The investigative team's statistician chose a chi-square test for the hypothesis. Using Table 2-8, what test would you have chosen?

Displaying Statistics: Tables. Tables facilitate communication of statistical data and, if planned appropriately, can guide data collection and analysis. Experienced researchers construct *dummy tables,* or outlines of tables, before they collect data. They fill in the tables as they collect data, and they analyze and write the results from the completed tables. The tables will be modified for publication, but the basic data are readily accessible in an organized format.

Tables are helpful in communicating large amounts of data, such as sample characteristics, in a succinct manner. To communicate clearly, a

TABLE 2-8. *Guide to Selected Inferential Statistics for Testing for Differences Between Groups*

	Level of Measurement of Dependent Variable		
TYPE(S) OF GROUP(S)	*NOMINAL*	*ORDINAL*	*INTERVAL/RATIO*
One sample (comparing distribution of variable to a hypothesized distribution)	Chi-square test for goodness of fit	Sign test Wilcoxon matched pairs Signed rank test	*Means:* Unknown population variance: one sample t-test, $df = n - 1$ Known population variance: one sample Z-test *Proportions:* One-sample Z-test for proportions
Two independent groups	Chi-square tests Fisher exact test	Median test Mann-Whitney U test	*Means:* Two-sample t-test for independent samples $df = n_1 + n_2 + 2$ *Proportions:* Two-sample Z-test for proportions
More than two independent groups	Chi-square tests	Extension of median test Kruskal-Wallis test	*Means:* One-way analysis of variance (one-way ANOVA)
One group—before/after, or two related groups (matched pairs)	McNemar test	Wilcoxon matched pairs Signed-rank test	*Difference scores:* Paired t-tests for paired data (t-test for related samples) $df = n - 1$ where n = number of pairs
One group with fewer than two repeated measures. Or fewer than two related groups (matched triplets, etc.)	Cochran Q test	Friedman test	Repeated measures analysis
Two groups before/after	Adaptation of data for Chi-square tests Adaptation of data for Fisher exact tests	Adaptation of data for Mann-Whitney U test (if scores can be subtracted)	*Mean changes:* Two sample t-test for independent samples, $df = n_1 + n_2 - 2$ One-way analysis of variance *Means:* Analysis of covariance
More than two groups before/after	Adaptation of data for Chi-square tests	Adaptation of data for Kruskal-Wallis test (if scores can be subtracted)	*Mean changes:* One-way analysis of variance *Means:* Analysis of covariance

Note: Lower level tests may be used for higher level data, but some loss of information may result.

table must have an explicit title that specifies its contents. The table should be understandable without reference to the text.

A *crosstabulation* is a special type of table that allows for the visual inspection of a relationship between variables. We examined crosstabulations when we looked at the relationship between tampon use and TSS (see Table 2-3).

Displaying Statistics: Figures.   Figures, or pictorial representations, also facilitate communication of statistics. Figures are generally reserved for important concepts or findings. Like tables, figures can be planned beforehand. Their final form, of course, will be dictated by the actual results.

Different figures have different uses. The nature of the data and the purpose of the display will guide the selection of figures. For instance, *bar charts* are helpful in showing discrete categories of data. *Pie charts* show the parts of a whole. *Scatterplots* help depict relationships between ordinal or interval/ratio variables. *Line graphs* can emphasize trends over time. *Flow charts* help explain sequential steps, such as complex sampling procedures.

It is important to become familiar with the purposes of various types of charts and graphs. In community health practice, an effective graphic

TABLE 2-9.   *Number and Percentage of Families Using EPSDT After Intervention*

Intervention Group	Total	Using EPSDT	
		NUMBER	PERCENTAGE
Families with Telephones			
Control	154	5	3.2
Mailed intervention	147	12	8.2
Phone call	150	23	15.3
Home visit	148	30	20.3
Families Without Telephones			
Control	151	10	6.6
Mailed intervention	153	15	9.8
Home visit	145	10	6.9
Total	*1048*	*105*	*10.0*

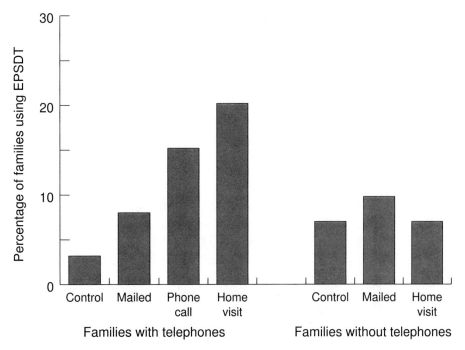

FIGURE 2-4
Percentage of families using EPSDT after intervention.

presentation of a health problem may make the difference between fund-ing or no funding for a program request. Personal computer programs enable nonartists to make visually pleasing and effective figures.

APPLICATION

The EPSDT investigators constructed numerous *dummy tables* for the variables in the study, for example, for statistics to describe the sample of families, such as the numbers and ages of children, and for rates of EPSDT use according to inter-vention group. As data collection proceeded, the investigators filled in the tables. Table 2-9 is one of them in its completed form.

The investigators also planned to construct figures for their central findings. They decided that a bar chart showing the rate of EPSDT use for each study group would help illustrate the results of test of the hypothesis. Figure 2-4 shows what this figure looked like midway through the study.

Components of Informed Consent

1. Invitation to participate in study
2. Assurance that subject has right to refuse to participate and that refusal will not place subject in jeopardy
3. Assurance that subject has the right to withdraw from participation and that withdrawal will not place subject in jeopardy
4. Explanation of purpose of study
5. Explanation of study procedures (as they relate to subjects)
6. Description of potential risks, discomforts, inconveniences, or threats to dignity involved in study
7. Description of any costs to subjects of participating in study (including expenses for elements of participation such as travel)
8. Explanation of benefits of study (as they relate to subjects)
9. Description of any compensation to be expected, whether monetary or otherwise
10. Disclosure of any available alternatives
11. Assurance of confidentiality or anonymity
12. Statement regarding contact person and an offer to answer questions
13. Description of any compensation available in the event of injury resulting from participation
14. Concluding statement noting that subject indicates by signature (or, in certain studies, by return of completed questionnaire) that he/she has read the information and has decided to participate

Step 7: Ensure the Protection of Human Subjects

Before the study can proceed, investigators must ensure that the methods include protections for human subjects. Such protections must be in place whether the research involves direct participation by human subjects or simply a review of existing data for humans (such as medical records and tissue specimens collected for another purpose). A review board or a designated individual in the health agency will generally assess whether the protections are adequate. The researcher must allow adequate time for the review, which can take a few days to a month. If multiple agencies are involved, each may require a review. Key aspects to consider in protecting human subjects are discussed below.

Many community health studies deal with existing data or with surveys that do not identify individuals. In such cases, the requirement to protect human subjects may include only an assurance of *anonymity,* meaning that the researcher will not have knowledge of the individual identities of subjects, or an assurance of *confidentiality,* meaning that the researcher will not disclose individual identification either intentionally or unintentionally.

In studies involving direct participation by human subjects, federal guidelines mandate that *informed consent* be obtained from individual subjects. The basic components of informed consent are summarized in the accompanying display. These components must be presented to subjects in language that is clear, unambiguous, and appropriate for their age, educational level, and level of understanding. Special restrictions apply to minors and individuals whose ability to provide informed consent may be compromised.

In studies that test ways to improve services or access to services in governmental programs, federal law allows a researcher to apply for a waiver of informed consent (Code of Federal Regulations, 1991). A waiver can simplify research in community health settings, but it does not mean that human rights can be ignored. Subjects still cannot be forced to participate. All reasonable protections, including confidentiality, must be maintained even though the full components of informed consent are not discussed.

APPLICATION

In the EPSDT study, the investigators requested a waiver of informed consent. The research was for the purpose of improving access to EPSDT services, and requiring full informed consent might actually mislead parents to think that EPSDT services were a form of research on children. Parents were allowed to refuse an educational intervention, just as they might refuse any service. The study included many protections for confidentiality. For example, data were kept in locked cabinets, and computer passwords were regulated and changed frequently. The participating state and county agencies approved the study procedures and granted a waiver of informed consent.

Step 8: State the Limitations of the Study
At this point, nearly all the details of the study have been planned. Given real-life resources and constraints, compromises undoubtedly have been

made between what is desired and what is possible; no study is perfect. Now, the imperfections should be reviewed as a whole and stated explicitly.

In effect, the statement of limitations serves as a final check on the validity of the study methods. It provides an opportunity to reconsider aspects of the study that should and still can be revised. Every effort should be made to remedy the limitations before the study begins. The statement of limitations also helps ensure that the validity of the future results will not be overestimated by the researcher or by others.

Throughout this chapter, limitations have been discussed in terms of individual aspects of study methodology. In identifying the limitations of a study as a whole, it is helpful to consider the limitations in terms of threats to the internal and external validity of a study.

Internal validity refers to the validity of the results within the context of the study, or the confidence with which it can be said that the results can be attributed to the factors considered in the study and not to factors that were not considered. A true experiment with controls for possible confounding variables is the surest way to ensure the internal validity of a study. However, *no* study is perfect. In stating the limitations of a study, a researcher should describe aspects of research methodology, specific to the study, that fail to control for threats to internal validity.

The following are a number of classic threats to internal validity.

1. Selection bias.
The results may be influenced by over- or underrepresentation of certain characteristics in the sample.

2. Test effects.
The results may be influenced by the measures used in the study. For example, in a study of blood pressure medication, improvement in blood pressure may be attributable to changes in health behavior resulting from having the blood pressure measured regularly during the study rather than to the medication.

3. History.
The results may be influenced by events that occur outside the realm of the study. For example, in studying Agent Orange and birth defects, research findings were confounded by possible life events and

exposures that occurred between the father's exposure to Agent Orange and the subsequent birth of a child with a defect.

4. Maturation.

The results may be influenced by changes that occur due to time itself. Children normally grow and develop; wounds normally heal; problems simply get better over time. In studying a program's impact on infant mortality, researchers must consider that, without a program, the U.S. infant mortality rate usually improves each year.

5. Mortality.

The results may be influenced by the loss of subjects through death, migration, or disinterest. The subjects who remain at the end of the study may be quite different from those who do not.

6. Hawthorne effect.

The results may be attributable to the fact that people sometimes act differently under research conditions than they do in real life. In particular, subjects may want to please the researcher.

7. Novelty effect.

A procedure or intervention may be appealing simply because it is new. It may lose its appeal (and effectiveness) when implemented in practice after the research study.

8. Regression to the mean.

Statistically, subjects who initially have very low or very high values on a variable are likely to have a less extreme value if tested again. For example, a subject who scores 99% on a test has very little room for an increased score (100%) but much room for a decreased score (from 98% to 0%).

External validity refers to the validity of the results outside the study; that is, the confidence with which the results from the sample can be generalized to the population. Use of a probability sample of adequate size is the surest way to control for threats to internal validity. However, even a study using a probability sample is limited in generalizability to the population from which the sample was drawn. Consider, also, that regardless of the quality of the sampling method, if internal validity is poor, external validity also will be poor. That is, if the findings are not valid within the study, they cannot be valid outside the study. In stating limitations regarding external validity, aspects of the sample or population that limit the generalizability of the findings should be described.

APPLICATION

The EPSDT study used an experimental design and a probability sample of households in six rural counties from 1990 to 1992. Despite careful planning, the study had a number of limitations; two are listed below. The first one represents a threat to internal validity; the second, a threat to external validity. Can you think of other limitations?

1. The study itself was expected to heighten interest in EPSDT in the study counties. Personnel in these offices might promote EPSDT more during the study than they did before the study or would after the study.
2. Because the population from which the random sample was drawn consisted only of families meeting the study criteria in six rural counties, results cannot be generalized to other areas or other populations.

Step 9: Conduct a Pilot Study

The purpose of a pilot study is to test the instruments and procedures on a small group. The pilot study may reveal unanticipated problems that can be remedied before the study is implemented on a large scale. If no problems are identified, the study may proceed as planned. The researcher must keep in mind that approvals must be obtained from the necessary review boards *before* conducting a pilot study.

APPLICATION

After obtaining approval from the review boards, the investigators conducted a pilot study with 100 families in one of the six counties. The pilot study showed that the instruments had high reliability and that the procedures were feasible to implement. It also provided data about the time needed to implement each intervention. This information was useful in planning how many nurses were needed to conduct the study. Data trends, though insufficient for definitive analysis, suggested that the interventions might be improving EPSDT use. Thus, the pilot study verified the need to pursue further study, as planned, with a larger sample.

Step 10: Implement the Methodology

By this time, the methods have been planned, documented, and tested in a pilot study. Therefore, this step is straightforward. The researcher simply follows the research plan all the way through data analysis.

APPLICATION

The EPSDT investigators implemented the methods as planned. They used a computer to select random samples from the sampling frame and to randomly assign subjects to intervention and control groups. Using detailed protocols and valid and reliable instruments, they conducted the interventions and collected data as planned. They calculated descriptive statistics and performed chi-square tests. They constructed tables and figures to display the findings (e.g., refer again to Table 2-9 and Figure 2-4).

Step 11: Interpret the Results

Step 12: Communicate the Results

After the data are analyzed, the results must be interpreted and then communicated to audiences who can use the information. Interpretation and communication, of course, are two separate steps; in other words, the results cannot be communicated until they have been interpreted. Nevertheless, the steps are intertwined. When done well, interpretation and communication of research findings demonstrate a synthesis of the researcher's understanding of a number of factors, which are described in the following paragraphs.

Comprehension of Basic Principles of Epidemiology, Demography, and Research.   The results of a study must be interpreted in view of the validity and limitations of the methods used to collect the data, and the findings must be presented to the audience in this light.

Understanding of the Specific Statistical Measures Used.   This is part of the researcher's understanding of the basic principles of epidemiology, demography, and research, but it also implies specific knowledge of the statistical measures actually used in the study. This chapter has presented the advantages and disadvantages of some of the most common statistical measures of health. These and other measures must be interpreted in respect to their purposes and limitations.

Familiarity with All Aspects of the Data.   Researchers sometimes make the mistake of focusing on one particularly interesting finding, to the exclusion of other results. This may lead to misinterpretation. Other results may contradict the particular finding or indicate a trend not apparent from an isolated piece of data.

Knowledge of Theory and Past Research.   You have learned that a research study must be planned in view of existing theory and research. The results must also be interpreted and explained in this context. If a finding is not compatible with existing knowledge, the researcher must explore possible reasons for the inconsistency. The researcher also should address further research needs that have been identified by the study.

Awareness of Influences of the Real World on the Results.   It is possible to become so immersed in a study that the context of the real world is forgotten. The researcher has an obligation to be aware of and report real-life influences on the data. For instance, was a particular statistic (such as mean, rate, and so on) influenced by deviant values from one particular segment of the sample? In a multiclinic setting, were the records from a particular clinic not documented as reliably as the rest?

Awareness of Influences of the Study Results on the Real World.   The researcher should also consider the results in terms of their potential impact on the real world. Sometimes in their preoccupation with statistics, researchers confuse *statistical significance* with real-life or *clinical significance*. With large enough samples, almost any difference may be statistically significant. But, for instance, does it make a real-life difference if one group has a mean diastolic blood pressure of 76 mm Hg and another has a mean of 82 mm Hg, even if the difference is statistically significant? Conversely, a small sample may result in lack of statistical significance, not because there is no true difference but because the statistics are not sensitive to the difference. For example, in a small study, the difference in diastolic blood pressures between a group with a mean of 84 mm Hg and a group with a mean of 98 mm Hg might not be statistically significant. The lack of statistical significance should not blind the researcher to the potential need for intervention in the group with the *clinically* higher blood pressure.

Communication to Appropriate Audiences. A study is incomplete until the findings are communicated; otherwise, the research has not fulfilled its purpose of providing new knowledge. The researcher's knowledge of the potential influence of the results will help identify the audience to whom the results should be communicated. The information should be directed toward groups that can use and apply the results—those that can do something with the new knowledge. Communication may be in the form of local, regional, or national presentations; professional newsletters; or professional journals. For assistance in planning how to report your study findings, you may wish to refer to publications by Selby, Tornquist, & Finerty (1989a, 1989b), Tornquist (1986), or Zotti, Selby-Harrington, & Riportella-Muller (1994).

APPLICATION

Midway through the EPSDT study, preliminary analyses showed that all the interventions produced higher rates of EPSDT use than the control procedures. Among families with phones, home visits were the most effective intervention, followed by phone calls and mailed pamphlets. Among families without phones, however, home visits were not more effective than mailed pamphlets. The researchers were puzzled by the latter finding, which was inconsistent with earlier research. Therefore, they interviewed 110 parents who had received various interventions in the study and found that, indeed, the parents preferred to receive health information by mail.

The analyses also showed that the cost per effect (that is, per child receiving EPSDT care as a result of the intervention) for a home visit was much higher than the cost per effect for a phone call or mailed pamphlet; thus, the use of home visits for the sole purpose of encouraging parents to use EPSDT would not be cost-effective. Because home visits would not be cost-effective and phone calls could not be used for families without phones, the researchers identified the mailed pamphlet as having the greatest promise of being feasible for widespread use in practice.

The researchers also considered the fact that, although the *relative* impact of the interventions was great, the *absolute* impact was small. The highest rate of EPSDT use for an intervention group was 20% (compared with 3%–7% for the control groups); the researchers wanted to improve this rate. Therefore, while they continued to analyze data for the remainder of the study, the researchers also planned new interventions for future study. The findings of the current study, as well as statewide concerns about populations with low literacy, guided them to develop a new mailed pamphlet intended for use by people with limited reading skills.

The investigative team communicated the study findings, tempered by the limitations of the study, to other professionals who could use the findings. They made presentations to staff from agencies dealing with health, social services, and Medicaid, and they also made presentations at regional and national conferences (see Stearns et al., 1992; Tesh, Selby, Stearns, & Riportella-Muller, 1993). As various parts of the study were finalized, the investigators published the findings in public health and nursing journals (see Richardson, Selby-Harrington, & Sorenson, 1993; Selby et al., 1990; Selby, Riportella-Muller, Sorenson, Quade, & Luchok, 1992; Selby-Harrington & Riportella-Muller, 1993).

Summary

In this chapter you have been introduced to demography, the broad science of populations; epidemiology, the specific science of population health; and research principles applicable to community health. You have learned that research is an integral part of community health practice. Research directs all phases of community health practice: assessment, diagnosis, planning, implementation, and evaluation. In this chapter, you saw how community health investigators applied the intertwined concepts of demography, epidemiology, and research to study a health problem in community health practice. What began as a clinical concern in several public health clinics resulted in a study with findings that have implications not only for the specific clinics but also for researchers and clinicians nationally.

Be assured that you are not yet expected to conduct research with implications for the health of the nation. Nevertheless, after studying this chapter, you should be able to apply epidemiologic, demographic, and research principles to your community health practice. When you are ready to begin a research study of your own, this chapter will help guide you through the research process. For more detailed information on epidemiology, demography, or research, you may wish to consult the reference list.

REFERENCES

American Educational Research Association (AERA), American Psychological Association (APA), & National Council on Measurement in Education (NCME). (1985). *Standards for educational and psychological testing.* Washington, DC: American Psychological Association, Inc.

Becker, M. H., Haefner, D. P., Kasl, S. V., Kirscht, J. P., Maimon, L. A., & Rosenstock, I. M. (1977). Selected psychosocial models and correlates of individual health-related behaviors. *Medical Care, 15,* 27–46.

Centers for Disease Control. (1980, September 19). Follow up on toxic shock syndrome. *Morbidity and Mortality Weekly Report, 29,* 441–445.

———. (1981, June 30). Toxic shock syndrome—United States, 1970–1980. *Morbidity and Mortality Weekly Report, 30,* 25–33.

———. (1983, August 5). Update: Toxic shock syndrome—United States. *Morbidity and Mortality Weekly Report, 32,* 398–400.

Centers for Disease Control and Prevention. (1993, September 10). Public health focus: Physical activity and the prevention of coronary heart disease. *Morbidity and Mortality Weekly Report, 42,* 398–400.

Code of Federal Regulations, Federal Register. (1991, June 18). Federal policy for the protection of human subjects: Notices and rules, Part II. Title 45CFR. Washington, DC: Office of the Federal Register, National Archives and Records Administration, U.S. Government Printing Office.

Cook, T. D., & Campbell, D. T. (1979). *Quasi-experimentation: Design and analysis issues for field settings.* Boston: Houghton Mifflin.

Cravens, G., & Mair, J. L. (1977). *The black death.* New York: Dutton.

Crichton, M. (1969). *The Andromeda strain.* New York: Alfred A. Knopf.

Davis, J. P., Chesney, P. J., Ward, P. J., LaVenture, M., & the Investigation and Laboratory Team. (1980). Toxic shock syndrome: Epidemiologic features, recurrence, risk factors, and prevention. *New England Journal of Medicine, 303,* 1429–1435.

Dunne, T. L. (1978). *The scourge.* New York: Coward, McCann, & Geohegan.

Fitz-Gibbon, C. T., & Morris, L. L. (1987). *How to design a program evaluation.* Newbury Park, CA: Sage Publications.

Green, L. W., Krueter, M. W., Deeds, S. G., & Partridge, K. B. (1980). *Health planning: A diagnostic approach.* Palo Alto, CA: Mayfield.

Hammett, M., Powell, K. E., O'Carroll, P. W., & Clanton, S. T. (1992). Homicide surveillance, 1979–1988. *Morbidity and Mortality Weekly Report, 41,* SS–3, 1–33.

Lilienfeld, D. E., & Stolley, P. D. (1994). *Foundations of epidemiology* (3rd ed.). New York: Oxford University Press.

MacMahon, B., & Pugh, T. F. (1970). *Epidemiology: Principles and methods.* Boston: Little, Brown & Co.

Mausner, J. S., & Kramer, S. (1985). *Epidemiology: An introductory text.* Philadelphia: W. B. Saunders.

Morley, W. E., Messick, J. M., & Aguillera, D. C. (1967). Crisis: Paradigms of intervention. *Journal of Psychiatric Nursing, 5,* 531–544.

Morrison, A. S. (1992). *Screening in chronic disease* (2nd ed.). New York: Oxford University Press.

Munro, B. H., & Page, E. B. (1993). *Statistical methods for health care research* (2nd ed.). Philadelphia: J. B. Lippincott Co.

National Center for Health Statistics. (1993, September 28). Annual summary of births, marriages, divorces, and deaths: United States, 1992. *Monthly Vital Statistics Report, 41*(13), 1–33.

Pender, N. J. (1987). *Health promotion in nursing practice* (2nd ed.). Norwalk, CT: Appleton & Lange.

Polit, D. F., & Hungler, B. P. (1991). *Nursing research: Principles and methods* (4th ed.). Philadelphia: J. B. Lippincott Co.

Remington, R. D., & Schork, M. A. (1985). *Statistics with applications to the biological and health sciences* (2nd ed.). Englewood Cliffs, NJ: Prentice-Hall.

Richardson, L. A., Selby-Harrington, M. L., & Sorenson, J. R. (1993). Guidance for using a pilot study: An example of research on minority children. *Journal of National Black Nurses' Association, 6*(2), 44–55.

Rogers, C. (1969). *Freedom to learn.* Columbus, OH: Charles E. Merrill Publishing.

Roht, L. H., Selwyn, B. J., Holguin, A. H., & Christensen, B. L. (1982). *Principles of epidemiology: A self-teaching guide.* New York: Academic Press.

Selby, M. L., Gentry, N. O., Riportella-Muller, R., Quade, D., Legault, C., & Monahan, K. (1990). Evaluation of sampling methods reported in selected clinical nursing journals: Implications for nursing practice. *Journal of Professional Nursing, 6*(2), 76–85.

Selby, M. L., Riportella-Muller, R., Sorenson, J. R., Quade, D., Stearns, S., & Farel, A. (1992). Nursing interventions to improve EPSDT utilization: The Healthy Kids Project. *Search, 16*(1), 3–4.

Selby, M. L., Riportella-Muller, R., Sorenson, J. R., Quade, D., Sappenfield, M. M., Potter, H. B., & Farel, A. M. (1990). Public health nursing interventions to improve the use of a health service: Using a pilot study to guide research. *Public Health Nursing, 7*(1), 3–12.

Selby, M. L., Riportella-Muller, R., Sorenson, J. R., Quade, D., & Luchok, K. L. (1992). Increasing participation by private physicians in the EPSDT program in rural North Carolina. *Public Health Reports, 107*(5), 561–568.

Selby, M. L., Riportella-Muller, R., Sorenson, J. R., & Walters, C. R. (1989). Improving EPSDT use: Development and application of a practice based model for public health nursing research. *Public Health Nursing, 6*(4), 174–181. Reprinted in Spradley, B. W. (1991) *Readings in community health nursing* (4th ed., pp. 323–336). Philadelphia: J. B. Lippincott.

Selby, M. L., Tornquist, E. M., & Finerty, E. J. (1989a). How to present your research. Part I: What they didn't teach you in nursing school about planning and organizing the content of your speech. *Nursing Outlook, 37*(4), 172–175.

———. (1989b). How to present your research. Part II: The ABC's of creating and using visual aids to enhance your research presentation. *Nursing Outlook, 37*(5), 236–238.

Selby-Harrington, M. L., Mehta, S. M., Jutsum, V., Riportella-Muller, R., & Quade, D. (1994, January/February). Reporting of instrument validity and reliability in selected clinical nursing journals, 1989. *Journal of Professional Nursing, 10*(1), 47–56.

Selby-Harrington, M. L., & Riportella-Muller, R. (1993). Easing the burden on health departments: A cost-effective method for public health nurses to increase private sector participation in the Early and Periodic Screening, Diagnosis and Treatment (EPSDT) program. *Public Health Nursing, 10*(2), 114–121.

Singleton, R. A., Straits, B. C., & Straits, M. M. (1993). *Approaches to social research* (2nd ed.). New York: Oxford University Press.

Snow, J. (1936). *Snow on cholera, being a reprint of two papers by John Snow, M.D., together with a biographical memoir by B. W. Richardson, M.D., and an introduction by Wade Hampton Frost, M.D., 1936.* New York: The Commonwealth Fund.

Spielberger, C., Gorsuch, R., & Lushene, R. (1968). *The state-trait anxiety inventory.* Palo Alto, CA: Consulting Psychologists Press.

Stearns, S., Selby, M. L., Riportella-Muller, R., Sorenson, J., Farel, A., & Chaudhary, M. A. (1992, November). *Increasing use of EPSDT through outreach interventions.* Paper presented at the meeting of the American Public Health Association, Washington, DC.

Tesh, A. S., Selby, M. L., Stearns, S. C., & Riportella-Muller, R. (1993, January). *Nursing interventions to improve use of health services for indigent children.* Poster presented at the Third Primary Care Research Conference, Agency for Health Care Policy and Research, Atlanta, GA.

Tornquist, E. M. (1986). *From proposal to publication. An informal guide to writing about nursing research.* Menlo Park, CA: Addison-Wesley Publishing Company.

Zotti, M. E., Selby-Harrington, M. L., & Riportella-Muller, R. (1994, May/June). Communicating research findings to readers of clinical nursing journals: Guidance for prospective authors. *Journal of Pediatric Health Care, 8*(3), 106–110.

3

Ecological Connections

Robert W. McFarlane

Judith McFarlane

Objectives

The community health nurse needs to have an understanding of the principles and applications of human ecology as they affect human health. After studying this chapter, you will be able to

- Understand the ecological mechanisms that facilitate the migration of pollutants from their sources to human populations
- Apply this ecological knowledge to the promotion of health and the identification of human health problems of environmental origin

Introduction

No person or community is an independent entity. Each is intimately linked to the environment, frequently in ways we have never imagined. Thus, the environment influences health, directly and indirectly, through subtle, indirect pathways. Conversely, human activities affect the health of the environmental system. One aspect of *human ecology* is the study of these linkages. This chapter will explore the ways in which interconnections, transport mechanisms, and constant change combine to affect health.

Political action in the United States during the 1970s produced new legislation and strengthened a number of existing laws protecting human populations and the environment. Pollution-control efforts concentrated on reducing the quantities of pollutants emitted by major point sources, such as smokestacks or water-discharge pipes. These pollutants affected large numbers of people over broad areas of the nation. The success of these efforts can be gauged by the measurable reduction of the major air and water pollutants that has been achieved in our environment.

The current challenge is to control pollutants from nonpoint sources—pollutants that are released in smaller quantities from innumerable locations. These arise from agricultural activity, urban development, motor vehicle operation, and the disposal of solid wastes, among other sources. They are present in our homes and workplaces as well as at industrial sites. These pollutants may be released in smaller quantities and may affect fewer people than the point-source contaminants, but many are potentially more toxic. Many exhibit carcinogenic, mutagenic, or teratogenic effects.

The carcinogenic potential of hazardous pollutants in air, water, and solid waste is perceived by the public as a major health problem. An effective public policy must be developed to define and reduce any significant risks to public health that may arise from exposure to hazardous substances. Determining *if* and *when* and *how* human exposure to potentially hazardous substances should be regulated will be an essential, yet difficult, governmental task. Risk management decisions are always complex and almost always involve some degree of uncertainty that cannot be resolved with the available scientific facts.

The difficulties of creating a public policy are further compounded by the observation that everyone does not respond in the *same way* to the *same exposure* to the *same chemical substance*. The effects of a given substance may be magnified in some people by a concurrent exposure to other chemicals or minimized in other people because of genetic characteristics. The cost of providing complete protection to everyone may not be justified if the benefits would apply to only a small fraction of the exposed population. Further, the existence of health problems unrelated to pollution can complicate evaluation. For instance, in a milieu in which voluntary substance abuse and obesity are major community health problems, it is difficult to determine the limits of regulated exposure to an environmental risk.

In recent history, the interdependency of the human species and the natural world has been too frequently overlooked or ignored. As we seek ways to alleviate problems associated with health, it is imperative to be cognizant of nature's operating principles. The "laws of nature" have not been repealed, and knowledge of these laws is vital to understanding the origin of health problems and in successfully designing strategies to reduce them. The law of gravity is particularly important to

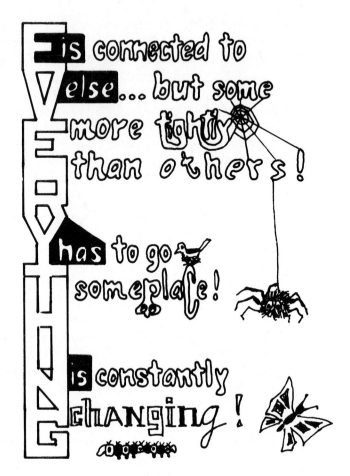

FIGURE 3-1
The basic laws of ecology.

the ecological system. Everything that goes up, including pollutants, must come down, and everything dumped on the surface of the earth must ultimately flow downhill. Water and even land masses, such as mountains, move slowly to the sea. It is imperative that we learn to design with nature, exploiting these principles to advantage, rather than expending resources in a useless struggle, for nature always wins.

It is important to remember three commonsense observations that are frequently overlooked because of their inherent simplicity (Figure 3-1).

Everything is connected to everything else, but some things are con-nected more tightly than others. This observation is the least obvious, and it will be the objective of this chapter to demonstrate its validity. As we go from a climatically controlled workplace to a correspondingly pleasant home, insulated from the vagaries of the weather even while en route, it is easy to forget that working in a climate-controlled environment is a very recent phenomenon, restricted to a minority of the world population. As we select foodstuffs from the bounty of 24-hour supermarkets, we seldom stop to wonder where a particular item came from; what chemical abuses it may have suffered during its growth, harvest, or transportation; or what unsuspected surprises may lurk beneath the protective cellophane.

Everything has to go someplace. Although this observation is readily acknowledged, "someplace" is generally considered synonomous with "away" and is not considered to be a problem until the "away" becomes your living space. This may produce the now familiar "NIMBY" reaction (not in my back yard!). As human populations and industrial develop-ment grow, pollutants are produced in greater quantities and dispersed over longer distances. At the same time, unpopulated areas are dimin-ishing. Some pollutants are conspicuous and readily detected. Others, perhaps more insidious, are detected only when sought; the search fre-quently requires elaborate instrumentation and methodology.

Everything is constantly changing. Although constant change is uni-versally recognized, the nature and rate of change are generally unap-preciated. The natural environment undergoes continual change. Some changes seem irreversible, permanent, or barely detectable from our per-spective in time (for example, geologic transformations and continental drift). Other changes are cyclic (such as the seasonal climate) or transient (floods or droughts). However, changes produced by the actions of human beings have become more prominent. Significant human-induced changes began with the domestication of animals and the development of agriculture. These led to the growth of large human settlements, soon fol-lowed by deforestation and the depletion of local resources. The rate of change increased greatly as muscle power was replaced by mechanical power and renewable energy resources (wood, wind, and water) were replaced by energy derived from fossil fuels.

During the last few decades, human impacts have reached an unprecedented intensity and now affect the entire world, owing to a vastly increased population and higher per capita consumption. The nature of change has also been altered as development projects redirect rivers, create lakes, alter sedimentation patterns, and introduce new crops, in addition to producing agricultural-industrial air, water, and soil pollution. The desire to control the environment often creates conflicts between our goals and natural environmental patterns. In the quest to increase production, people often deflect natural flows of energy, bypass natural processes, sever food chains, simplify natural systems, and consume large energy subsidies in order to maintain the equilibria in artificial systems. The pursuit of short-term gains often results in irreversible environmental degradation. Humanity has become a geologic agent and is rapidly altering both the face of the earth and the planet's capacity to support human populations.

When exploring these interconnections, it may be useful to remember that only one rule has no exceptions: There are exceptions to every rule.

Energy and Nutrients

All living organisms require both nutrients with which to build and maintain their bodies and energy to drive the chemical reactions that permit them to function. The nutrients are continuously recycled by way of natural processes and are used over and over again. The energy literally arrives from outer space and cannot be recycled.

The sun is the only significant source of energy in our solar system. A substantial portion of the sunlight that reaches the earth is reflected back into space (the same phenomenon of reflecting light permits viewing of the moon and other planets). The light that is absorbed by the earth is transformed into a lower energy state. Eventually all of this energy will be radiated back into space as heat. Our existence is dependent upon what is done with this energy before it leaves the earth.

This process of absorption is a familiar one because our bodies absorb heat from the sun in the same way. When outdoors in winter, we may consciously seek to position ourselves in direct sunlight to warm ourselves by absorbing this free energy, and in summer we seek shade and rapidly overheat when exposed to the sun. Our absorption can be modified through varying the color of our outer garments, using white or light colors to reflect sunlight and black or dark colors to increase absorption.

Consider another example: An automobile is parked with all its windows closed. Sunlight passes through the windows and strikes the dashboard, steering wheel, and seat covers. The energy of the sunlight is absorbed and transformed into infrared energy, or heat. This lower form of energy cannot pass through the windows as readily as the visible wavelengths of light. Thus, heat builds up inside the automobile, and those objects that absorbed the most energy have the quickest rise in temperature. The interior of the car will become much warmer than the outside environment, and the car will radiate heat long after the source of light is removed at sundown. This is often called the *greenhouse effect.*

The earth's unique atmosphere has the same effect. Heat radiating from the surface of the earth is trapped by the atmospheric gases. Uneven heating of the earth's surface (caused by the sun heating/lighting one side at a time) creates air and water currents. These currents distribute the heat more evenly and moderate extreme temperature fluctuations (typical of objects in space that lack an atmosphere, such as our moon).

The previous examples illustrate two effects of sunlight: a transformation of energy, from visible lightwaves to invisible heat, and a displacement in time and place, with the effects of absorption felt long after the source of illumination is gone and the heat displaced considerable distances by air and water masses.

Living organisms exist by capturing the physical energy of sunlight and transforming it into the energy of chemical bonds in organic molecules. This process, *photosynthesis,* is unique to green plants. Therefore, humans and all other animals are totally dependent upon the productivity of the plant world for survival. When animals eat green plants, they release the energy stored in the chemical bonds and use it to power their own activity. Both plants and animals are capable of respiration, which releases the energy stored in organic molecules.

The laws of thermodynamics apply to these biological energy processes. The first law states that energy may be transformed from one type of energy to another, as from light to chemical bonds to heat, but it is never created or destroyed. The second law specifies that no process involving an energy transformation will occur spontaneously unless there is a degradation from a concentrated form into a dispersed form; that is to say, no energy transformation is 100% efficient (Figure 3-2). Thus, although living organisms are successful in channeling the energy of sunlight into a series of chemical reactions that store and release energy in small, manageable amounts, the end result is always the same: the release of heat to the environment and eventually to outer space.

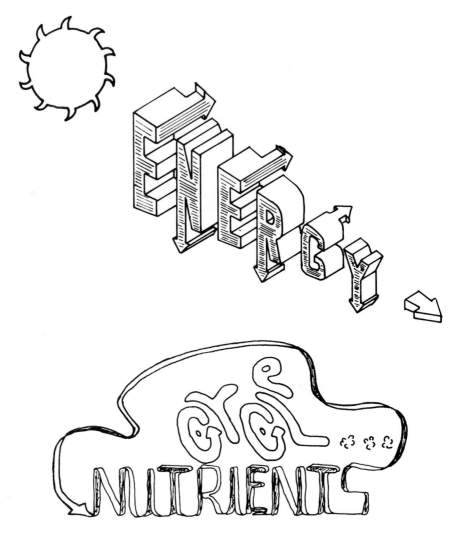

FIGURE 3-2
Energy degrades and nutrients cycle.

This process is at work constantly, as when the metabolic heat of our bodies is released in expired air, urine, and feces or radiated from our body surfaces. The time delay in these biological processes may be considerable, as the amount of energy bound up in organic fuel (such as wood) and fossil fuel (coal, petroleum, and natural gas) attest. Today's primary fuel sources were produced by biological activity under environmental conditions that no longer exist on earth. It is important to note that biological energy transformation is a flow-through process. Energy enters the earth's environment, is stored and used, and departs in a transformed state. Energy is never cycled.

Nutrients behave in a very different manner. The chemical elements of living organisms circulate from the environment to the organisms and, following death of an organism, back to the environment. These paths, known as *biogeochemical cycles,* exhibit varying degrees of complexity and time scales. Most elements cycle from a sedimentary reservoir in the earth's crust, and a given molecule may have a limited geographic range. A molecule absorbed from the earth may enter plant tissue and persist until the death and decomposition of the plant. If the plant is eaten, the molecule may move a short distance as part of the animal before returning to the earth when the animal decomposes. Other substances cycle as gases from an atmospheric or hydrospheric reservoir, and these may be distributed globally, particular examples being nitrogen, oxygen, carbon dioxide, and water.

At this point you may ask what all this has to do with health. The essential point is that human beings have complex and elaborate chemical and homeostatic mechanisms that function to acquire and retain nutrient- and energy-containing molecules from the environment. Any toxic or undesirable chemicals that mimic required nutrients or are otherwise incorporated into these natural cycles and pathways will also be transported into our bodies. Frequently it is not a question of whether a given chemical will find its way into our bodies but rather how long will it take, how much will be acquired, and how long will it persist in both our bodies and the environment. Two decades after the pesticide dichlorodiphenyltrichloroethane (DDT) was banned from use in the United States, it is still present in measurable quantities in all people examined.

The Organization of Life

The capture and use of energy by living organisms is accomplished by the high degree of organization characteristic of all levels of the biological world. Subatomic particles combine to form atoms. These atoms link to create molecules. More atoms can be added to produce macromolecules, which are vitally important to organisms. Macromolecules can be assembled into organelles, the essential components of cells. Cells replicate to form a mass of tissue and initiate specialization. Several types of tissue can unite to create an organ. A number of organs can function together as an organ system. The aggregate of the organ systems becomes the free-living organism.

Furthermore, hierarchal organization continues. A group of individuals of any one kind of organism comprises a population. The composite of all the populations of all the different kinds of organisms occupying a given area comprises a community. (Note an essential difference here: Health professionals consider only people when describing a community, whereas ecologists include all organisms.) Because organisms do not live in a vaccuum, the physical components of the world must also be considered. The living community functions together with the nonliving (abiotic) environment to form an ecosystem.

The ecosystem is the basic functional unit in ecology. It includes both biotic communities (organisms) and the abiotic environment, each influencing the properties of the other and both necessary for maintenance of life. Within an ecosystem, the flow of energy and materials follows distinct pathways. Green plants capture the energy of sunlight and manufacture energy-rich organic compounds. Animals eat the plants or eat other animals that have fed on plants. This transfer of energy from plant to animal to another animal is known as a food chain. At each transfer, a large proportion (usually 80% to 90%) of the energy manufactured or eaten by an organism is consumed by that organism in respiration and is not available for transfer to another animal. Humans and other animals typically consume many different kinds of food. Food chains are rarely simple; they are generally extensively interconnected with one another in a "food web."

The productivity of an ecosystem can be measured by determining the rate at which radiant energy is captured and stored as organic substances that can be used as food materials. High rates of productivity occur when physical factors are favorable and energy subsidies outside the system reduce the cost of maintenance. For example, saltwater marshes have very high productivity because rivers carry nutrients downstream to reach the marsh and tidal action circulates these materials within the marsh and flushes out the waste products. Thus, water power and tidal energy subsidize productivity of the marsh ecosystem, benefiting local marine organisms that concentrate their larval and juvenile growth stages in these regions of high productivity. Humans receive direct benefit from this productivity in the form of harvested seafood but frequently view such a marsh as a mosquito-ridden wasteland convenient to the beach, begging to be drained, filled, and covered with condominiums. The subsequent disappearance of the seafood is viewed as another perversity of nature, unconnected to the devastation of the ecosystem.

In complex natural communities, organisms whose food is obtained from plants through the same number of steps are considered to belong to the same trophic level. A given species may function at more than one trophic level according to the source of energy actually eaten. For example, humans function at the second level when eating plant material, the third level when consuming beef, and the fifth level when dining on carnivorous fishes such as tuna or salmon. Understanding the trophic concept and energy loss between trophic levels is important when problems of human nutrition are considered. As food becomes scarce, food chains must be shortened to avoid energy loss. Staple foods are commonly highly productive grasses—cereals, rice, corn, and so forth. It is inefficient to use such plant foods to produce meat for human consumption. Cattle are efficient converters of nonedible grasses (nonedible, that is, for humans, who lack the necessary digestive enzymes) to meat and have evolved a complex four-chambered stomach (which incorporates bacteria that help break down the food) for this purpose. Affluent societies circumvent nature's energy-efficient food chains by feeding corn to cattle to increase the fat content of beef intended for human consumption. Although more delectable, this marbled beef subsequently creates new health problems.

Food webs and trophic levels are phenomena associated with ecosystems. The physical boundary of a given ecosystem is often indistinct. Even such a discrete habitat as a pond is used by species that alternate between aquatic and terrestrial environments. Minerals can reach the pond from anywhere within its watershed, an area typically much larger than the pond itself. Other chemicals can reach the pond from hundreds of miles away, as the spread of pollutants that create acid rain has taught us. Many food webs overlap several ecosystems. A cursory survey of a pantry shelf or supermarket will easily demonstrate the widespread food-transportation system that has been developed to ship staples, fruits, and delicacies across continents and oceans. Pollutants and toxins readily accompany these foodstuffs.

Primitive humans were aware of humanity's niche in the biological community and exploited numerous plants and animals in pursuing the hunter-gatherer mode of existence. Agricultural humans focused on a few domesticated species and began to regard other plants and animals as weeds and pests. The increased productivity of cultigens permitted larger human populations but also led to dependence on a less diverse nutrient base. Technological humans, particularly urbanites, have forgotten their dependence on natural ecosystems and agro-ecosystems. The quest to further increase agricultural production and control pest organisms by chemical means has added new threats to health in the name of feeding human populations.

Ecological Interactions and Health

Interactions between organisms are particularly important in the cause, transmission, and persistence of disease. Infectious diseases fall into several broad categories, depending upon the number of organisms involved. The simplest consists of only two members, a pathogen and its host. Smallpox is such a system; the virus is the pathogen, and a human is the host. Infected individuals who recover are no longer susceptible to reinfection. The immune mechanisms can be stimulated with a vaccine and, through this action, the host becomes immune to the pathogen. As the potential host population is reduced (by way of vaccination), the pathogen is unable to persist and will eventually become extinct.

Many diseases include a third party, a vector that transmits the pathogen from host to host without becoming infected itself. For example, the pathogen that causes the bubonic plague is a bacterium that is transmitted to humans (and other animals) through the bite of a flea. The bacterium is maintained in populations of rodents of various kinds. The rodents provide the reservoir wherein the bacillus persists; the fleas are merely vectors of transmission from an infected rodent to an uninfected rodent or to a human being. Humans are secondary hosts, but when the bacillus is introduced into a crowded human population, the results can be devastating, as has been demonstrated by the epidemics that occur every few centuries. These epidemics have disappeared on their own, not as the result of human countermeasures.

Pollution

Pollutants are the residues of things humans make, use, and throw away. Nondegradable pollutants either do not degrade or degrade very slowly

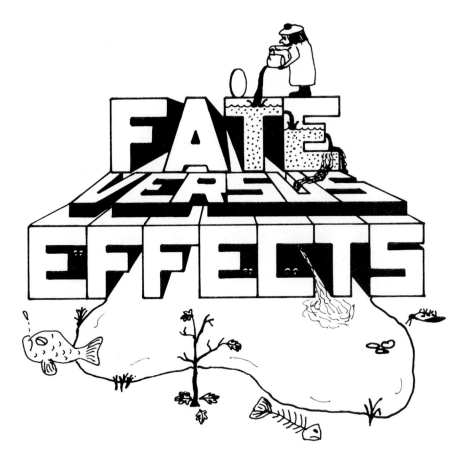

FIGURE 3-3
Fate versus effects of a pollutant.

in the natural environment. Biodegradable pollutants can be rapidly decomposed by natural processes unless input exceeds decomposition or dispersal capacity. Degradable pollutants that provide energy or nutrients may increase the productivity of an ecosystem by providing a subsidy when the rate of input is moderate. However, high rates of input can cause productivity to oscillate, whereas additional input may poison the system completely.

When any pollutant is introduced into the environment, we must be concerned about both the *fate* of the pollutant (where it goes and how it gets there) and its *effect* on humans or any of the ecosystems upon which we depend (Figure 3-3). We must always keep in mind that any effects that pollutants have on other species are early warning symptoms that something is amiss in the ecosystem and that humans may well be the next to be affected. There are five mechanisms of particular concern.

Major Pollutant Mechanisms

Transport

Transport of the pollutant, once introduced into the environment, is generally accomplished by way of wind patterns or aquatic systems. Pollutants can be dispersed aerially as particulates or in a gaseous state; they can travel long distances before falling to earth as dust or being carried in rainwater. Ironically, the construction of taller smokestacks to relieve local pollution generally results in greater dispersal, thus enlarging the area affected without diminishing the amount of pollutant released. Once air pollutants have settled to earth, they frequently continue their movement by traveling along waterways. Following a single heavy rainfall, stormwater runoff can mobilize more suspended particulates than may be transported during the rest of the year. Dissolved pollutants may be transported long distances before settling onto the bottom sediments through some precipitatory mechanism.

Pollutants generally exert greater influence on aquatic ecosystems than on terrestrial environments. Air pollutants may enter a person's lungs or settle on vegetation and then be eaten with the plants. Water, though, is nature's best solvent, and many pollutants go into solution in aquatic ecosystems, with the result that aquatic animals and plants live in a weakly polluted soup. Many chemicals enter the biota directly through the skin or across gill surfaces, for there is no escape from a dissolved pollutant. The effects of a given one-time polluting event, such as an accidental spill, are therefore exerted for a longer time in aquatic ecosystems. Not only is a greater portion of the pollution incorporated into and cycled within the biotic nutrient pool, but material that settles into the sediment can also be resuspended and redistributed with every major storm event. The dispersion of pollutants is also more restricted in aquatic systems than in terresterial ones because movement is always downstream, until the pollutants reach the ocean. The efficacy of ocean transport has been demonstrated by the ubiquitous spread of several insecticides throughout the world; their area of distribution even includes the Antarctic continent.

Transformation

Transformation of a pollutant within an ecosystem takes place in many ways. Harmful substances can be rendered innocuous or even helpful during the biodegradation process. But occasionally a relatively harmless substance is transformed into a noxious form. A classic example is the transformation of metallic or inorganic mercury, which is relatively immobile, into methylmercury by microorganisms living in aquatic sediments. Methylmercury is readily incorporated into detrital food chains, which may terminate with human consumption of contaminated fish and shellfish, producing the neurological disorder known as Minamata disease. Nonbiogenic chemical transformations are more common in the environment; for example, one such transformation is the conversion of sulfur dioxide and nitrous oxides in the atmosphere to form sulfuric and nitric acids and create acid rain.

Bioaccumulation

Bioaccumulation refers to the introduction of substances into ecological food webs. Chemicals that behave in a manner similar to essential elements are most susceptible to rapid uptake and retention. Chiefly because of human beings and their activities, the ecologist must now be concerned with the cycling of nonessential elements. For example, the radionuclides of strontium and cesium, whose chemical behavior is analogous to calcium and potassium, respectively, are introduced into the environment by nuclear reactors and represent a potential health hazard.

Biomagnification

Biomagnification results when the accumulation of a pollutant greatly exceeds the rate at which an organism eliminates it. The pollutant is concentrated in organisms at a low trophic level, where it is further concentrated and passed to the third level, and so forth. For example, polychlorinated biphenyls (PCBs) are a large class of 209 separate chemical compounds that held many industrial applications before 1976, when they were banned in the United States. Each of these compounds has a different type and degree of toxicity, bioaccumulates at different rates, and behaves differently when free in the environment. In the 1970s these PCB compounds were associated with adverse health effects in people eating fishes from the Great Lakes. The PCBs were acquired by phytoplankton that quite innocuously acted as tiny scavengers of the pollutant, reaching levels of only 2.5 parts of PCB per billion parts of phytoplankton. These were then eaten by zooplankton, which in turn were eaten by larger zooplankton, in which PCB concentrations increased nearly 50-fold, reaching 123 parts per billion. The zooplankton were eaten by small fishes, rainbow smelt, with PCBs increasing 9-fold to 1 part per million. Next, the smelt were eaten by lake trout, which reached 5 parts per million PCB, and finally consumed by humans (or other end-chain carnivores). At each step, the PCBs were sequestered in the fatty tissue of the carrier and stored. The final concentration of PCBs in herring gull eggs, which are rich in stored fat and sometimes consumed by humans, was 124 parts per million, or 50,000 times greater than the original concentration in the phytoplankton.

Synergism

Synergism is the simultaneous action of separate substances or agencies that together produce a greater total effect than the sum of their individual effects. It is common to discover that a given substance behaves in one fashion in a controlled laboratory environment and quite another when introduced into a natural ecosystem, where it interacts with a number of physical and chemical properties of the environment.

Toxic Substances

In recent years, *toxic substances* have received a great deal of attention in governmental regulations and the news media. Any chemical can be toxic, including table salt, sugar, and the chlorine in drinking water. Toxic substances are generally considered to be any chemicals or mixtures of chemicals, either synthetic or natural, that are poisonous to humans or plants or animals under expected conditions of use and exposure. There are four major categories of toxic substances. *Pesticides* are lethal chemicals specifically designed to kill weeds, fungi, insects, mites, rodents, and other pests. Four pesticides have been banned from further use in the United States: DDT, aldrin, dieldrin, and chlordane. *Industrial chemicals* are particularly numerous, and a few have proven especially dangerous (for example, asbestos, benzene, vinyl chloride, and PCB). A number of *metals* such as arsenic, lead, cadmium, and mercury have also proven to be very toxic in the environment. The fourth category includes those substances with isotopes that emit various types of *radiation,* such as strontium, cesium, iodine, and so forth.

There are nearly 60,000 different chemical substances in commercial use in the United States today, manufactured or processed by 12,000 establishments; 98% of these chemicals are safe. Fifty-five thousand firms generated 290 million tons of hazardous waste in 1981. More than 17,000 hazardous waste disposal sites have been identified, and hundreds of these sites represent a substantial threat to human health. In 1987, the first year of the EPA Toxics Release Inventory, 19,278 manufacturing facilities reported 22.5 billion pounds of toxic substances released to the environment or transferred to other facilities for treatment and disposal. Almost half, 9.6 billion pounds, of these toxic chemicals were released to U. S. surface waters.

Chemical toxicity occurs when a chemical agent produces detrimental effects in living organisms. The effects of a toxic substance can be immediate or long-term and can harm selected tissues or the entire organism. Both the toxicity of the substance and the expected exposure to the organism must be considered to define the anticipated risk. Neurotoxins are likely the most significant toxic substances in both prevalence and severity that pose a risk to human health. Epidemiologically, a relatively small fraction of major neurologic disorders are inherited; most neurological diseases appear to be associated with environmental factors. Many commercial chemicals used in very large amounts and known to persist in the environment have neurotoxic properties. In fact, insecticides, designed to have neurotoxic properties, are manufactured for deliberate release into the environment.

Pollutants and Human Population Size

All of the environmental processes described so far can influence human health. Any pollutant or toxic substance introduced into the environment is subjected to these processes, many of which lead directly to human beings. Pollution of the environment occurs when these pollutants overwhelm the capacity of the environment to assimilate them without being thrown out of balance. Thus, pollution is a rate function involving a quantity of pollutant introduced over a period of time. This rate is directly correlated to population size.

It can be said that all pollution is the result of population growth. A single family, living on a subsistence level in the wild, burning wood as their fuel and discarding rubbish and human wastes on the landscape, would seldom be a polluting factor in their environment. The population of a small village would denude the landscape of wood fuel, pollute the air with smoke from numerous wood fires, and litter the ground with rubbish and human wastes randomly dispersed. Cities, with more numerous inhabitants, totally overwhelm the environment with rubbish and human wastes, fostering the development of sewage and garbage disposal systems. Industrial development increases the number of pollutants and environmental insults. Our past practice for handling pollutants has been to just dump them, taking further action only when the natural systems have been overwhelmed. We need to reverse this practice and remove the bulk of pollutants before inflicting them upon nature. Then the natural ecosystem can work for us by removing the final bit of pollution that always proves so difficult and expensive to neutralize.

Demographic changes can rapidly alter the stress inflicted upon the environment. As population grows, the stress increases. If the population moves, both the nature and the intensity of an environmental problem can shift. For example, the recent decline of industrial productivity in the northeastern United States has resulted in a shift in the population caused by the exodus of workers (particularly younger families) and an improvement in the surface water quality. The growth of population in the south, especially the arid southwest, is both increasing water pollution as well as straining overall water supply.

The solution to one environmental problem may be the creation of another. Pollutants do not disappear. Sulfur that is scrubbed out of power plant smokestack gases ends up as a sludge stored on the ground, where it may threaten water quality. Pollutants removed from wastewaters by precipitation end up in the bottom sludge, which also requires disposal. Unfortunately, if the sludge is burned, the pollutants may be released into the air, to settle and become incorporated into the water or land once again. If the sludge is buried in a landfill, it may threaten surface water or groundwater supplies. Sewage treatment plants that aerate water as part of the process may discharge substantial amounts of volatile toxic substances to the air. *Everything has to go someplace.*

In summary, virtually any pollutant that is introduced into the environment will subsequently be transported away from its point of entry. It may be transformed into another chemical form, either less or more hazardous. It will probably be accumulated by biological organisms, possibly becoming magnified in its concentration. It is likely to react with other chemicals or physical processes and to produce unanticipated effects. Distinct and efficient chemical cycles and pathways that have evolved over millions of years ensure that toxicants will enter biological systems and eventually reach humans or other organisms on which they depend. *Everything is connected to everything else* and *everything has to go someplace.* There is nowhere to hide. The only solution is to stop the pollution.

Interconnections

Humanity's attempts to intervene in natural processes seldom go smoothly and frequently produce effects far removed from the immediate intervention site. Some of the most profound effects have been experienced in attempts to control or eradicate diseases. The following example reveals some unexpected connections.

Malaria is caused by four species of *Plasmodium,* a single-celled sporozoan parasite. During the first stage of the disease, elongate sporozoites in the blood penetrate cells within the liver. The sporozoites multiply asexually to produce numerous merozoites. During the second stage of the disease, the merozoites leave the liver and enter red blood cells. The merozoites reproduce, again asexually, within the red blood cells and erupt, with the progeny invading new red blood cells and continuing the cycle. These eruptions eventually synchronize to 48-hour or 72-hour cycles, depending on the *Plasmodium* species involved. The shock of the simultaneous release of the merozoites can produce chills in the victim, followed by a high fever caused by toxins released with the merozoites. Some merozoites become gametocytes, capable of sexual reproduction.

The human immune system functions by being able to recognize the chemical antigens of an infectious agent and producing specific antibodies to combat it. The malarial pathogen presents three different stages (sporozoite, merozoite, and gametocyte) with three different antigens. Antibodies that counter one antigen are not effective against the other two stages. Also, the antibodies will be effective only when the various parasite cells are free in the bloodstream. Once they have entered either liver cells or red blood cells, they cannot be attacked by the antibodies. Thus, an effective vaccine would have to work against all three stages.

Mosquitoes are found in abundance virtually everywhere in the world. More than 1500 species are known, and a few tropical and subtropical species are involved in the transmission of human diseases.

Larval mosquitoes develop in water, and many species are quite adaptable in their choice of breeding sites, using water that collects in abandoned tin cans, rubber tires, and so forth. Adult male mosquitoes suck plant juices for their nourishment and do not bite animals. Adult females require a blood meal to provide nutrients for their eggs. Various species bite reptiles, birds, and mammals (including humans) to obtain the blood. When a female *Anopheles* mosquito bites a human who is infected with malaria, the malarial gametocytes may be drawn up into the digestive system of the insect. The gametocytes are transformed into gametes within the stomach of the mosquito, where they unite to form a zygote and then burrow into the cells in the wall of the stomach. The resulting oocyte produces numerous new sporozoites, which migrate to the salivary glands of the mosquito. When the female mosquito next bites a human, some sporozoites may be injected into the wound by way of saliva. Mosquito saliva contains an anticoagulant to keep the blood flowing until the mosquito has drunk her fill.

This complicated procedure is the only mechanism by which the malaria parasite is transmitted indirectly from one human host to another. It cannot be transmitted by direct human contact (although it has been transmitted by means of blood transfusion and intravenous drug abuse), nor is it passed from one mosquito to another. It persists only by using the mosquito vector to complete its complex lifecycle. Malaria is a widespread and debilitating disease. It has been estimated that each year, worldwide, 250 million people fall ill with this disease, and more than 1 million die. It causes anemia, fever, spleen enlargement, and miscarriage; contributes to high infant mortality; and causes in its victims a greater susceptibility to many kinds of infection. The eradication of malaria has been a top priority goal of the World Health Organization (WHO) for many years.

As the primary hosts of the malarial parasite, humans represent three distinct populations according to their susceptibility to the disease. Some people are susceptible to being infected with the disease, some are already infected, and some are immune to infection. Newborn infants may acquire some antibodies from their mothers, but these do not persist. Children from one to four years of age are highly susceptible to malaria and constitute most of the deaths from the disease. Older children and adults can develop partial immunity to small numbers of the malarial parasites, but when large numbers are present, the parasites tend to overrun this limited immunity.

Temporary artificial immunity to malaria can be created with the continuous intake of drugs. The South American Indians discovered that the bark of the cinchona tree yielded quinine, which was effective in preventing and treating malaria. The famous gin and tonic, made with quinine water, is reputed to have been developed by the British to ameliorate their daily intake of quinine in malarial regions. Quinine was replaced by quinacrine hydrochloride, which had the side effect of coloring the eyes yellow. The drug in present use is chloroquine, which prevents DNA replication and RNA synthesis in the parasitized red blood cells. For prevention and suppression of malaria, chloroquine must be taken on a weekly basis.

Mosquitoes have no immune system to counteract invasion by malaria parasites. Uninfected females become infected by biting an infected human. Infected mosquitoes never recover from the infection and continue to transmit the parasite to subsequent victims. Malaria can be maintained in areas of low human population density if the mosquito population density is high. However, mosquitoes do have high rates of reproduction. Efforts to eradicate malaria have focused on eradicating the mosquito or at least lowering mosquito populations to the point where they were no longer effective vectors of the disease.

The weapons of choice for this worldwide campaign were insecticides. A favorite was DDT, a chlorinated hydrocarbon that attacks the central nervous system. Although synthesized in 1874, it was not used as an insecticide until 1939. It is a broad-spectrum pesticide, affecting many organisms in addition to the target species. DDT was used widely during World War II to protect U.S. troops from malaria, typhus, and other insect-borne diseases. DDT was inexpensive to manufacture and easy to handle. Its long-lasting residual effect was hailed as one of its chief advantages.

Within a dozen years, unwelcome side effects began to appear. Eggshell thinning in birds began as early as 1947. Fishes, crabs, shrimps, and oysters accumulated lethal concentrations of DDT even at very low levels of exposure. Citizen opposition to widespread use, particularly aerial spraying, began in 1957. Domestic *production* of DDT peaked at 188 million pounds annually in 1963 but declined to 60 million pounds in the 1970s. Domestic *consumption* peaked at 79 million pounds in 1959 and declined to 20 million pounds by 1971. In 1972 the Environmental Protection Agency (EPA) suspended virtually all uses of DDT in the United States on the grounds that continual use would pose an unacceptable risk to humans and the environment.

DDT was more persistent in some environmental systems than others. Residues in soil degrade slowly. In arid areas, the time required for one half of the DDT to wash out or break down exceeds 20 years. Eventually, DDT breaks down in the environment to DDD or DDE, which are even more potent. DDT applied to soils can evaporate into the air and move long distances (it has even been recorded in antarctic snow). Rainfall and surface runoff transport DDT to streams, rivers, estuaries, and oceans.

The Food and Drug Administration established a maximum allowable concentration of DDT in foodstuffs at 5 parts per million (ppm). By the 1960s several species of fish from the Great Lakes as well as the Atlantic and Pacific Oceans exceeded this level. The National Human Monitoring System tracked selected chlorinated hydrocarbons in human adipose tissue from 1970 to 1983. DDT has been found in more than 99% of all human tissues sampled. Total DDT (including DDD and DDE) in human fatty tissues peaked at 8 ppm in 1971. DDT is concentrated in fatty tissues of the body and frequently contaminates milk and dairy products. At one point the DDT content of human milk exceeded the 5 ppm level, rendering breast milk unfit for human consumption.

Since DDT was banned in the United States, the level of DDT in food organisms and wildlife has slowly, but steadily, declined. DDT residues in human fat slowly declined to 1.7 ppm in 1983, the final year of the survey (see Figure 3-4).

DDT provides vivid evidence of worldwide environmental transport mechanisms. DDT has spread throughout the world and has been found in both arctic fishes and antarctic penguins, far from any site of direct DDT aplication. In addition, DDT has been directly implicated in the precipitous decline of brown pelican and peregine falcon populations. Both species occupy positions at the end of long food chains in which DDT is concentrated at each transfer level. DDT interferes with calcium metabolism, causing the birds to produce eggs with abnormally thin shells that frequently crack during incubation, thus failing to hatch. Consequently, both bird species are now classified as endangered. Both of these cases reveal only the tip of the iceberg, for DDT contamination is widespread throughout their food web.

Through the use of these pesticides, the war against malaria appeared to be succeeding for a number of years, with spectacular reductions being made in the prevalence of the disease. Many agencies and governments felt that the benefits gained far outweighed the envi-

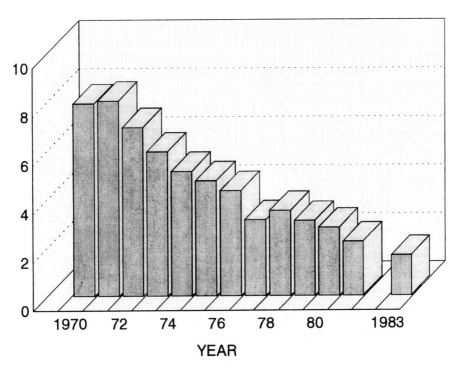

FIGURE 3-4
DDT residues in human adipose tissue.

ronmental costs. However, in recent years the prevalence of malaria has soared to precontrol levels in the very areas that enjoyed the greatest success. The mosquitoes are no longer affected by the insecticides and, in some regions, the malarial organisms within their human hosts no longer respond to chemotherapy. Human endeavors have encountered the reality of biological adaptation.

One explanation for this biological adaption is variability, which is exhibited by all organisms. This is recognized readily in humans, for we not only look different as individuals, but our chemical makeup, reaction to drugs, and even taste sensors also respond differently to a given stimulus. In a parallel fashion, not all targeted organisms will succumb to a given pesticide. In any large population, there always seem to be a few organisms that survive various stressors. Thus, when an area is treated with an insecticide, the majority of the mosquito population, perhaps more than 99%, will die. But the resources that originally supported that mosquito population may be unaffected, and some of the natural enemies and predators of mosquitoes may also have been killed by a broad-spectrum pesticide. So the few mosquitoes that survive find themselves in an advantageous situation: Their resources are intact, their enemies are gone, and they can reproduce and grow in number as they please. But one significant change has occurred. Assuming that the characteristic that permitted them to survive the pesticide is inheritable, all of their progeny will also possess this characteristic. This means that the new generation will be stronger than the previous one and will not be susceptible to that pesticide.

This description of adaptation is an oversimplification, but the principle is valid. It is applicable equally to the development of drug- or antibiotic-resistant strains of microorganisms. In fact, this has occurred with malaria organisms in some parts of the world, where chloroquine-resistant strains have arisen. Just as the overuse of antibiotics leads to antibiotic-resistant pathogens, the overuse of insecticides leads to insecticide-resistant insects. When the strength and frequency of insecticide applications are increased, insecticide-resistant insects develop all the more quickly.

Widespread insecticide application can have even broader effects. Malaria was a serious, prevalent disease in Borneo, where in some areas over 90% of the population suffered from enlarged spleens. In 1955, WHO began a successful program of malaria control. Two insecticides, DDT and dieldrin, were sprayed inside the thatched-roof houses to eradicate two species of mosquitoes that were transmitting the malaria. The insecticides also reduced the populations of small parasites of a moth species. The parasites avoided thatch that had been sprayed with DDE and were killed outright by dieldrin. Freed from their parasites, the population of moth larvae expanded rapidly and consumed large quantities of thatch in the housetops. The insecticides were also picked up by cockroaches and geckos (small lizards that lived in the houses and fed upon insects). Both cockroaches and geckos were captured and eaten by the domestic cats kept by the villagers. The cats proved to be particularly susceptible to the insecticides, and many of them died.

With the cat population drastically reduced, two species of rats, native to the forests and plantations, then invaded the villages. These rats were potential carriers of plague, typhus, and leptospirosis. Thus, while the villagers had gained protection from malaria, they were subsequently exposed to much more virulent pathogens. To redress this imbalance, surplus cats were transported from urban areas to the villages, some even being packed into special containers and parachuted into remote villages.

These examples demonstrate the reality of extensive ecological interconnections. Environmental transport mechanisms have distributed DDT all over the globe. DDT has been transformed into its breakdown products, DDD and DDE, which are even more dangerous than their precursor. All three forms are accumulated by biological organisms and concentrated as they progress upward in ecological food webs. The concentration of DDT in higher food organisms is commonly 30,000 times greater than the concentration dissolved in water at a given site. Biological populations are both variable in their response to given toxicants and quick to produce toxicant-resistant populations that negate the temporary inroads gained by human actions. Once introduced into the environment, DDT and other pesticides may persist for decades, contaminating and killing numerous nontarget organisms. Humans are not exempt from these processes, and toxic chemicals that are released for very commendable reasons may return to haunt us for years to come. The pathways and interconnections are frequently unpredictable, even when the road is paved with good intentions.

The Complex Human Environment

The preceding section has described humans interacting with the physical world and other species in a simplistic fashion. The complete human environment is difficult to comprehend because of the multiplicity of interrelated elements. The delivery of health care sometimes goes awry because the influence of certain elements is underestimated or unappreciated. A conceptual model of the human environment from an ecological viewpoint can ofttimes illuminate the problem and guide efficient intervention.

An ecologic model (Figure 3-5), like most models, proposes a framework from which to study and understand a phenomenon. A complete enumeration of all salient components of human health would be too complex to illustrate; therefore, this model is limited to environmental variables. The *Environment* is the world that surrounds people wherever they go, whatever they do. An ecological approach to the study of

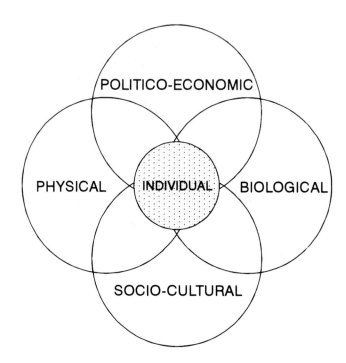

FIGURE 3-5
The environmental systems that affect each individual.

human health relates the biological, physical, sociocultural, and politico-economic components of a person's environment to any deviation in him or her from a state of health. The model can be applied to study the health of any defined subpopulation (for example, infants, children, adolescents, and the elderly) as well.

Environmental systems not only act on the individual person but also interact with one another, and a change occurring in one system will frequently affect others. Each system consists of components that act with and upon other systems to bring about equilibrium or disequilibrium within the system.

Change occurs within a system when one variable acts on a second variable to force alteration. Climate and topography are variables within the physical system that can act separately or in unison to cause change within the other systems. For example, food distribution (determined by a set of politicoeconomic variables) depends on the production ability of the land (determined by physical variables such as climate and topography), which in turn influence the selection and consumption of food (determined by sociocultural variables); all of these affect human growth (a biologic variable).

The environmental systems show both inter- and intradependence in function and effect. The systems (depicted as circles in Figure 3-5) interface with each other and overlap to form a network that encases the individual (the inner circle of Figure 3-5). At any time, all systems may impinge on the individual simultaneously.

Layered within the systems is a hierarchy of four subsystems: the individual, the family unit, the community (ecologically speaking, the human population), and the nation (Figure 3-6). Each subsystem is conditioned for the occurrence of illness by the environmental systems. When acted upon, the subsystems interact both *intra*dynamically and *inter*dynamically to mitigate or reinforce the conditioning influences of the systems' variables; in this way, the subsystems modify the systems. Each subsystem is also influenced by its developmental stage. For instance, an individual may react to an external perturbation differently as an infant, child, adolescent, adult, or elder. A family may be small or extended, with young or school-age children, semi-independent adolescents, or elderly parents to accommodate. A community may be small, homogeneous, and cohesive or large, diverse, and divisive. A nation may be agrarian, industrial, and poor or rich in human and natural resources.

To explain, a family with inadequate access to the basic needs of food and shelter (conditioned by politicoeconomic production and accompanying distribution policies) may act to change these impediments by migrating to an area of improved access to basic needs. Migration, in turn, can force change in intrafamily physical, biologic, sociocultural, and politicoeconomic composition of the community and nation.

Conceptually, both the subsystems and environmental systems are in a constant state of interaction (*everything is connected to everything else and is constantly changing*). Enumerating the variables within the systems and measuring the interaction among them is the key to operating the model. In Figure 3-6, the environmental systems and subsystems are displayed in a tabular arrangement, with variables boxed according to the systems most acutely affected by their interaction. Certain variables, such as migration and consumption of basic needs, equally interact with all systems as they affect the family and individual's functioning.

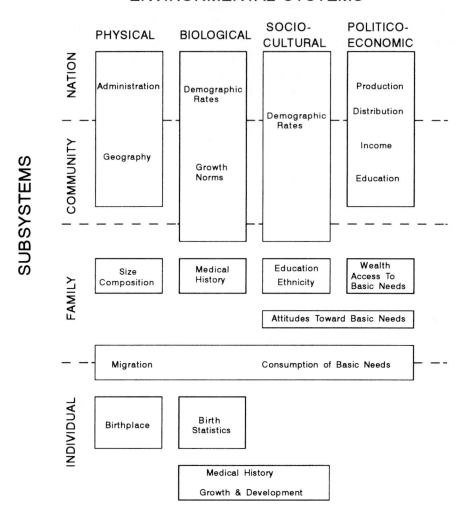

FIGURE 3-6
The environmental systems and subsystems affecting human health.

Other variables, such as birth statistics, (age at birth, sex, birth order, and condition) are primarily within one system, affecting one developmental stage (the child) of one subsystem (the individual). Lines encasing variables are not set boundaries; rather, they serve as a guide to identify the system and subsystem most affected by variable manipulation.

The purpose of the conceptual model is to offer a framework from which to select significant variables related to the health status of a chosen individual. The variables that appear in Figure 3-6 are a synthesis of the epidemiologic, demographic, and social health indicators consistently proposed, tested, and recommended as valid and reliable indices of child health. Application of this model is described in the regional case history that follows.

APPLICATION: A LOCAL CASE STUDY

Now that we understand what pollutants are and how they reach humans, how can this information be used to solve community health problems? The following scenario is offered as an example of such problem solving. The pollution episode was real; the embellishments and details are fictitious.

The Problem

A graduate nurse accepted a job with the Department of Public Health in Leadville. The town's primary industry and economic base was a small lead mine and smelter. The director of Public Health informed our nurse, during her first week on the job, that a local group of environmental activists had complained about the insidious, but undefined, health effects of the smelter operation and demanded that it be closed. The devastating economic impact that such an action would precipitate prompted the mayor and city council to exert pressure on the health department director. As the latest immigrant from academia, our community health nurse was selected to design and implement an investigation of the health effects of the smelter. The director's final words to her were "Do something, even if it is wrong!" Naturally, because this was not a budgeted item, the financial and staff support available to her were limited.

The First Goal

Our nurse decided that her first goal should be to determine if the lead smelter was affecting the health of the local residents. She knew nothing about lead as an environmental toxicant, but she was trained well in problem solving, so she forged ahead with confidence.

Available Information

Our nurse began by researching the health effects of lead in the environment and the environmental impacts of lead smelter operations. She learned that lead is ubiquitous in nature, being a natural constituent of the earth's crust. Because lead is an element, it cannot be destroyed and may be expected to persist indefinitely in the environment in some form. Current production of lead in the United States is 1.3 million tons per year, of which 50% is used in batteries, 20% in antiknock compounds for gasoline, and 6% in pigments and ceramics.

Lead's primary routes into the human body are ingestion of food and water and inhalation of atmospheric particles. Rocks and soils usually contain 10 μg to 30 μg of lead per gram of material. Natural groundwaters have 1 μg to 10 μg of lead per liter of water, which is below the safe drinking water standard of 15 μg per liter. There does not appear to be any biomagnification of lead during the movement of nutrients from soil to groundwater to organic matter in plants. There exists a definite, positive correlation between the concentration of lead in water and the concentration of lead in the blood of humans drinking the water. The amount of lead that will dissolve in water is dependent upon both hardness and pH. More lead will dissolve in soft water than in hard water, which contains more dissolved mineral salts. Accordingly, only 1 μg of lead will dissolve in a liter of moderately alkaline water at pH 9, but 10,000 μg of lead will dissolve in a liter of moderately acid water at pH 5.5. Seawater contains only 0.03 μg of lead per liter of water, but freshwater ecosystems average 23 μg per liter (ranging from 2 μg to 140 μg).

The toxicity of lead to aquatic animals is affected by the season of the year, water temperature and chemistry, animal size, and length of exposure. Chronic effects can be detected at 7.6 μg per liter, and acute effects are manifested at 450 μg per liter. Bacteria have been reported to convert inorganic lead to organic forms. Although algae may concentrate lead as much as 31,000 times above ambient water concentrations, there is no evidence of biomagnification in the food chain from aquatic vegetation to fish and shellfish. Fish do not constitute an unusually significant source of lead in the human diet.

Armed with this basic information, our community health nurse could identify and evaluate the ecological mechanisms that may affect lead accumulation by humans. She understood that lead is an ubiquitous but minor component in biogeochemical cycles, but these cycles appear to exert only a slight influence on human lead accumulation. Its ubiquity does create problems in designing epidemiological studies and interpretation of data. In regard to food chains, lead adhering to the exterior surfaces of food items is perhaps of more significance than lead contained within the food. Leafy vegetables with extensive surface area would be particularly important in this respect. The transfer of lead between trophic levels does not appear to be significant. Even so, lead is not biodegradable.

In regard to environmental transport, lead is extremely mobile along both atmospheric and hydrologic pathways, and virtually all human lead consumption is the direct result of such movement. Certain bacteria are able to transform inorganic lead to organic forms. Lead is also altered photochemically. Neither action is likely to contribute significantly to human accumulation or toxicity. Lead is readily accumulated into virtually all living organisms. There is little evidence of increasing biomagnification at higher trophic levels. The solubility of lead in water is significantly affected by the pH and hardness of the water, so synergistic effects are important. The status of essential nutrients such as calcium, iron, phosphorus, fat, and protein in a human being affects the extent of gastrointestinal absorption of ingested lead. Pregnant women have increased risk of iron and calcium deficiency and physiological stress, which may lead to a higher risk at a given lead exposure. There is no available information on the assimilative capacity of natural ecosystems for lead.

Having learned more than she ever wanted to know about lead in the environment, our community health nurse queried the appropriate offices of the EPA and the state health department. She learned that air emissions and water effluent from the smelter and mine have been continuously monitored and that the lead concentrations of each were below the prescribed federal and state guidelines. The community drinking water was also sampled regularly and always found to contain less than the 15 µg of lead per liter of water permitted. Both agencies reported that the smelter had recently upgraded its pollution-control devices and that company officials were conscientious in their control efforts. The local health office had received no reports of lead intoxication from the local hospital or private physicians. Thus, on the basis of existing information, there was no indication of a community health problem resulting from the lead.

TAKE NOTE

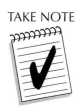

Our health professional realized that her efforts thus far had only addressed the possibility of acute lead toxicity in her community. She determined that her next step should be to search for chronic effects by means of a limited screening program. This created several questions: How could she select a target population? How could she reach them? Could she use any existing programs as an avenue of contact?

A *special risk* population is one exhibiting characteristics associated with significantly higher probability of developing a condition, illness, or other abnormal status due to exposure to a given toxic agent. Two such populations are definable for lead: preschool children and pregnant women. Our nurse's health department already had two programs that could provide ready access to these populations: a Well-Child Clinic and Maternal-Infant Care. Thus, she had two alternatives at this point, but she was also operating under certain constraints.

The primary goal was still to determine if a health problem existed, so she would not want to begin to use her meager resources until the problem under study was more clearly defined.

Her literature survey identified the highest-risk group to be children aged one to six years. These clients would be the most likely to exhibit the effects of lead toxicity. Pregnant women would require higher levels of lead before exhibiting toxic symptoms. Unborn fetuses are perhaps most susceptible to lead toxicity, but they are also the most difficult to assess. Infants show less effect than toddlers or preschoolers, perhaps due to their limited mobility and different diet. Thus, the preschool children participating in the Well-Child Care Program at the clinic would be the most rewarding group to investigate.

Survey Data

Our health worker learned from her literature survey that the amount of lead present in a blood sample is a good indication of body lead levels. She accepted 15 µg of lead per 100 ml of blood as her action level, in accordance with the U.S. Surgeon General's recommendation. This is the level at which a child is considered to be in potential danger of developing clinical lead poisoning. She arranged for the analysis of the blood samples and the cooperation of the clinic personnel who run the Well-Child Care Program in obtaining a capillary tube sample of blood from each of the 100 children in their program.

Remembering that each datum of information collected costs additional money to process and analyze, what other information could our nurse justifiably collect with each blood sample? She limited her choices to just six pieces of information: (1) the child's *name,* to identify each sample; (2) the child's *address,* to determine the relationship of the residence to the smelter location and to aid in relocation of the client; (3) the child's *age,* because age is known to correlate to lead uptake and toxicity and will be a general indicator of the child's activity pattern; (4) the child's *sex,* because the sex role of the child may influence lead uptake; (5) the *pica history* of the child (*pica* is the mouthing of unusual items such as dirt and paint chips, both of which are potential routes of lead ingestion); and (6) the *occupation and worksite* of adult members of the household, to identify families associated with the smelter.

Survey Results

The collection and analysis of the 100 blood samples produced the following results: All 100 children had detectable levels of lead in their blood, 24 had more than 15 µg of lead per 100 ml of blood, and 10 had more than 20 µg of lead. All children with blood lead at a level greater than 20 µg had one or more household adults employed at the smelter, but not all children with household adults employed at the smelter had blood lead greater than 20 µg.

Action Taken

Having demonstrated that a *chronic* lead toxicity problem existed, the community health nurse notified the health director of the results. She also noted that blood lead levels of 60 µg or more dictated immediate chelating treatment and that levels of 80 µg or more should be accompanied by demonstrable metabolic toxicity. The health director mobilized an immediate treatment program for all children with blood lead levels greater than 60 µg and ordered continuation of the screening program and investigation of the route of lead uptake by the children.

The Second Goal

Our health professional now shifted her focus to determining the route of lead uptake by the affected children. She decided that a matched sample investigation would be most appropriate. She proceeded to match each family of an above-threshold (20 µg) child to a family with a below-threshold child of similar sex and age. She was able to obtain 20 matched pairs in this manner. Having selected the families for further investigation, she had to determine what samples and information to collect.

Second Survey Data

The nurse decided to obtain blood samples from all of the children in the matched sample, to verify the original blood lead data; all of the involved siblings, to determine if other children in the families had elevated levels; and all household adults, for comparative purposes. Samples of tap water, house paint, yard soil, and house dust were also collected to assist in identifying the source of the lead uptake.

Second Survey Results

The blood levels of the children previously sampled were nearly identical to the original data, verifying the original analyses. The blood levels of siblings were strongly correlated with those of the children originally sampled. The fathers of all children with blood lead levels greater than 20 µg per 100 ml of blood also had blood levels above 20 µg and required chelation treatment. The mothers of all families had blood lead levels below 15 µg. No families inhabited houses with leaded paint. There was no difference in the lead content of yard soil between above-threshold and below-threshold families. Similarly, there was no difference in the lead content of the tap water. All families were serviced from the city water supply, and all samples were below the 15 µg per liter limit.

Household dust lead concentrations from above-threshold families averaged 2600 µg of lead per gram of dust; the concentrations from below-threshold families averaged 400 µg per gram, with less than a 2% probability that this significant difference was attributable to chance alone. The blood lead level of the children was strongly correlated with the level of lead in household dust. Geographic analysis revealed that all families resided nearly equidistant from the smelter, which was located eight miles from the town. Prevailing winds would transport emissions away from, rather than toward, residential areas. Smelter employees who were members of below-threshold families held administrative or clerical positions and were not directly involved with the smelting process. Smelter employees who were members of the above-threshold families were directly involved with the smelting process.

Interpretation, Verification, and Remedy

Our community health nurse deduced from the second survey results that the origin of the lead affecting the children might be their fathers' workclothes. Subsequent investigation proved this to be the case. The workclothes were worn home and cleansed by the family. The solution to this problem was to provide showers and clothes lockers for the workers at the plantsite. Workclothes were then provided by the company and laundered in a special facility at the site. The homes were thoroughly cleansed, and blood lead levels were eventually lowered to and maintained at normal values for that geographic locality. An unidentified health problem was discovered and corrected, without closing down the plant or causing severe economic disruption.

APPLICATION: A REGIONAL CASE STUDY

The Problem

The following study concerned children with infection and the environmental variables they shared. Much is known about the effects of infection; the morbidity and mortality statistics are salient testimony to its impact on child growth, development, and survival. Surprisingly little is known, however, about the ecological milieu that shrouds infected youngsters or the causal paths by which the environmental variables interact to determine child health.

Epidemiologic studies of infection are plentiful, but their focus is usually on the incidence and seriousness of the problem, with little attention to the associated social or cultural forces. Similarly, sociologic analyses of infection focus on behaviors and attitudes, usually skirting the biologic as well as the economic and political factors. The objective of explaining this study was to demonstrate the usefulness of an ecologic model to identify and quantify the physical, biologic, sociocultural, and politico economic variables related to infection among children.

Health statistics for children in rural communities, especially youngsters of indigenous heritage, reveal that they have more problems than urban children. For example, in Chile, infant mortality rates in rural communities are more than twice those of urban communities. When risk is matched for ethnicity, indigenous children have a far higher risk, which is reduced somewhat if they live in urban areas but still remains substantially higher than that of nonindigenous children living in rural areas. The chance for indigenous children to attain the same mortality rate as nonindigenous children is directly correlated to years of maternal schooling.

In developing countries, income determines food consumption. With inadequate income, nutrient intake suffers. *Malnutrition,* defined as a deficiency of the essential nutrients required to support normal physiologic functions, has startling effects on health. The Pan American Health Organization found that a preexisting nutritional deficiency or immaturity (defined as a severe growth deficit) was the underlying or associated cause of death in 57% of deceased preschool children in the Americas. Infection was the leading (58%) cause of death, and 61% of those children who died of infection also had a nutritional deficiency. Malnutrition and infection demonstrate a synergistic and compounding relationship. *Infection,* a state in which microorganisms reproduce and cause damage to the host, is a radically different and more lethal process in a child than in an adult. Malnutrition and infection affect the vast majority of children in developing countries.

When a community seeks to maximize its resources of health personnel and capital goods to service the greatest number of children, it requires a tool that will (1) appraise the impingement of biopsychosocial variables that surround the child and (2) establish the relationships that link these variables to health status indicators, such as the presence or absence of infection. Because infection is usually a short-term problem, whereas malnutrition is a chronic state of ill health, age-specific prevalence rates of infection are considered crucial indicators of health status and were used to measure health condition in this study.

Population and Methods

The Multinational Andean Genetic and Health Survey assessed the health status of the indigenous population living in Chile's northern province of Tarapacá.

Northern Chile is geographically divided into three ecologic zones—the lowland coast, mountainous sierra, and highland altiplano—which differ radically in topography and climate. Associated with the differences are biotic changes that determine the types of agroeconomics, and thus lifestyles, that can be practiced. The health status of 988 children and 1108 adults in 12 communities was determined; these people represented 70% to 90% of the people in any given village.

The International Classification of Diseases codes were used. Children with one or more diagnoses of infection were considered "infected"; children with one or more noninfectious disorders were categorized as "noninfected"; and children without coded diseases were considered "well" and "free of disease." Additionally, family health variables were abstracted from census data collected concurrently. Family wealth was scored according to the number of animals and amount of acreage owned. Four anthropometric measurements—weight, height, arm circumference, and subscapular skinfold—were used to study the relationship between growth and present health status. From known surnames, ethnicity was determined: non-Aymara (Spanish), Mestizo (mixed Spanish and indigenous), or Aymara (indigenous).

The people studied were primarily agriculturists who derived their livelihood from the land. Inhabitants of the highlands had little arable land, but large expanses of grazing pasture were available. They used their livestock (goats, llamas, and alpacas) to convert the inedible (to humans) natural vegetation into animal products (meat, milk, cheese, and fibers) suitable for human use. Conversely, residents of the sierra had more arable land, more irrigated fields, more diverse livestock (adding sheep and cattle) and agricultural crops, and thus more available foodstuffs. Coastal residents had the least arable land (desert stream floodplains) but benefited from a favorable climate and subsidized irrigation. Plant production was high and diverse on the coast, but animal products were restricted.

Population Characteristics

The physical examinations of children of all three ecologic zones revealed that 40% of them had one or more infections, 18% exhibited one or more noninfectious disorders, and 42% were well and free of disease. Infection did not decrease appreciably with age. Non-Aymara children living on the coast were most likely to be well and free of disease, whereas highland children had the highest rates of infection. The prevalence of noninfectious disorders showed little ethnic variability and no appreciable difference between coast and altiplano regions.

A complex clustering of interacting variables prevailed at the family level. Some, such as the number of persons in the household, influenced child health directly (the larger the family, the more potential reservoirs for the incubation and transmission of infection). Other variables exerted their influence indirectly, acting through a web of interrelationships. A primary problem in understanding the ecologic determinants of child health is deciding how to assess the extent to which a given variable acts within the family's environment, directly or indirectly, to affect health status. Analysis of socioeconomic variables (maternal age, education, and health; paternal occupation and health; and family wealth) revealed that well children were likely to have a mother with secondary education and that infected children were likely to have a mother with no education.

Additionally, children with one or more infections were more likely to be cared for by a mother who was also infected, who was younger than 35, and who had minimal or no education. A large number of infected youngsters in the altiplano resided in homes below the median wealth index, but neither wealth nor the father's occupation differentiated the health status of coastal or sierra children. Only among sierra children did the father's health correlate significantly to the child's health. Most early child and maternal health factors varied as a function of region but not of ethnicity.

When compared to well youngsters, infected children consumed fewer foods, and regionally, altiplano children consumed the fewest foods. Region of residence with associated access to food, shelter, education, and health care proved more connected to child health than culture and associated lifestyle behaviors. Child health was determined by environmental factors operant at the individual, family, and community level.

Model Application

Most children in *developing* nations (and some children in *developed* nations) reside in abject poverty, resulting in inadequate dietary intakes and significant prevalence of infectious disease. The dilemma facing health workers and planners in all countries is how to use existing resources to the greatest benefit of the largest number of children. To promote child health, causal determinants of infection and malnutrition as well as cost-effective interventions must be identified. The problem is how to define and measure the crucial variables of child morbidity.

Most assessment models are linear, unidirectional, and not designed to look beyond the child or immediate family for health indicators. The ecological determinants responsible for the prevalence, severity, and duration of the infection-malnutrition cycle are practically unknown. In developing countries, almost all pediatric morbidity data are obtained from hospital records; consequently, they offer uncertain direction for regional or community health planning, especially in rural areas where people have limited or no routine access to medical care.

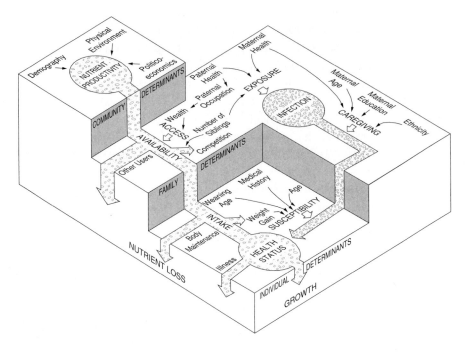

FIGURE 3-7
The ecological determinants of child health.

The Chilean study used an ecologic model to sort physical, biologic, socio-cultural, and politicoeconomic variables that impinged on child health. Descriptive and multivariate analyses were used to delineate the variables that exerted an appreciable effect on child health. Using ecologic concepts and the variables found to be important links to child health, a model of the ecological chain of events has been constructed (Figure 3-7). This "ecologic map" begins with the geographic region of residence—the community.

The region, or community, surrounds the child with a given set of physical forces, including climate, water supply, and topography. These forces interact with demographic structure and political and economic organization to determine the nutrient productivity of the land. Food production in any region is conditioned by economic forces (resources allocated to food production and food distribution), social forces (land tenure), and political edicts (policy and legal implication of land ownership and use). These forces unite and determine the quantity and quality of land used for food production; the persons and technology applied to the land to maximize production; and the diversity, nutritive value, and distribution of the produce. The physical, biological, sociocultural, and politicoeconomic forces within each region that determine the quantity and quality of nutrients available to the family for consumption.

The family consists of a clustering of interacting variables, many of which serve as gates, acting to impede or facilitate members' access to available nutrients. Simultaneously, infection-risk factors abide within the household, variables that mitigate or accentuate the child's risk of illness. Both nutrient intake and infection risk concurrently determine health status, which is reflected in growth patterns.

The web of interconnection continues even further. Paternal health influences paternal occupation, which determines family wealth and, in turn, defines purchasing power and access to available nutrients. The number and age of siblings influence both access to food (through competition) and infection risk (through exposure). In addition, poor maternal health not only exposes the child to illness but also acts as a deterrent to adequate care giving. Care giving is also affected by maternal ethnicity, age, and education. Each factor determines the mother's knowledge and experience regarding basic health-promoting acts, such as hygiene practices, appropriate weaning foods, and needed nutrients and physical care during illness. Obviously, when the care giver is impaired by lack of knowledge or poor health, the child's risk of infection increases.

The child is a composite of risk factors that interact with familial and regional variables to set his or her health status and subsequent growth. The quantity and quality of nutrients consumed by the child determine weight gain and nutritional status. Weight gain is a product of both nutrient intake and a risk variable for infection. The malnourished child has impaired immunocompetence and is prey to infection. Also influencing a child's weight gain are weaning age and weaning foods; both affect the child's nutritive status and susceptibility to infection. Finally, the child's age and past medical history decrease or accentuate susceptibility to infection. In this study, it was the young, preschool children, ill within the last two weeks, who experienced the bulk of morbidity.

For most children, the interaction of nutritive intake and infection determines growth. Infection is wasteful and has a negative effect on nutrient absorption, metabolism, and use. As a result, the child loses weight, and growth is halted or retarded. Low nutrient intake equally retards growth. Children have greater nutritional needs relative to body mass; the younger the child, the more kilocalories per kilogram of body weight are needed for normal metabolism and growth. The risk of infection is high for all children, especially for infants and preschool-age youngsters, regardless of their nutritional status; however, when adverse infection-risk factors combine with marginal nutrient intake, the result is morbidity and delayed growth.

Policy Implication

Current assessment of world health indicates that lack of basic needs is the primary barrier to wellness. To provide basic needs and improve access to and availability of human services (for example, education, health, sanitation), most countries have focused on providing selected basic needs to designated groups, such as school feeding programs or prenatal care. Unfortunately, regard for the environment, from which the needs arose, is usually omitted. To focus on selected needs without assessing the environment from which the needs arose ignores the complex interrelationships of the biopsychosocial system and negates the structure that created the health problems. Basic-needs intervention programs that do not address ecologic dynamics can create an illusion of success and allow continuation of social and political inequalities that are themselves major contributors of poor health.

Child health is ecological and relates to the total environment that surrounds children, the physical ecosystem, as well as social, political, and economic organizations. Each system determines the production, availability, and distribution of resources and the eventual access of children to basic needs, which, in turn, dictates both health and growth. Children's health and nutrition problems will not be improved substantially until measures are instituted to eradicate poverty.

Using an ecological model to identify and sort the determinants of infection among children in northern Chile, researchers found that the region of residence consistently emerged as a significant correlate of health. *Region* embraces politicoeconomic factors as well as a set climate and demographic state that determine nutrient productivity and access. Once the child acquires food, whether the nutrients are used to maintain and promote growth or are degraded by infection that retards growth and development depends on the family milieu, especially the mother's health, age, and education. Additional risk factors include family wealth, ethnicity, and paternal health. No one risk factor can be addressed independently of the others. Infection is promoted or hindered by a maze of intercorrelated variables, and to address only one or two does little more than vibrate the web of causation.

The root determinants of child health lie deep in the social, economic, and political fiber of the people. Child health cannot be improved independently of changes in the environment surrounding the child. To focus on selected prevention programs (such as improved nutrition or adequate housing) without simultaneously attending to the environment from which the deficits arise (such as existing political and economic policies) negates the determinant values of health and is an inappropriate use of time, money, and personnel.

Reflections

Where does this knowledge of ecological processes leave us? As practitioners of community health, how does this information aid us?

First, we must be aware that the health of any population can be affected by its surrounding environment. Next, be skeptical of any claims of perfect disposal schemes for pollutants; they do not exist. Remember that pollutants can travel long distances undetected. Water treatment systems usually precipitate pollutants to a bottom sludge. Eventually the sludge must be cleaned out. If it is burned, will the pollutants go back up the smokestack, only to settle into another watershed? If it is buried in a landfill, will they remain in place or seep into a groundwater reservoir, only to surface at your kitchen faucet? Everything—including pollutants—has to go someplace, and it may be difficult to keep them in any one place.

Finally, as a consumer or a public advocate, do not demand perfect disposal schemes. Demand honest and realistic estimates of the risk that invariably accompanies any plan, no matter how appealing. Beware of flowcharts that indicate perfect control of pollutants at all stages of the cycle. Remember that it is people who handle pollutants, and the *people factor* can overwhelm every other part of any plan. It is people who load, transport, and dispose of pollutants. It is people who operate and maintain pollution control systems. It is people who give illegal orders for "midnight dumping and roadside disposal." In some instances, particularly involving the ultimate disposal of nuclear wastes, we may be planning caretaking operations that exceed the realm of past human experience. Our oldest civilizations generally have not persisted for more than 5,000 years, and individual nations typically survive for far shorter periods. Can we honestly listen to glib talk of storing radioactive materials that will require maintenance for 10,000 years or longer—and take such plans seriously?

REFERENCES

Commoner, B. (1971). *The closing circle—nature, man and technology.* New York: Bantam Books.

Council on Environmental Quality. (Issued annually since 1970). *The annual report of the Council on Environmental Quality, Executive Office of the President.* Washington, DC: U.S. Government Printing Office.

———. (1981). *Environmental Trends.* Washington DC: U.S. Government Printing Office.

McFarlane, J. (1985). Use of an ecologic model to identify children at risk for infection and to quantify the expected impact of the risk factors. *Public Health Nursing, 2*(1), 2–22.

———. (1990). Ecologic determinants of the health of Aymara children. In W.J. Schull & F. Rothhammer (Eds.) *The Aymara: Strategies in human adaptation to a rigorous environment.* (pp. 87–100). Boston: Kluwer Publishers.

Odum, E.P. (1989). *Ecology and our endangered life-support systems.* Sunderland, MA: Sinauer Associates, Inc., 1989.

Storer J.H. (1953). *The web of life.* New York: The New American Library.

U.S. Environmental Protection Agency. (1976). *Quality criteria for water.* Washington DC: U.S. Government Printing Office.

———. (1987). *The Toxics release inventory: A National perspective.* Washington, DC: Office of Toxic Substances.

U.S. General Services Administration. (1983). Code of Federal Regulations. Title 40—Protection of the environment, part 50. National primary and secondary ambient air quality standards, part 129. Toxic pollutant effluent standards, part 141. National interim primary drinking water regulations, part 143. National secondary drinking water regulations. Washington, DC: U.S. Government Printing Office.

4

An Advocacy Approach to Ethics and Community Health

Sally Gadow
Carole Schroeder

Objectives

After reading this chapter, you should be able to
- Describe the universalist tradition in primary health care
- Describe advocacy as an alternative ethical model for health care
- Begin to apply an advocacy approach to your practice with the community as partner

Introduction

Traditional health care ethics have tended to emphasize issues involving the individual client rather than the community. To broaden that narrow focus, current discussions of health care ethics include attention to issues of public policy. The conclusion that a health professional might draw from this dichotomy is that nothing of ethical interest happens in the region of health care that falls between the care of individuals, at one extreme, and the formulation of policy, at the other.

Most people, however, live their lives at neither extreme. Their primary experience happens elsewhere. People think and act in a lifeworld, a primary situation consisting of places, projects, and relationships: In other words, they live in communities. Community health care as a distinct ethical domain is largely unexplored, yet it may be more important ethically than either individual clients' care or public policy. Primary health care engages people where they live, in communities. Thus, it is an intimate practice, and intimacy entails the potential for significant harm as well as benefit. Health care at the primary level has the power to affect people's lives in radical, pervasive, and often unseen ways.

One approach to community health ethics would be to define the community as client, but this has two limitations. The first is that this approach ignores significant differences between an individual and a community. The second limitation is that defining communities as clients creates the potential for a traditional client-professional relationship, characterized by client dependence, passivity, and neediness in conjunction with professional authority, expertise, and invulnerability. In that model, "clients are constructed as deviant, and service provision has the character of normalization" (Fraser, 1989). A community as client is subject to the same repressive forces faced by an individual client, for example, a gendered or racialized definition of community or a professionalized definition of health. Functioning as official interpreters of community health, primary health professions could become "therapeutocracies," removing clients' powers to interpret their own needs (Fraser, 1987). However, defining the community as a partner rather than as a client of the professional offers a different ethical approach, that of advocacy.

An ethic of advocacy calls for the formation of partnerships between professionals and community members in order to enhance community self-determination. In these partnerships, professionals and communities form relationships to help the latter discern their values and needs and to develop an encompassing health narrative that includes all views. Unique and nongeneralizable, the narrative is specific to the community that develops it, for it expresses the particular health values of the people involved. Unlike other ethical models, the aim of the partnership is improved community health *as defined by the members of the community* rather than as defined by the professional. By interpreting community as partner and primary health care as intrinsic to the life of a community, advocacy mandates that everyone in the community be represented, not just those with political or professional authority.

Although many professionals value the inclusion of diverse views in health care decisions, enacting that value is limited in practice by a universalist ethical tradition that frames service delivery in the United States.

Implications of Universalism for Community Health Care

The universalist tradition that frames service delivery in the United States effectively prohibits community self-determination in health. That tradition views people as identical, equal, and autonomous, thereby excluding individuals whose autonomy is different or diminished. Significantly, these are usually the people most affected by decisions regarding community health: the poor and uninsured, single women with children, people lacking transportation, alienated teenagers and gang members, homebound elderly people, and homeless persons. Yet the inability of these groups to participate in the public arena and to influence decisions affecting their health must be challenged in a system so committed to abstract equality that actual inequalities are invisible.

Historically, universalism emerged from the search for a single set of principles on which a system of justice could be grounded. The effect of basing justice on principles of rationality, equality, and neutrality has been to privilege the autonomous and disembodied self and to create the notion of a "generalized other" (Benhabib, 1992). This tradition has three important implications for health professionals: authorization of a single definition of the good (in this case, health), exclusion of the private domain from the service arena, and professional self-identification as expert authority and needs interpreter.

Single Definition of Health

Universalism assumes that a single morality or view of the good is valid, rather than validating many moralities based on different conceptions of the good. Operating out of the universalist tradition, professionals assume a stance of authority and certainty, believing that the general professional definition of health is valid for all. This belief renders professionals incapable of recognizing the particularity of communities and the various meanings of health within a single community. By ignoring contextual, personal, and cultural meanings of health, professionals generalize an abstract model of health across communities. Generalized models often fail to meet the diverse needs within communities and thus fail to be used. Rather than reexamining abstract assumptions about health, many professionals label groups of people as "noncompliant," assuming that failure to use services represents lack of interest in (the professional meaning of) health.

Exclusion of the Private Domain

The separation of public and private domains, which is inherent in universalism, allows subtle exclusion of people who do not fit current definitions of public needs. For example, in the United States, spheres of family/intimacy historically have been deemed outside the public realm. Privatization of family/intimate relationships has excluded them from attention. Because the lives of women and children are conducted primarily through those spheres, domestic violence, child abuse, child care, and most reproductive concerns traditionally have been relegated to the private realm. Until the women's movement brought these issues to public awareness, they were considered too intimate for public attention. Renegotiating the traditional boundaries between public and private domains is one way to begin addressing the health care needs of an entire community.

The Professional as Normalizer

A further implication of universalism is the professional's self-identification as expert authority and thus as community normalizer. The notion that the professional is the bearer of expert and authoritative knowledge that the community lacks is rarely questioned in modern health care; as a result, little recognition is given to communities as experts regarding their own health needs. Instead, individuals, families, and communities are viewed as deviant, passive, and in need of normalization. The resulting hierarchy privileges the professional interpretation, while disempowering communities' interpretations of their own needs. Moreover, the professional's self-identification as expert authority fosters a sense of invulnerability that distances professionals from the people they serve and destroys the possibility for mutuality in relationship.

Because professional knowledge can lag behind social changes, health care delivery is often based on invalid assumptions. For example, despite the fact that the traditional ideal of the two-parent family (husband working, wife providing child care and homemaker services) is no longer the norm in many communities, the model continues to express for many professionals the "normal" family. Consequently, health professionals may view single mothers as failed families, needing psychological intervention instead of affordable child care, housing, health care, and well-paying jobs. Due in part to an outdated ideal of family, therefore, professional attitudes can effectively silence the community of families headed by single mothers before they even attempt to speak.

Another example of the failure of universalism is the current obstetrical approach to childbirth in which professional goals override personal meanings. The medicalization of pregnancy and birth emphasizes (and sometimes legislates) production of a normal fetus as having priority over the rights or experience of the mother. Emerging from universalism and the entrenched view of professional as expert authority, this view does violence to women's personal meanings of pregnancy and birth and results in underutilization of prenatal and birthing services.

An analysis of obstetrical literature suggests that medicine defines childbirth in terms of a manufacturing metaphor in which the fetus is a product (Martin, 1992). In that definition, the pregnant woman is marginal, an obstacle to be removed from the center of the situation and replaced by an expert who externally narrates and technologically produces the desired outcome (a healthy fetus). No longer is the woman central to the birthing experience: "The control over knowledge about the pregnancy and birth process that the physician has through instruments...devalues the privileged relation she has to the fetus and her pregnant body" (Young, 1984, p. 46).

The medical narration of childbirth is particularly evident in services offered to women receiving public assistance and those experiencing complicated (high-risk) pregnancies. Despite the fact that the efficacy of some obstetrical practices, such as childbirth position, enemas during labor, and shaving the mother's pubic area, has not been demonstrated, other choices rarely exist for these women regarding their care. In addition, the medical narrative of pregnancy fosters a woman's feelings of failure: Having failed to obtain private medical care and to maintain a healthy pregnancy, she has failed to be a "normal" woman, has become a "problem," and so has abrogated any right to assert herself over the management of the pregnancy and delivery.

Not surprisingly, many of these women also "fail" to obtain or comply with prenatal care regimens offered through public assistance programs and high-risk clinics. Particularly alarming is the fact that the U.S. infant mortality rate is significantly higher than the rates in most developed countries. Buried in that statistic is the fact that the number of infant deaths in African-American families is nearly three times the number in Caucasian families. This fact further attests to the failure of a health care system based on universalism to meet the needs of particular women and infants.

By critically reevaluating universalism in light of these implications for health care, professionals can redefine themselves and their values in order to relate to communities in other ways. An ethical framework of advocacy offers an alternative to universalism.

Advocacy: An Ethical Framework

The term *advocacy* has many uses in the literature of health care ethics (Bernal, 1992; Winslow, 1984). Its meaning here is a professional's commitment to enhance client autonomy and to assist clients in voicing their values (Gadow, 1990).

Advocacy as a moral position is derived from the nature of ethics itself, namely, the possibility of choice. Ethics is reflective inquiry motivated by the question, What is the right decision in this situation? If that question is allowed no more than one answer, dictated by a force claiming greater legitimacy than the questioner (a force such as religious, legal, or scientific authority), choice is impossible and ethical inquiry is futile. In answering questions about value, ethical inquiry is the alternative to force. Any form of force that preempts free reflection silences ethical inquiry.

Health questions, like all questions about the direction of human life, involve decisions about value. The very concept of health is based upon decisions (often at a level neither client nor professional recognizes) to value some functions, abilities, experiences, and outcomes over others. Certain outcomes—life rather than death, for example—may represent such a crucial value for a culture that they become institutionalized as an element of health and take on the appearance of fact instead of value, of necessity rather than choice. But a single person refusing the "fact" and insisting on a different outcome is sufficient to illustrate the value basis of health.

To summarize the two points that are the basis for advocacy:

- Health decisions are based on values.
- Value questions can be addressed only when choice exists.

Advocacy, in minimal terms, means that a client's freedom of choice should not be infringed on. The professional, while obligated to act in the client's best interest, is not permitted to interpret that interest contrary to the client's definition. In positive terms, advocacy has broader implications that extend beyond respect for self-determination. Enhancing client autonomy involves not only respect for but also engagement with clients in expressing their values as unique persons.

An individual can express her uniqueness only if her values are clearly in her mind, having been reexamined in the context of her health concern. Yet that clarification is the most difficult just when it is most important, when a health situation threatens to overturn existing values. In those circumstances, the person has the alternatives of (1) revising her values to incorporate the new situation or (2) recreating the situation to conform to her values. In either case, her decisions will be based on her values. Paradoxically, the situation—if serious enough—may call for a decision affecting the very center of a person's world at the same time that the personal world has tilted disturbingly.

Paternalism makes too much out of this tilt; consumerism, too little. *Paternalism* is the commitment to professional decision making *for* clients, based on the belief that need renders a person incapable of rational judgment. Client autonomy is by definition impaired; hence, professionals are obligated to impose their expertise. Consumerism, on the other hand, is the commitment to professional *non*involvement in client decisions, based on the belief that rationality transcends a tilted personal world. Autonomy is undiminished by illness or injury; therefore, the professional's obligation is to respect the right of self-determination by not intruding in a client's decision making.

Advocacy differs from both of these positions in that it emphasizes the ambiguity intrinsic to health concerns. Client decisions about values are neither the insuperable tasks that the paternalist assumes they are nor as facile as the consumerist believes. Advocacy accepts the likelihood that for most people, significant health alterations require reorientation and a new version of personal autonomy. The professional's role is to participate with clients in developing autonomy in the new situation by helping them to discern their values. On the basis of that reflection, clients can reach decisions that express their own reaffirmed or revised values. Only in this way, when the self is engaged and expressed, can a client make decisions that are *self*-determined rather than merely *not* determined by others.

A client is an embodied self, and part of self-determination involves the relation between self and body. Disruptions in health often create a sense of the body as an objectlike other, alien to the self. Clinical categories and interventions further objectify the experience of embodiment. As a result of objectification, the body seems to become the property of institutions like science, medicine, or law, without a felt connection to the person. At the same time that objectification overwhelms experience, the subjectivity of humiliation, fear, or pain can further isolate persons from their familiar world; in the subjectivity of extreme pain, the world can disappear altogether (Scarry, 1985).

In advocacy, the health professional involves the client in establishing a self-body relation that reconciles the extremes of subjectivity and objectness. The body may retain the meaning of "other" to the client, but advocacy assists a client in freely deciding how to interpret the otherness of the body—perhaps as crony, sage, or intimate adversary. The specific character of the body-as-other is not crucial, as long as its meaning includes more than objectness (that is, includes the body as self or subject) (Gadow, 1980). This interpretation makes the new self-body relation analogous to the intersubjective relation between persons.

The meaning of the body-as-subject offers enhanced client autonomy, because new complexity has emerged in the individual, making new choices possible. Besides the body, other aspects of the person—emotional, intellectual, spiritual, and interpersonal—can also enrich the individual if given voice. In this view, the person is a *community* of interests and subjectivities, each offering a different perspective.

As in any community, however, a hierarchy often exists, so only a few voices are heard on most issues. Whether in the individual or in the community, hierarchy entails the suppression of views and constriction of choices. Because the primary discourse excludes them, excluded views find expression only in dissident forms such as protest or revolt. Advocacy is the participation with individuals in recognizing seemingly alien views as their own (and furthermore, legitimate) voices in decision making. In this way, advocacy assists in amplifying clients' perspectives and, thus, available choices.

Ultimately, self-determination is the freedom to interpret experience and determine meaning for oneself. Advocacy is participation with clients in reaching practical decisions, but at a more fundamental level, advocacy involves participation with a client in deciding the *meaning* of an experience. The greater the diversity of views available, the more choices open to an individual in deciding how to interpret an experience. Engagement with clients at the level of existential choice is the primary means whereby advocacy can enhance autonomy.

It is this existential engagement that distinguishes advocacy from consumerism and paternalism and suggests a client-professional partnership that is foreign to both of those positions. Advocacy is a partnership in which professional and client compose a mutually satisfactory interpretation of their situation. In the partnership, both persons are moral agents, freely accepting or declining the interpretation that each offers, until they reach a meaning that both affirm. The meaning they compose can be considered a narrative, an interpretation that—to their satisfaction—coherently connects all of the elements of the situation. Ultimately, advocacy becomes participation with clients in coauthorship of a health narrative.

The connection between advocacy and authorship is based on the view that every situation represents a narrative or story, a humanly constructed set of meanings that make sense out of phenomena (Carr, 1986). Because no situation has predetermined, unalterable meanings, none has a literal or correct meaning. Other interpretations are always possible. That ambiguity, the absence of final meanings, makes freedom possible. Ambiguity is the space where choice exists, imagination operates, and new narratives can be created.

However, paternalism imposes on clients its own interpretation of their experience, whereas consumerism is indifferent to the narrative that clients adopt. Only advocacy as partnership is based on a mutuality without either imposition or indifference. Both persons have a stake in the narrative they compose, and both are present as particular persons, not as abstract categories that assign expertise to the professional and vulnerability to the client. Each has a different expertise, equally essential to the narrative. And each is vulnerable. In fact, the professional is often more vulnerable than the client, who, lacking recourse to the certainty and authority that professionals claim, may already excel at accommodating ambiguity.

The meaning that persons create through advocacy can be termed a *relational narrative*. This relational narrative is different from narratives derived from impersonal sources like science or policy. Advocacy as coauthoring a relational narrative is an example of communicative or discourse ethics. In contrast to ethics based on abstract principles, communicative ethics is a dialogical model involving concrete, contextual deliberations among particular persons. The narrative that a client and professional compose claims no universal validity: "Discourse ethics is not one more thorough experiment in universalizability but an ethics of practical transformation through participation" (Benhabib, 1986).

In summary, advocacy aims to enhance and express client autonomy through client-professional creation of a relational health narrative. What are the implications of this ethical model for primary health care, for a practice in which the community is the *partner* of the professional?

Implications of Advocacy for Community Health

In an ethic of advocacy, no longer does a single authoritative point of view dominate. Instead, morality becomes contextual, the product of mutual interaction and a willingness to reason from the other's point of view (Benhabib, 1992). That willingness is the basis for a community health ethic in which service recipients have an equal voice in the development and delivery of care. When community is defined as partner, univocal decisions are not valid, for all views become legitimate influences in decision making. In an advocacy approach, practitioners become free to engage with a community as a particular partner rather than as an abstract aggregate and to act on the belief that true expertise regarding health resides in the community itself.

The aim of advocacy is to enhance community self-determination through construction of a unique health narrative that guides delivery of services. Fundamental to construction of a health narrative is knowledge about the community's needs and values. Therefore, research methods congruent with advocacy become as important as care delivery models. Participatory research methods, expanded public health nursing, school-based neighborhood clinics, and nurse-managed care centers are but a few examples of a community health ethic in which the professional and the community are partners.

Participatory Research

Utilizing principles of participatory research is a means of increasing community self-determination and control. Participatory research calls for the involvement of local people to collectively investigate problems, analyze information, and act as a community. Basic to participatory research is the concept of collective or community knowledge and the building of relationships as the basis of collective problem solving. In order to use participatory principles, professionals are obligated to relate to community research subjects as equals. In this way, both professionals and community members begin to see that each group possesses an area of expertise that can benefit the other (Lather, 1986).

Ethnographic assessment of problems and solutions is one means of approaching communities as equal participants in health care. Traditional needs assessments are typically conducted from the perspective of researchers living outside the community, using secondary data such as epidemiological, historical, registry, and census data. In contrast, in ethnographic analyses of communities, professionals may live in communities for weeks and months at a time, interviewing diverse community members and participating in community life. Information from community members is considered primary data; by living and participating in the community, professionals are less likely to apply disembodied, abstract knowledge to a generalized other.

Focus groups are another means of ensuring community participation in decisions affecting community health. Focus group techniques are a naturalistic method of qualitative research designed to elicit views from the participant's perspective rather than from the researcher's framework (DesRosier & Zellers, 1989). The groups provide a forum for generating innovative solutions to chronic problems. Gathered in a group to discuss health values and needs, community members are considered the primary informants of the research process. Most importantly, this method mandates inclusion of representatives of all persons affected by the analysis. Open-ended questions are used to elicit information, such as

> What is it like living in your community?
> What are your community's strengths? Weaknesses?
> What is health for your community?
> What does health mean for you?

Members of different focus groups bring their results back to the community for analysis in neighborhood meetings. That information is then used to assist in construction of the health narrative that will guide the development and delivery of services in the community.

Public Health Nursing

The reinterpretation of community health using a model of advocacy involves construction of a health narrative that encompasses all views. But how are views to be expressed by those who historically have been excluded from participation (such as mothers lacking child care and transportation, adolescents, gang members, or the working poor)? The disenfranchised often have little trust in professionals and little belief that their own participation can make a difference in their lives. More effective involvement of public health nurses could build on nurses' already established ability to reach marginalized individuals and families. Public health nurses have a long tradition of empowering those outside the public arena. They are closer to families and their problems than professionals who deliver services out of clinics and hospitals. Because they visit people in their homes, they are experienced in approaching clients from a position of shared power. One nurse characterized her practice as mutual disclosure: "You don't have all your professional hoopla as a shield. . . . You have no uniform, no stethoscope around your neck, no little gadgets to assert your authority. It's you and that person listening to each other" (Zerwekh, 1992).

Public health nurses' expertise in locating "disappearing" families is well documented. Ideally situated as advocates for individual and family health and skilled in building trusting relationships, nurses have a sound understanding of local needs and services. Already experienced as advocates for individual and family health, nurses in a community advocacy model could translate their special knowledge from family services into the larger context of community partnerships.

School-Based Clinics

Expansion of existing school-based clinics into comprehensive neighborhood health and social service centers is another means of delivering care to people in their own locale. Most families are already associated with schools, and by integrating social, health, and educational services into neighborhood centers, school-based clinics could increase underserved families' access to public services (Uphold & Graham, 1993). Because schools are based in neighborhoods, underrepresented people's access to health care services can be increased; people lacking time and transportation can more easily participate when decision making and service delivery occur close to their homes.

Nurse-Managed Centers

Community nurse-managed centers are an especially promising means of actualizing an advocacy ethic in community health practice. They are unique in providing clients with direct access to nurses without first requiring a referral fee. Because their focus is maintenance of health rather than diagnosis and treatment of disease, they deliver a wide range of primary services such as wellness maintenance, assessment and screening, education and counseling, symptom management, medical services, and support of home care rather than hospital care. Guided by a health narrative developed by professionals and community members together, these centers could become models for comprehensive delivery of primary health care based on advocacy.

One example of such a center is the Denver Nursing Project in Human Caring, a nurse-managed outpatient center for persons with HIV/AIDS. The center was conceived in 1988 by nurses concerned that the health and social needs of persons with HIV/AIDS were not being met in the acute care system. The advisory board includes persons affected by the disease and local health professionals. Three local hospitals and the University of Colorado School of Nursing contributed to the center's initial operations. In 1990 and 1993, federal funding was obtained from the U.S. Department of Health and Human Services, Division of Nursing, to increase community access to nurses and expanded services at the Denver center. Services include assessment and referral, education for self-care, maintenance of home care rather than hospital care, prevention and management of symptoms, support and counseling, and alternative health treatments (less than one fourth of services are traditional medical services such as blood, fluid, and medication administration; laboratory tests; and so on). Due to the chronic nature of HIV/AIDS, assistance in negotiating the health and social service system is emphasized as a means of client empowerment.

Collective decision making operates at the center, and a rotating, elected board of clients meets frequently to provide input into all programs offered by the center. Unilateral power relationships of professional privilege and authority are not tolerated; instead, persons utilizing the center are considered experts in interpreting their own needs. In initial interviews, clients are asked to "tell the story of living with HIV." In this way, aspects of the situation that *the client* deems meaningful become the starting point for care planning.

Mutual engagement between nurses and clients for the purpose of client empowerment is a focus of the center, using a partnership model of nursing care. Based on the results of focus groups conducted at the center in 1990, the partnership model evolved out of expressed client and staff needs, rather than unilateral professional interpretation of needs (Schroeder & Maeve, 1992). Clients have been involved in all phases of planning, implementing and evaluating the care partnerships.

Despite affiliation with institutions that endorse the medical model of disease intervention, the center endorses no single medical narrative of HIV/AIDS as authoritative. Instead, health is individually defined and actualized by clients and nurses through their personal partnerships. This model of community nurse-managed care has proven to be a well-utilized (as well as cost-effective) method of delivering meaningful service at the community level (Schroeder, 1993).

Conclusion

Although the public demand for health care reform is no longer ignored by legislators or health professionals, little will actually change unless the traditional values of universalism and authority underlying community health care are renegotiated by the very professionals who have been mandated to change. Rather than new external structures, a new internal ethic is necessary to guide the efforts of health care reform. An advocacy model of community health returns power to communities through partnerships of professionals and representatives of *all* members of a community. Through partnership, professionals and communities develop a health narrative that expresses the diverse values of the community regarding health. Unique and nongeneralizable, the narrative guides service delivery and reform within the community that participated in its development as partner.

REFERENCES

Benhabib, S. (1986). *Critique, norm, and utopia: A study of the foundations of critical theory.* New York: Columbia University Press.

———. (1992). *Situating the self: Gender, community and postmodernism in contemporary ethics.* New York: Routledge.

Bernal, E. W. (1992). The nurse as patient advocate. *Hastings Center Report, 22*(4), 18–23.

Carr, D. (1986). *Time, narrative, and history.* Indianapolis: Indiana University Press.

DesRosier, M., & Zellers, K. (1989). Focus groups: A program planning technique. *Journal of Nursing Administration, 19*(3), 20–25.

Fraser, N. (1987). What's critical about critical theory? The case of Habermas and gender. In S. Benhabib & D. Cornell (Eds.), *Feminism as critique* (pp. 31–56). Minneapolis: University of Minnesota Press.

————. (1989). *Unruly practices: Power, discourse and gender in contemporary social theory*. Minneapolis: University of Minnesota Press.

Gadow, S. (1980). Body and self: A dialectic. *Journal of Medicine and Philosophy, 5*(3), 172–185.

————. (1990). Existential advocacy: Philosophical foundations of nursing. In S. Spicker & S. Gadow (Eds.), *Nursing images and ideals: Opening dialogue with the humanities* (pp. 79–101). New York: Springer Publishing Company.

Lather, P. (1986). Research as praxis. *Harvard Educational Review, 56*(3), 257–277.

Martin, E. (1992). *The woman in the body: A cultural analysis of reproduction*. Boston: Beacon Press.

Scarry, E. (1985). *The body in pain: The making and unmaking of the world*. New York: Oxford University Press.

Schroeder, C. (1993). Nursing's response to the crisis of access, costs and quality in health care. *Advances in Nursing Science, 16*(1), 1–20.

Schroeder, C., & Maeve, K. (1992). Nursing care partnerships at the Denver Nursing Project in Human Caring: An application and extension of caring theory in practice. *Advances in Nursing Science, 15*(2), 25–38.

Uphold, C., & Graham, M. (1993). Schools as centers for collaborative services for families: Visions for change. *Nursing Outlook, 41,* 204–211.

Winslow, G. R. (1984). From loyalty to advocacy: A new metaphor for nursing. *Hastings Center Report, 14*(6), 32–40.

Young, I. M. (1984). Pregnant embodiment: Subjectivity and alienation. *Journal of Medicine and Philosophy, 9,* 45–62.

Zerwekh, J. (1992). Laying the groundwork for family self-help: Locating families, building trust, and building strength. *Public Health Nursing, 9*(1), 15–21.

5

Cultural Competence in Partnerships with Communities

Judith C. Drew

Being the other is feeling different; it is an awareness of being distinct; it is consciousness of being dissimilar. Otherness results in feeling excluded, closed out, precluded, even disdained and scorned. . . . On the one hand being the other frequently means being invisible. . . . or inevitably seen stereotypically. For the majority, otherness is permanently sealed by physical appearance. For the rest, otherness is betrayed by ways of being, speaking, or of doing.

(Madrid, 1988, pp. 10–11, 16).

Arturo Madrid tells his story of being different, of its significance and its consequences. His poignant expressions of "otherness" are wake-up calls for us. Our sensitivities may be sharpened if we consider that in any place at any time we might just be an "other."

Objectives

This chapter focuses upon the concepts basic to cultural interpretations of differences among people; how those differences are revealed in client-provider interactions; and how awareness, understanding, and changes in our sensitivity and functioning can make us and our institutions more culturally competent. After studying this chapter, you should be able to

- Discuss the concepts of diversity, ethnicity, culture, and cultural health care systems
- Acknowledge the influence of culture and ethnicity upon health beliefs, illness behaviors, and client-provider relationships

- Rediscover your own cultural identity and its role in shaping who you are
- Value the significance of culturally competent providers and institutions

Introduction

Since 1965, changes in immigration patterns and birth rates have influenced U.S. population demographics. Experts suggest that the population of diverse racial and ethnic groups will continue to grow at a rapid rate through the middle of the 21st century, when decendents of European whites will become a designated minority (Congress & Lyons, 1992). In appreciation of these trends, health care providers will interact more frequently with clients of diverse ethnic affiliations whose health beliefs, languages, and life experiences differ greatly from their own. Diversity is a fact of human existence and must be celebrated. Celebrating diversity comes from an awareness of one's own ethnic and cultural backgrounds, an understanding of how they influence everyday life, and an appreciation for the rich beauty that the tapestry of American peoples exhibits.

Beyond awareness and understanding, health care providers must develop skills to work with culturally diverse clients, their families, and their communities. Many believe that these skills are learned rather than innate and that they require commitment and nurturing. Such an imperative also suggests that programs and services be designed so that they are available, acceptable, and appropriate to the cultures they seek to serve (Adams, 1990). This "cultural competence" demands that practitioners and delivery systems understand a client's, family's, and even a community's perception of their health needs (Cross, 1987), including their health status and acceptable sources of help during vulnerability and illness. Therefore, the following sections of this chapter present concepts that will assist you in building cultural competence, beginning with an enlightened awareness of diversity, ethnicity, and culture and illustrating their influence on individuals' and communities' health and illness beliefs and practices. Self-assessment and an analysis of client-provider interactions are presented as learning experiences with implications for practice. After all, successful health promotion outcomes and intervention strategies depend on our abilities to competently reach and work with the diverse communities we serve.

Diversity, Ethnicity, and Culture

Derived from the Latin *divertere, diversity* implies the condition of being different or having differences. There is no attempt made here to imply a ranking, ordering, or prioritizing of differences; they simply exist. How we look at and deal with differences in human attributes can either build bridges or construct barriers with individuals in and across groups and communities. Rather than thinking of differences as sources of conflict, we should view them as part of a whole process of social and individual identity. A celebration of differences can become commonplace when we understand that the principle strengths upon which our country is built suggest a tolerance for individual uniqueness and a collective creativity. Recognizing that each of us differs in what we think is functional in our lives, we must understand that those who act differently from the mainstream are not deficient in something or "disadvantaged"; they are rich in a different culture and "other-advantaged" (Dervin, 1989; Lyons, 1972).

Nurses admit to knowing little about the backgrounds, beliefs, and values of the people they serve. Asking clients to teach us about themselves will extend to others our sensitivities about being different and will empower others to share their own awareness. Taking the time to value both the differences and commonalities across American ethnic and cultural groups will provide us with valuable insights into the human experience and enable us to build bridges between providers and the growing numbers of diverse clients.

Given current population reports, it is estimated that one out of every four persons in the United States is a member of an ethnic minority (May, 1992). In its purest form, the term *minority* implies a condition of difference based on enumerating an identifiable characteristic. Wirth (1945) has suggested that a minority is "a group of people who, because of their physical or cultural characteristics, are singled out from others in the society in which they live, for differential and unequal treatment, and who therefore regard themselves as objects of collective discrimination" (p. 347). Health care providers need to appreciate the special histories of ethnic minority groups, how their identities are preserved, their variant subcultures, and their unique coping structures—all of which have been challenged by change, exploitation, and prejudice (Moore, 1971). Despite consistent attempts to improve health care to ethnic minorities, statistics reveal that white European-Americans still have higher life expectancy rates at most ages (Devore & Schlesinger, 1991). We still have a long way to go to improve services to groups of Americans who are at great risk. To do this, we must understand that differences exist between the health care providers and care recipients and that those differences are rooted in our heritage, ethnicity, and culture.

Whether ethnicity is associated with minority or majority populations, ethnic groups are composed of persons who share a unique cultural background and social heritage that is passed from one generation to another. Ethnicity should be understood as a social differentiation that engenders in us a sense of self-awareness and exclusivity, a sense of belonging. Our ethnicity gives us a membership in a distinct social group and differentiates us from those in other groups. Our distinction is often based on such cultural criteria as a common ancestry; shared history; a common place of origin; language, dress, and food preferences; and participation in rituals, networks, clubs, or activities (Holzberg, 1982). For example, when members of an Italian-American family gather at a wedding, the nature of the celebration expresses the ethnic culture in many ways. The ceremony and the formalities are representative of "the way things are done." At the celebration that follows the exchanging of vows, the guests may feast on antipasto, linguini, chicken marsala, and cappuccino. Soon after, the accordian player might strike up the Tarantella, an Italian folk song. Young and old alike may grasp hands and promenade as they laugh and sing. Late in the evening, the elders may be heard sharing stories about "the old country" with excitement and pride. Although the members of this group may have emigrated at different times and may have been born in America, they share common bonds based on native language, history, and values. The passing of these beliefs, values, knowledge, and practices takes place through the rituals of sharing and participating in cultural events and celebrations.

It may be helpful to think of your own ethnic culture. What group(s) do you identify with and why? What are your common bonds? What cultural rituals do you celebrate and with whom? What are the purposes and meanings of your gatherings and celebrations? What types of things are shared and learned when people get together? What types of foods are prepared for the event? Are there dances, special rites, or ceremonies? Each of us can probably identify several shared beliefs, values, and practices that make us members of unique collectives, and many of us strive to preserve our rich cultures and histories by passing them on to each successive generation. Foods, languages, and other bonds of common ancestry are the cultural aspects of ethnicity that serve to offer consistency and structure to life and provide individuals with abilities to interpret life events as significant and meaningful (Royce, 1982).

In health and illness, an ethnic group's shared beliefs, symbols, and customs serve as common reference points that members use to judge the appropriateness of their decisions and actions (Kleinman, 1978). However, attention must be given to the variations within and between generations that are sometimes attributed to acculturation, socioeconomic status, and education (Congress & Lyons, 1992). Caution should be taken by all health care providers not to generalize beliefs and practices to every member of an ethnic group or culture. Although ethnicity captures the larger cultural component of human experiences, we must not permit our awareness of a culture to erode its members' individual identities and dignity.

Culture, Health and Illness, and Nursing

Ethnic culture is the medium through which an individual's beliefs, standards, and norms for health and illness behaviors are structured, learned, shared, practiced, and judged. Cultural beliefs give meaning to health and illness experiences by providing the individual with culturally acceptable causes for illness, rules for symptom expression, interactional norms, help-seeking strategies, and determining desired outcomes (Harwood, 1981; Kleinman, 1980). For example, when you awake before school with a dryness in your throat and cramps in your stomach, several beliefs about what could be wrong and how you should act in response to what is wrong are set into action. What is causing this to happen to me? What can I do about it? Should I stay home from school? Whom should I call to help me? What will people think if I stay home today? The answers to these questions and the actions you take are learned and are influenced by the experiences you have had with your family and the larger ethnic aggregate. In some cultures, a special home-remedy tea can be taken for specific complaints of dry throat and cramps, and going to work or school is an expectation. Other cultural groups may expect you to be visited by a healer, stay home from work or school, and tell no one else about your problem.

Noted psychiatrist and anthropologist Arthur Kleinman studied members of many diverse ethnic groups to gain an understanding of the links between cultural beliefs and health and illness behaviors and actions (Kleinman, 1980). The findings of his studies are especially helpful in guiding community practitioners who interact with clients in their homes and various types of community institutions. He found, like other researchers, that cultural beliefs based in shared meanings, values, and norms are the basic guidelines that individuals use for recognizing that something is wrong, interpreting what it might be, and organizing a plan of appropriate actions (Kleinman, 1986). For example, before action is taken in response to a problem, individuals and family members must first agree that the symptoms represent a problem. Next there is an examination of all possible and probable causes, which may range from behaviors and foods to violations of cultural norms. Once a cause is identified, a plan of action is made, and appropriate treatment is determined. In addition, how we act when we are "ill" is determined by our ethnic culture. Some cultures have specific norms for sick role behavior, whereas other cultures suggest that you continue to carry out your everyday role to the best of your abilities. In this overall illness recognition and management process, cultural beliefs influence the reasons the client formulates to explain the illness, the language and terms used for communicating the health problem, the choice of whom one talks to about the problem, the range of acceptable healing alternatives, how choices are made, and expectations for treatment outcomes (Helman, 1984; Kleinman, 1980; Mechanic, 1986).

For those of us in the nursing profession, culturally sensitive health care continues to be a central focus of a holistic and humanistic philosophy that guides our practice (Aamodt, 1978; Leininger, 1978; Munet-Vilaro, 1988). Because *nursing* is defined as the diagnosis and treatment of human responses to actual or potential health problems (American Nurses' Association, 1980), the role of cultural beliefs in guiding a client's health practices and responses to illness episodes is an important nursing concern (Whall, 1987).

The goal of culturally sensitive care can only be achieved through conscious efforts at gaining knowledge of different groups' ways of explaining, understanding, and treating health problems. Certainly, gaining this knowledge and putting it to use will take some time, but it is important for practitioners to learn the strategies presented in this chapter for eliciting from clients their cultural models for health, illness, and help seeking. We have a responsibility to elicit and understand the health and illness beliefs and behaviors of ethnic group members served by the community. Eliciting these beliefs requires skill and sensitivity, and understanding requires a sincere commitment that is revealed to coworkers as well as clients.

Cultural Health Care Systems

Basic to successful interactions between clients and providers is the understanding that we are all different from one another, with different ethnic and cultural backgrounds and, therefore, different health and illness beliefs and practices. There's that word again: *different*. But despite our differences, we come together at a mutually agreed-on place to achieve a common goal: to maintain or regain health. The dilemma presented here is that health means different things to each of us; we recognize it and measure changes in it differently, act in diverse ways when faced with these changes, and seek different methods for achieving similar outcomes. The settings where we meet and interact with each other may take on different veneers and titles, but they are all what Kleinman has called "cultural health care systems" (Kleinman, 1980). The simple fact that culture influences health and illness beliefs and behaviors serves as a constant reminder to us that wherever clients and providers interact, there is a system, and it is influenced by the beliefs, values, norms, and standards that each of us brings to it.

Cultural health care systems are made up of individuals experiencing and treating illness and the social institutions where interactions between clients and providers take place (Kleinman, 1980; Kleinman, 1986). Each cultural health care system can have as many as three recognized sectors, most commonly referred to as *popular, folk,* and *professional.* Typically, the popular sector is composed of ordinary people, families, groups, social networks, and communities. The lay practitioners and healers comprise the folk sector, whereas the professional sector is composed of the licensed health professionals (Kleinman, 1980). Let us look at the popular, folk, and professional sectors in some detail.

Popular

The popular sector of cultural health care systems is made up of informal healing relationships that occur within one's own social network.

Although the family is at the nucleus of this sector, health care can take place between people linked by kinship, friendship, residence, occupation, or religion (Helman, 1984). In the U.S., there are as many versions of the popular sector as there are ethnic cultures. In neighborhoods where many ethnic groups have settled, popular sectors of health care systems are found to have several different ways of managing health and illness. Despite these differences among the ethnic groups, all of the people who make up the popular sector participate in making decisions about health and illness experiences.

In the popular sector, the process of defining oneself as ill begins with a self-diagnosis confirmed by significant others based on the implicit standards of what it means to be well (Angel & Thiots, 1987; Eisenberg, 1980; Helman, 1984). Consequently, a person is defined as ill when there is agreement between self-perceptions of impairment and the perceptions of those around him (Helman, 1984; Weiss, 1988). The social, ethnic, and cultural values upon which the illness judgment is based focus on the experience of discomfort, failure to function as expected, and a change in physical appearance. Whether or not a symptom is recognized as significant or normal is also influenced by the occurrence, persistence, and prevalence of the symptoms among group members (Angel & Thiots, 1987; Helman, 1984).

Once a symptom is recognized as significant, decisions about appropriate actions must be made. These decisions are also usually based on beliefs, standards, and norms passed along from previous generations. For example, decisions about seeing a doctor for a health problem, as opposed to taking care of the symptoms at home, are made by the affected individual in collaboration with family and the social network. If the symptom is commonly observed in other members of the family or community and home remedies have successfully treated the problem, then going to the doctor is not a priority. Within this sector, both the recipient and the provider share similar assumptions about health and illness. Therefore, misunderstandings are rare, and the healer's credentials are based on experience rather than professional education and licensure (Chrisman, 1977; Kleinman, 1980).

Folk

The folk sector of cultural health care systems includes the interaction between a client and sacred and secular healers. Most healers share the same basic cultural values, beliefs, and world views about health, illness, and treatment as their constituents, and family members are included in the diagnosis and treatment of the individual. Healers in this sector use a holistic approach that includes the analysis of the client's relationship with other people, with the natural environment, and with supernatural forces (Helman, 1984). Treatment rituals and recommendations are prescribed to correct the imbalance and to promote healing. Healers have little formal training, although some have served an apprenticeship with another healer. Most are believed to receive healing powers through family position, inheritance, signs, revelations, or gifts (Helman, 1984; Lewis, 1988).

Within the folk sector, illnesses are defined as syndromes from which members of a group suffer and for which their culture provides a cause, a diagnosis, preventive measures, and regimes of healing (Rubel, 1977). For example, Latinos refer to *susto,* which is a condition of fright caused by a traumatic experience (Rubel, 1977).

Professional

In contrast, the professional sector of cultural health care systems is made up of organized health professionals who are formally educated and legally sanctioned (Kleinman, 1980). Unlike the popular and folk sectors, the clients and the providers in the professional sector typically differ in their social and cultural values, beliefs, and assumptions. Based on these differences, as well as the unfamiliar surroundings and rules of the institutions where care is given in the professional sector, the client-provider relationship is frequently one of mistrust, suspicion, and conflict.

Unlike the multidimensional illness orientation of the popular and folk sectors, the professional system embodies the unidimensional disease orientation of biomedicine (Allan & Hall, 1988; Blumhagen, 1982; Chrisman, 1982; Kleinman, 1980; Young, 1982). In the biomedical view, disease is a physiologic and psychologic abnormality; this view is exclusive of and counter to the popular, holistic view of illness as a meaningful experience perceived and constructed in sociocultural context (Allan & Hall, 1988; Angel & Thiots, 1987; Theiderman, 1988). Some of us have prepared a home remedy for a sore throat problem or have applied a poultice to relieve a headache or a persistent cough. These are examples of actions taken, in the popular sector, in response to symptoms that are interpreted as part of a meaningful illness experience.

Sore throats, headaches, and persistent coughs are interpreted by the professional sector as meaningful in the context of disease. Specifically, each symptom is viewed as having a real or potential role in a serious disease process, and treatment is focused on finding a scientifically tested remedy.

Decision Making

People who become ill make choices about whom to consult in the popular, professional, or folk sectors of the cultural health care system. There is overwhelming evidence to suggest that those choices are influenced by the individual's subjective definition of the illness, its meaning, and its expected course (Andersen, Kravitz, & Anderson, 1975; Bishop, 1987; Fabrega, 1974; Mechanic, 1979; Rundall, 1981; Sharp, Ross & Cockerham, 1983; Zola, 1966). Attitudes toward different types of providers and decisions about whom one should seek for help vary according to how the symptom is interpreted and what it means to that person as a significant life event (Bishop, 1987; Cheung, 1987; Sharp, Ross, & Cockerham, 1983; Zola, 1973).

Forming these decisions is also a function of shared, family- and culture-based learning (Mechanic, 1982). Remember back to your childhood days and a significant episode of not feeling well and answer these questions:

- Who decided what was wrong with you?
- What were the interpretations of your symptoms?
- Who made the decision about what to do for you?
- With whom did this person consult?
- Did the meanings of your symptoms and who was consulted have anything to do with the selected treatments?
- What were the expected outcomes from your treatments?
- How were those outcomes evaluated?

Just as important as finding answers to your own health and illness beliefs and practices is investigating the significance of these factors and processes in your clients' illnesses.

In developing a help-seeking pattern, most individuals establish a therapeutic network that may include informal relationships with persons and providers from some or all of the three sectors of cultural health care systems. Different types of providers, including family members and folk healers, may be used concurrently or in sequence depending on the client's perception of the cause of the problem, course of the illness event, and desired healing outcomes (Angel & Thiots, 1987; Helman, 1984; Kleinman, 1980; Mechanic, 1982). Typically, individuals make their help-seeking choices based on prior learning, symptom significance, compatibility between the philosophies of the sectors, and evaluation of the treatment outcome (Blumhagen, 1982; Chrisman, 1977; Kleinman, 1980; Young, 1982). It seems logical that clients, in the process of seeking help, may involve a network of potential consultants ranging from informal structures in the nuclear family to select laypersons and professionals (Friedson, 1961; Roberts, 1988).

Conflict Among Sectors

Given our diverse cultural backgrounds, we should not be surprised to find that research across many health-related disciplines provides evidence that barriers, conflicts, and misunderstandings among the system's sectors are in part related to the differences in cultural beliefs about illness causation and management (Chavez, 1984; Chrisman, 1977; Friedson, 1961; Garro, 1982; Kleinman, 1980; Press, 1980; Roberson, 1987).

Although we may never have viewed conflicts through Kleinman's (1980) perspective before, we have all encountered conflicts between providers and clients. We may have even *been* the clients! Have you ever gone to the doctor only to find that he or she recommended a method of treatment that was not what you expected? Have you ever found that a medication prescribed by the doctor for your problem is something that you would rather not take? None of us is a stranger to these types of conflicts. We find that even after offering students in undergraduate and graduate nursing programs a greater knowledge of ethnicity and culture, the conflicts in beliefs and practices between sectors and resultant barriers to effective health care remain unresolved. The lack of progress in reducing barriers can be linked to professional providers' relative inattention to the popular sector of cultural health care systems. Have you ever heard a professional provider say, "This client is difficult" or "This client is noncompliant with his medicines and he won't follow his diet"? Perhaps you have spoken such comments yourself without thinking that what has been prescribed or recommended may not be compatible with the client's beliefs about treatment. The problem could be more basic than a mere treatment conflict; perhaps the client and provider have incongruent beliefs about what is wrong and what caused the symptom of illness. In the popular or folk sector, illness is sometimes thought to be a somatization of a client's uneasiness with either a stressful relationship, the natural environment, or supernatural forces. This is an example of how cultural beliefs about the cause and management of an illness provide the client with a foundation for interpreting the illness experience as meaningful.

Because belief systems in the popular and folk sectors have often been termed as "unorthodox," "lay," "subjective," or "nonscientific" (Roberson, 1987) and have been associated with non-Western societies, the client's preference for such healing practices has often been dismissed by some professional health care givers. This is problematic because if the treatment does not fit the client's beliefs about the cause and the appropriate management of the problem, what is recommended by a professional may not be followed by the client.

If these problems are to be resolved, we need to understand and accommodate the ideologies and practices of diverse individuals. As professional providers, we must consider the significance of illness interpretations and meanings for the clients we treat, thus facilitating a more comfortable and secure client-provider relationship (Helman, 1984; Kleinman, 1980; Rubel, 1977; Tripp-Reimer, 1982; White, 1982). We must focus on the popular sector if working relationships are expected to have successful outcomes. Conflicts, misunderstandings, and barriers to effective health care will be reduced only by commitment to gain knowledge about the popular sector, where health beliefs and health practices are activated (Kleinman, 1980) and where 70% to 90% of all illness episodes are recognized and treated (Zola, 1972). The nursing profession's commitment to health and holism and its capacity to understand complex sociocultural responses to real and potential health problems make it the most logical choice for a professional sector element to act as a client advocate in facilitating interactions between the sectors. Appropriate advocacy must be based on the ability to understand the popular sector's realities and to translate and negotiate between the system's sectors with the goal of reducing barriers to culturally sensitive care (Chrisman, 1982; Weidman, 1980). In doing so, nursing will lead the charge for cultural *competence* among providers and will model the application of those attributes for health care institutions.

Without a doubt, differences are sources of conflict and misunderstanding in client-provider relationships (Angel & Thiots, 1987; Blumhagen, 1982; Good, 1977; Kleinman, 1980). A detailed understanding of cultural health care systems will provide us with many reasons for the existence and resolution of real and potential barriers between providers and laypersons in the caregiving process. Beyond a basic understanding of the ingredients for conflict, this paradigm of differences should be used by providers, partners, and communities as a guide for becoming culturally competent.

The Culturally Competent Provider

Cultural competence implies an awareness of, sensitivity to, and knowledge of the meaning of culture and its role in shaping human behavior (McManus, 1988). If *culture,* broadly defined, is socially transmitted beliefs, values, ways of knowing, and patterns of behavior characteristic of a designated population group (Kleinman, 1980; Wood, 1989), then *cultural competence* is the ability to express an awareness of one's own culture, to recognize the differences between oneself and others, and to adapt behaviors to appreciate and accommodate those differences (Dillard et al., 1992; McManus, 1988; May, 1992). Culture includes more than race and ethnicity and may take into consideration a person's gender, religion, socioeconomic status, sexual orientation, age, environment, family background, and life experiences (Dillard et al., 1992).

Cultural competence depends on the development of an attitude among health care providers. It is a process that begins with one's willingness to learn about cultural issues (Dillard et al., 1992), proceeds with the commitment to incorporate at all levels of care the importance of culture, and is operationalized by making adaptations in services to meet culturally unique needs (May, 1992). Although some practitioners may have specific knowledge of the languages, values, and customs of other cultures, the most challenging tasks are understanding the dynamics of difference in the helping process and adapting practice skills to fit the client's cultural context (McManus, 1988).

Developing an awareness and acceptance of cultural differences is required as a first step in the process of becoming a culturally competent individual (McManus, 1988). We have already established that there is extensive documentation that many ethnic minorities have beliefs and practices about health, illness, and treatment that differ significantly from the Western, scientific medical paradigm around which the U.S. health care delivery system is structured (Angel & Thiots, 1987; Kleinman, 1980; Devore & Schlesinger, 1990; Eisenberg, 1977; Zola, 1972). However, negatively labeling people because the provider believes them to differ from him/her and the mainstream is unacceptable. Differences must be explored and understood so that barriers to seeking health care can be reduced. Quality health care must be available, accessible, acceptable, and culturally appropriate to the populations, communities, and individuals we serve. Understanding differences begins with an awareness that they exist and continues with a willingness to accept them. In the sections that follow, there are suggestions for exercises to enhance your awareness of your own culture.

Cultural Awareness Exercises

Remember that a major component of cultural competence is an acknowledgment and awareness of one's own culture and a willingness to explore one's own feelings and biases (Dillard et al., 1992). Each person is responsible for building an awareness of how culture influences his or her own ways of thinking and making decisions. Included in this awareness must be an acknowledgment of how day-to-day behaviors reflect cultural norms and values perpetuated by our families and larger social networks. To develop this awareness, Hutchinson (1989) suggests that we ask ourselves several questions that will direct our exploration of our cultural heritage and how our daily interactions are influenced by that culture. Sample questions include the following:

- What ethnic group, socioeconomic class, religion, age group, and community do I belong to?
- What about my ethnic group, socioeconomic class, religion, age, or community do I wish I could change and why?
- What experiences have I had with people different from me?
- What were those experiences like, and how did I feel about them?
- What is there about me that may cause me to be rejected by members of other cultures or ethnic groups?
- What qualities do I have that will help me establish positive interpersonal interactions with persons from other cultural groups?

One strategy used in teaching diversity awareness to health professions students is a cultural assessment project that serves as a purposeful self-examination and as an exercise in appreciating differences. The project asks you to begin by identifying your own cultural beliefs and values about health and illness, education and vocation, foods, religion, and role expectations. (You can do this now as you read this section.) Once you've done that, think through your responses and make notations about how you remember being taught some of those values, practices, expectations, habits, and traditions.

- Where and how was knowledge about your heritage passed on to you?
- Who are the persons in your network responsible for influencing and shaping the lives of the young people?

Proceed with this project by seeking out someone known to you with a background, heritage, or ethnicity different from your own.

- Ask that person's permission for an interview and then ask him or her the same things you asked yourself in establishing your basic cultural richness.
- When you have the data you set out to compare with your own, sit down and analyze what sociocultural similarities and differences the two of you have.

This exercise is particularly beneficial to the beginner who has not ventured into self-awareness projects from a cultural beliefs and values perspective. Having analyzed similarities and differences, proceed with your analysis and focus on predicting potential areas of conflict between the two views as well as the positive, congruent strengths. These may be as simple as food preferences and celebrated holidays or as complex as preferred vocations, generational hierarchies, and healing rituals. You may complete this practice assignment by asking (if this "other" were your client):

- What potential strengths in similarities between us should I build upon to begin interactions with this client?

As the cultural assessment project points out, all interacting parties bring with them unique histories, communication styles, and learned expectations. Together, these contribute to potential misunderstandings and misinterpretations that manifest the dynamics of difference. Therefore, strategies of relating with clients must include eliciting information about their health and illness practices as well as basic ethnic and cultural norms. Specific knowledge about the culture is necessary for the relationship to be structured within the helping framework. Bringing down barriers and facilitating the negotiation of individualized plans of care will support positive health outcomes for all clients. The ultimate goal in planning collaborative approaches to illness treatment is to preserve the dignity of the client and to foster health promotion and healing programs that are likely to meet with compliance because they support rather than offend the clients. Additional information about eliciting the client's cultural health and illness beliefs follows later.

Eliciting Health and Illness Beliefs

We have explored the idea that cultural health beliefs are the major determinants of an individual's recognition and management of an illness experience. Although these beliefs exist independently of and prior to a given episode of illness (Kleinman, 1980), they are activated when one has to cope with and explain a particular experience or situation (Blumhagen, 1982; Gillick, 1985). Therefore, as practitioners, we should expect that it is appropriate to elicit cultural health beliefs when (and not before) an illness experience becomes a reality. According to several researchers, time and experience with an illness are necessary for the client to work the set of beliefs into a functioning set of reasons for the illness, directions for sick role behavior, and options for achieving healing (Blumhagen, 1982; Chrisman, 1982; Good & Good, 1981; Kleinman, 1980; Young, 1982). The significance of learning and knowing ethnic interpretations of health and illness is to allow the practitioner to further clarify the sources of beliefs from which clients formulate their illness realities (Roberson, 1987).

With respect to the health problem at hand, this process begins with eliciting the client's subjective explanations for the cause, duration, and characteristics of symptoms. Further discussion should include exploring the client's expectations for acceptable treatments, outcomes of the treatment, and the substance of the provider-client interaction (Berlin & Fowkes, 1983). Adaptations of Kleinman's (1980) original set of questions are offered by Randall-David (1989) as useful for asking clients their perspectives about health and their experiences. Answers to these questions further increase the cultural competence of the provider:

- What do you think caused your problem?
- Why do you think it started when it did?
- How long do you think it will last?
- What have you done about your problem?
- With whom did you discuss your problem?
- What kind of help and from whom would you like to receive help for your problem?
- How will you know when your problem is getting better?

Additional questions formulated by this author for purposes of conducting explanatory model research include

- What do you call your problem?
- What worries you most about having this problem?
- How did you come to know that you were having a problem?

Answers to these questions may take time and will take conscious effort to collect and use. However, the process is well worth the time and commitment as we gain a greater understanding and respect for all clients' health beliefs and practices. This understanding can lead to both improved client-provider relationships and treatment outcomes. An analysis of the answers to these questions and much introspection will enable health care providers to understand the complexities of cross-cultural interactions (McManus, 1988).

Adapting Skills

It is necessary to develop critical skills as a provider so that cultural assessments can be elicited and appropriate sociocultural care can be delivered in conjunction with prescribed treatment interventions. This implies a contextual understanding that treating the illness and understanding what it means to the individual is as important as working to resolve the disease process (Kleinman, 1988). Although nurses study communication strategies as part of their educational preparation, the cognitive skills necessary to understand another's cultural beliefs and backgrounds need cultivation, refinement, and practice.

Sound *physical and psychosocial assessment skills, sensitive interviewing skills, active listening, neutral body language,* and *self-awareness* are the basic attributes required of culturally competent providers.

Several of these attributes can be built using the contents of this chapter, but it is expected that the practitioner seek out continuing education that will expand the skills necessary for thorough data collection. For example, physical assessment of people of color may be a learning need for some, whereas spending more time in a cultural self-assessment and an analysis of potential conflicts between providers and clients may be a priority for others.

In addition to the need for sensitive interviewing, active listening is a learned skill that requires a lot of practice and critique. It is helpful if you can audiotape an interview that employs role playing between you and a "client" so that you and a colleague can critique your style. Use the following questions to evaluate your progress toward becoming a skilled interviewer:

- Am I using slang or jargon language that is only understood by other professionals?
- Are the questions I ask presented so rapidly in sequence that the client has no time to think and organize a response?
- Do I paraphrase a question so many times that it has lost its original intent?
- Are the questions I ask so long that the focus is diluted beyond recognition?

Sometimes the reasons our questions seem to go unanswered are related to our interviewing skills, styles, and competencies. For example, are you comfortable with pauses, or do you have the need to always hear a speaking voice, even if it is your own? Are you asking appropriate follow-up questions that will probe a client's response to an earlier question? It is important for you to value what the client is saying. Active listening and planning appropriate responses is one sure way of accomplishing the task.

You must also learn how to present yourself with neutral body language during interactions with clients. Not everyone likes being touched or having someone else in their space. Although we may think touch is important in healing, remember that it is of value to us, the providers, and may not be culturally appropriate to the clients we serve.

In addition to physical assessment data, eliciting patient and family explanations of health status and illness realities helps providers take the patient's perspective seriously in organizing clinical care strategies. In turn, the provider's effective communication style assists patients and families in making more useful judgments of when to enter into treatment, with which practitioners, for what treatments, and at what ratio of cost and benefit (Kleinman, 1988). It is imperative to approach health teaching and self-care training with the attitude that providers and patients are collaborators working toward the same goals of positive outcomes for the patient and the family. Negotiation among patients and providers over conflicts in explanations, interpretations, and understandings can reduce barriers to effective care and instill in the patient the provider's respect for alternative viewpoints and preferences. These strategies work together to close the gap between the patient and the provider (Kleinman, 1988) and are necessary to increase access to care and improve health for our entire nation.

The Agency

Cultural awareness, sensitivity, and competence are necessary accomplishments for all health care providers as well as the delivery systems of which they are a part. It makes no sense to have culturally competent practitioners in settings that are culturally ignorant. In services to individuals, families, and communities, culturally competent systems of care must acknowledge and incorporate the importance of culture, appreciate the dynamics of difference, and make a commitment to adapt services to meet unique needs (Cross, 1987; Roberts, 1990). Culturally competent programs and services will respect their clients' cultural beliefs as well as the staff members' beliefs and will include in their mission statements goals to maintain and improve the self-esteem and the cultural identity of employees and clients.

Several types of movements toward agency-level cultural competence have been reported in the literature. When success is measured by community acceptance and use, some are recognized as more successful than others. McManus (1988) reports that a simple outreach model suffers from rejection by ethnic minority groups because service agencies frequently deliver to diverse communities the same services offered to mainstream groups. This approach is perceived by many to be a form of color blindness that maintains barriers rather than removes them. A more meaningful and successful approach to agency cultural competence is mainstream support of local programs and services that employ and use staff who have similar cultural backgrounds to those for whom the services are intended (Gallegos, 1982; Barrera, 1978). This means that multilingual and multicultural services should be offered in some neighborhoods and communities. A needs assessment must be employed to identify the need for services, types of services, and the systems of service delivery that are most acceptable and efficient (Angrosino, 1978).

For many existing agencies and delivery systems, structures, services, and competencies must be modified or created to be consistent and compatible with the cultures they encounter in their client populations. Culturally competent services, systems, agencies, and practitioners possess the capacity to respond to the unique needs of populations whose cultures differ from dominant or mainstream America. To be culturally competent and to be fully utilized, services must be "available, affordable, accessible, appropriate, and acceptable" (Randall-David, 1989, p. 28).

An awareness that racial, ethnic, and minority groups have different needs, have been underserved, or have underused available services has created an interest in agency cultural competence. However, assessing the types of services identified as wanted and needed by target populations is crucial to the reception and use of services by people with culturally diverse backgrounds. Agencies striving for cultural competence must be able to accept the values of the community's ethnic cultures and to develop and refine services and skills for working with the local population (McManus, 1988).

Summary

Educators and providers must remember that ethnicity provides a sense of belonging to people in a pluralistic society: a celebration of differences in identity, strength, and survival. An understanding of ethnic culture is functional for coping with and appreciating differences. Research supports the roles of heritage and identity in influencing people's behaviors and attitudes and the perpetuation of ethnicity throughout generations. Cooperation with and respect for others with different heritages rather than eradication of differences, stimulation of conflict, and goals for sameness must be the focus of future practice and research. Cultural competence is an imperative for health promotion and successful outcomes for illness experiences. Many of the skills needed by providers are in place and available for enrichment through awareness, specialty and continuing education, and careful listening to what our clients teach us.

REFERENCES

Aamodt, A. (1978). The care component in a health and healing system. In E. Bauwens (Ed.), *The anthropology of health* (pp. 37–45). St. Louis: C. V. Mosby.

Adams, E. V. (1990). *Policy planning for culturally comprehensive special health services.* Rockville, MD: United States Department of Health and Human Services, Maternal and Child Health Bureau.

Allan, J. D., & Hall, B. A. (1988). Challenging the focus on technology: A critique of the medical model in a changing health care system. *Advances in Nursing Science, 10*(3), 22–34.

American Nurses' Association. (1980). *Nursing: A social policy statement.* Kansas City, MO: American Nurses' Association.

Andersen, R., Kravitz, J., & Anderson, O. (Eds.). (1975). *Equity in health services.* Cambridge, MA: Ballinger.

Angel, R., & Thiots, P. (1987). The impact of culture on the cognitive structure of illness. *Culture, Medicine, and Psychiatry, 2,* 465–494.

Angrosino, M. V. (1978). Applied anthropology and the concept of the underdog: Implications for community mental health planning and evaluation. *Community Mental Health Journal, 14*(4), 291–299.

Barrera, M. (1978). Mexican-American mental health service utilization: A critical examination of some proposed variables. *Community Mental Health Journal, 14,* 35–45.

Berlin, E. A., & Fowkes, W. C. (1983). A teaching framework for cross-cultural health care: Application in family practice. *The Western Journal of Medicine, 139*(6), 934–938.

Bishop, G. D. (1987). Lay conceptions of physical symptoms. *Journal of Applied Social Psychology, 17*(2), 127–146.

Blumhagen, D. (1982). The meaning of hyper-tension. In N. J. Chrisman & T. W. Maretzki (Eds.), *Clinical applied anthropology: Anthropologists in health science settings* (pp. 297–323). Boston: D. Reidel.

Chavez, L. R. (1984). Doctors, curanderos, and brujas: Health care delivery and Mexican immigrants in San Diego. *Medical Anthropology Quarterly, 15*(2), 31–37.

Cheung, F. M. (1987). Conceptualization of psychiatric illness and help seeking behavior among Chinese. *Culture, Medicine, & Psychiatry, 11,* 97–106.

Chrisman, N. (1977). The health seeking process: An approach to the natural history of illness. *Culture, Medicine, & Psychiatry, 1,* 351–378.

———. (1982). Anthropology in nursing: An exploration of adaptation. In N. J. Chrisman & T. W. Maretzki (Eds.), *Clinically applied anthropology: Anthropologists in health science settings* (pp. 117–141). Boston: D. Reidel.

Congress, E. P., & Lyons, B. P. (1992). Cultural differences in health beliefs: Implications for social work practice in health care settings. *Social Work in Health Care, 17*(3), 81–96.

Cross, R. L. (1987). Cultural competence continuum. *Focal Point: The Bulletin of the Research and Training Center to Improve Services for Seriously Emotionally Handicapped Children and Their Families, 3*(1), 5.

Dervin, B. (1989). Audience as listener and learner, teacher, and confidante: The sense-making approach. In R. E. Rice & C. K. Atkin (Eds.), *Public communication campaigns* (pp. 67–86). Newbury Park, CA: Sage.

Devore, W., & Schlesinger, E. (1991). *Ethnic-sensitive social work practice.* New York: Macmillan Publishing.

Dillard, M., Andonian, L., Flores, O., Lai, L., MacRae, A., & Shakir, M. (1992). Culturally competent occupational therapy in a diversely populated mental health setting. *The American Journal of Occupational Therapy, 46*(8), 721–726.

Eisenberg, L. (1977). Disease and illness: Distinctions between professional and popular ideas of sickness. *Culture, Medicine, and Psychiatry, 1,* 9–23.

———. (1980). What makes persons patients and patients well? *American Journal of Medicine, 69*(2), 277–286.

Fabrega, H. (1974). *Disease and social behavior: An interdisciplinary perspective.* Cambridge, MA: The MIT Press.

Friedson, E. (1961). *Patient's view of medical practice.* New York: Russell Sage.

Gallegos, J. S. (1982). Planning and administering services for minority groups. In M. Austin & W. Hersey (Eds.), *Handbook of mental health administration: The middle manager's perspective* (pp. 87–105). San Francisco: Jossey-Bass.

Garro, L. Y. (1982). The ethnography of health care decisions. *Social Science & Medicine, 16*(16), 1451–1452.

Gillick, M. R. (1985). Commonsense models of health and disease. *New England Journal of Medicine, 313*(11), 700–703.

Good, B. (1977). The heart of what's the matter: The semantics of illness in Iran. *Culture, Medicine, & Psychiatry, 1,* 25–58.

Good. B., & Good, M. J. (1981). The meaning of symptoms: A cultural hermeneutic model for cultural practice. In L. Eisenberg & A. Kleinman (Eds.), *The relevance of social science for medicine* (pp. 275–295). Boston: D. Reidel.

Harwood, A. (1981). *Ethnicity and medical care.* Cambridge, MA: Harvard University Press.

Helman, C. (1984). *Culture, health, and illness: An introduction for health professionals.* Boston: Wright.

Holzberg, C. S. (1982). Ethnicity and aging: Anthropological perspectives on more than just the minority elderly. *The Gerontologist, 22*(3), 249–257.

Hutchinson, I. (1989). *Strategies for working with culturally diverse communities and clients.* Bethesda, MD: The Association for the Care of Children's Health, Maternal and Child Health Bureau.

Kleinman, A. (1978). Clinical relevance of anthropological and cross-cultural research: Concepts and strategies. *American Journal of Psychiatry, 135*(4), 427–431.

———. (1980). *Patients and healers in the context of culture.* Berkeley: University of California Press.

———. (1986). Concepts & a model for the comparison of medical systems as cultural systems. In C. Currer & M. Stacy (Eds.), *Concepts of health, illness, & disease: A comparative perspective* (pp. 29–47). New York: Berg.

————. (1988). *The illness narratives: Suffering, healing, and the human condition.* New York: Basic Books, Inc.

Leininger, M. (1978). *Transcultural nursing: Concepts, theories, and practices.* New York: Wiley.

Lewis, M. C. (1988). Attribution and illness. *Journal of Psychosocial Nursing, 26*(4), 14–21.

Lyons, J. (1972). Methods of successful communication with the disadvantaged. In National Academy of Science, *Communication for change with the rural disadvantaged* (pp. 78–83). Washington, DC: Author.

Madrid, A. (1988). Diversity and its discontents. *Black Issues in Higher Education, 5*(4), 10–18.

May, J. (1992). Working with diverse families: Building culturally competent systems of health care delivery. *The Journal of Rheumatology, 19*(33), 46–48.

McManus, M. (1988). Services to minority populations: What does it mean to be a culturally competent professional? *Focal Point: The Bulletin of the Research and Training Center to Improve Services for Seriously Emotionally Handicapped Children and Their Families, 2*(4), 1–17.

Mechanic, D. (1979). Correlates of physician utilization: Why do major multivariate studies of physician utilization find trivial psychosocial and organizational effects? *Journal of Health and Social Behavior, 20,* 387–396.

Mechanic, D. (1986). The concept of illness behavior: Culture, situation, and personal predisposition. *Psychological Medicine, 16*(1), 1–7.

Mechanic, D. (Ed.). (1982). *Symptoms, illness behavior, and help seeking.* New York: Prodist.

Moore, J. (1971). Situational factors affecting minority aging. *The Gerontologist, 11,* 11–93.

Munet-Vilaro, F. (1988). The challenge of cross-cultural nursing research. *Western Journal of Nursing Research, 10*(1), 112–115.

Press, I. (1980). Problems in the definition and classification of medical systems. *Social Science & Medicine, 14B,* 45–57.

Randall-David, E. (1989). *Strategies for working with culturally diverse communities and clients.* Bethesda, MD: The Association for the Care of Children's Health.

Roberson, M. (1987). Folk health beliefs of health professionals. *Western Journal of Nursing Research, 9*(2), 257–263.

Roberts, S. J. (1988). Social support and help seeking: Review of the literature. *Advanced in Nursing Science, 10*(2), 1–11.

Roberts, R. (1990). *Developing culturally competent programs for families of children with special needs.* Washington, DC: Georgetown University Child Development Center, Maternal and Child Health Bureau.

Royce, A. P. (1982). *Ethnic Identity: Strategies of diversity.* Bloomington, IN: Indiana University.

Rubel, A. J. (1977). The epidemiology of a folk illness: Susto in hispanic America. In D. Landy (Ed.), *Culture, disease, and healing: Studied in medical anthropology* (pp. 119–128). New York: Macmillan.

Rundall, T. G. (1981). A suggestion for improving the behavioral model of physician utilization. *Journal of Health and Social Behavior, 22,* 103–104.

Sharp, K., Ross, C. E., & Cockerham, W. C. (1983). Symptoms, beliefs, and the use of physician services among the disadvantaged. *Journal of Health and Social Behavior, 24*(1), 255–263.

Theiderman, S. (1988). Workshops in cross-cultural health care: The challenge of ethnographic dynamite. *Journal of Continuing Education in Nursing, 19*(1), 25–31.

Tripp-Reimer, T. (1982). Barriers to health care: Variations in interpretation of Appalachian client behavior by Appalachian and non-Appalachian health professionals. *Western Journal of Nursing Research, 4*(2), 179–191.

Weidman, H. (1980). Comments on clinical anthropology. *Medical Anthropology Newsletter, 12,* 16–17.

Weiss, M. G. (1988). Cultural models of diarrheal illness: Conceptual framework and review. *Social Science & Medicine, 27*(1), 5–16.

Whall, A. (1987). Commentary. *Western Journal of Nursing Research, 9*(2), 237–239.

White, G. M. (1982). The role of cultural explanations in somatization and psychologization. *Social Science & Medicine, 16,* 1519–1530.

Wirth, L. (1945). The problem of minority groups. In R. Linton (Ed.), *The science of man in the world crisis* (p. 347). New York: Columbia University Press.

Wood, J. B. (1989). Communicating with older adults in health care settings: Cultural and ethnic considerations. *Educational Gerontology, 15,* 351–362.

Young, A. (1982). The anthropology of illness and sickness. *Annual Review of Anthropology, 11,* 257–285.

Zola, I. (1966). Culture and symptoms: An analysis of patient's presenting complaints. *American Sociological Review, 31,* 615–630.

———. (1972). Studying the decision to see the doctor. *Advances in Psychosomatic Medicine, 8,* 216–236.

———. (1973). Pathway to the doctor—from person to patient. *Social Science & Medicine, 7,* 677–689.

Part II

The Process of Community as Partner

6

A Model to Guide Practice

Objectives

Models that serve as guides for nursing practice, education, and research have
become important tools for community health nurses. This chapter, in which we
begin our examination of the nursing process as applied to the community as
partner, focuses on the use of one nursing model to guide practice. After completing this chapter, you should be able to

- Define *model* and *nursing model*
- Describe the purposes of a nursing model
- Begin to use a nursing model in practice

Introduction

Although nursing models have been in existence since the beginnings of
the profession, it was not until the 1960s that they were systematically
identified, studied, and explicitly applied to practice. Boundaries are
needed to define areas of concern for nursing, and a conceptual "map"
of the nursing process is a necessary guide for action. This is particularly
true when the nursing practice focuses on the entire community. The
community-as-partner *model* provides us with both the map and the
boundaries and will be used throughout this part.

Models

A conceptual model is the synthesis of a set of concepts and the statements
that integrate those concepts into a whole. A *nursing model* can be defined

as a frame of reference, a way of looking at nursing, or an image of what nursing encompasses. A nursing model is a representation of nursing, not a reality. Other types of models that are used to represent realities are model airplanes, blueprints, chemical equations, and anatomic models.

A model with which nurses identified for many years was the medical model, that is, a disease-oriented, illness- and organ-focused approach to patients, with an emphasis on pathology. However, reliance on the medical model excludes health promotion and the holistic focus that is central to nursing. Additionally, important aspects of care, such as psychological, sociocultural, and spiritual areas, are not included in the medical model. Thus, a nursing model should encompass all aspects of health care needs and incorporate long-range goals and planning.

As a representation of reality, a model can take numerous forms. Because they *describe* nursing, all nursing models are narrative; that is, words are the symbols that are used by nurses to define how they view their practice. And although all nursing models are described in words, many are clarified further through the use of diagrams or illustrations. The use of such images allows the model-builder to show relationships and linkages among the concepts in the model. Diagrams are an efficient and effective way of depicting nursing models. The diagram is often thought of as the model itself, with accompanying text then seen as the elaboration or explanation of the model.

The method chosen to depict a nursing model reflects the model builder's own philosophy and preference; no one method is accepted as the best. There are, however, certain components that must be included in any model of nursing. Table 6-1 presents these essential elements.

There is general agreement that four concepts are central to the discipline of nursing: *person, environment, health,* and *nursing. (Concepts* are defined as general notions or ideas and are considered to be the building blocks of models.) How each of the four concepts is defined will both dictate the organization of the model and be illustrated in that model. For example, health may be defined on a continuum with wellness at one end and death at the other, as a dicholomy wherein one is seen as well or ill, as the outcome of numerous biopsychosocial and spiritual forces, or as the interaction of these same forces. In the medical model, *health* has been defined traditionally as the absence of disease. Figure 6-1 depicts four ways to view health and illustrates these definitions. Notice that the diagrams vary widely, reflecting the fundamental differences among these views of health.

TABLE 6-1 *Essential Units of a Nursing Model*	
Essential Unit	**Description of Unit**
A goal of action	The mission or ideal goal of the profession expressed as the end product desired (a state, condition, or situation).
A descriptive term for the patient population	That concept that best isolates who or what is acted upon to achieve a goal, that is, those aspects of the person (as patient) or the organization or those aspects of their functioning toward which attention is to be directed; the target of action.
The actor's role	A descriptive label that indicates the nature of the nurse's (the actor's) actions on patients.
Source of difficulty	The origin of deviations from the desired state or condition.
Intervention focus	The kind of problems found when deviations from the desired state occur; the kinds of disturbances in patients that are to be prevented or treated. Mode is the major means of preventing or treating such problems (the kinds of levers that can be used to change the course of events toward the desired end).
Consequences intended	Outcomes of action that are desired, stated in more abstract or broader terms than the mission or including significant corollaries of the intended outcomes. Unintended outcomes may follow and may or may not be desirable.

(Data from Riehl, J.P., & Roy, C. 1980. Conceptual models for nursing practice (2nd ed.), p. 2. New York: Appleton Century-Crofts; from unpublished lecture notes of D. Johnson, UCLA, Fall 1975.)

What, then, are the uses of a model of nursing? Think for a moment of what a nursing model is to you—and how a model might be useful in your practice. Although you may not have formulated your own model of nursing, you have been influenced greatly in your education by the model or models upon which your nursing curriculum is based. Does your faculty subscribe to one particular nursing model? Just as the choice of a model creates a basis for curriculum planning and decisions, a model can also provide a basis for practice.

What is nursing to you? If you can express an answer to that question, you have begun to describe your model of nursing. A nursing model serves the following purposes:

- A map for the nursing process
  —Gives direction for assessment (What do you assess?)
  —Guides analysis
  —Dictates nursing diagnoses
  —Assists in planning
  —Facilitates evaluation

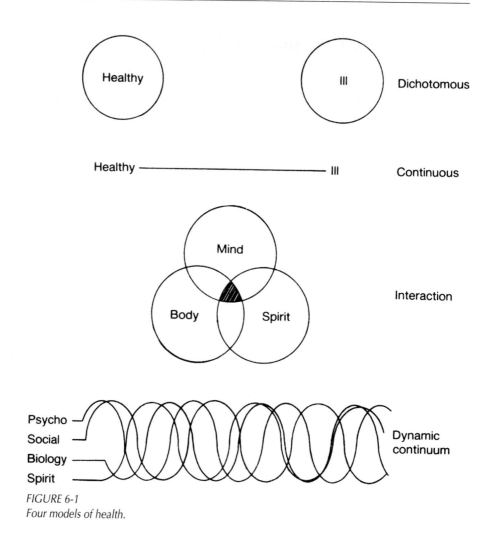

FIGURE 6-1
Four models of health.

- Provides a curriculum outline for education
- Represents a framework for research
- Provides a basis for development of theory

A model is nothing more—or less—than an explication of nursing. A model not only describes what *is* but also provides a framework for making decisions about what *could be*.

Community-as-Partner Model

Based on Betty Neuman's model of a total-person approach to viewing patient problems (1972), the *community-as-client model* was developed by the authors to illustrate the definition of public health nursing as the synthesis of public health and nursing. The model has been renamed the *community-as-partner model* to emphasize the underlying philosophy of primary health care.

Consider the community-as-partner model (Figure 6-2). There are two central factors in this model: a focus on the *community* as partner (represented by the community assessment wheel at the top, which incorporates the community's people as the core) and the use of the *nursing process*. The model is described in some detail to assist you in understanding its parts so that you may use it as a guide to your practice in the community. Refer now to Figure 6-3 for the following discussion.

The *core* of the assessment wheel represents the *people* that make up the community. Included in the core are the *demographics* of the population as well as their *values, beliefs,* and *history.* As residents of the community, the people are affected by and, in turn, influence the eight subsystems of the community. These subsystems are physical environment, education, safety and transportation, politics and government, health and social services, communication, economics, and recreation.

The solid line surrounding the community represents its *normal line of defense,* or the *level of health* the community has reached over time. The normal line of defense may include characteristics such as a high rate of immunity, low infant mortality, or middle-class income level. The normal line of defense also includes usual patterns of coping, along with problem-solving capabilities; it represents the *health* of the community.

The *flexible line of defense,* depicted as a broken line around the community and its normal line of defense, is a "buffer zone" representing a dynamic level of health resulting from a temporary response to stressors. This temporary response may be neighborhood mobilization against an environmental stressor such as flooding or a social stressor such as an unwanted "adult" bookstore. The eight subsystems are divided by broken lines to remind us that they are not discrete and separate but influence (and are influenced by) one another. (Remember that one of the principles of ecology is that everything is connected to everything else. This also applies to the community as a whole.) The eight

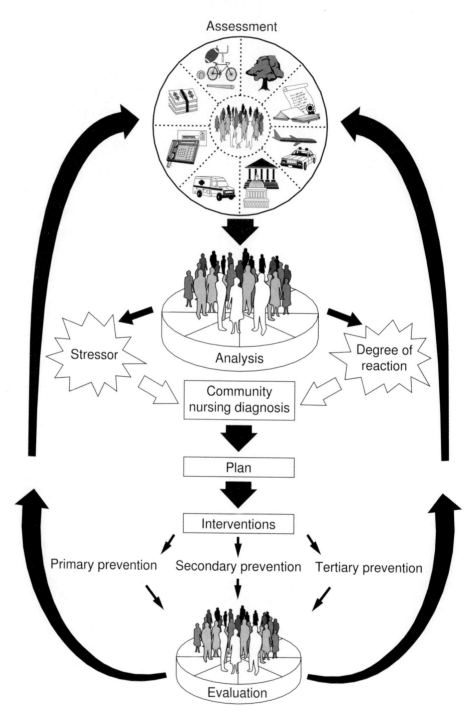

FIGURE 6-2
Community-as-partner model.

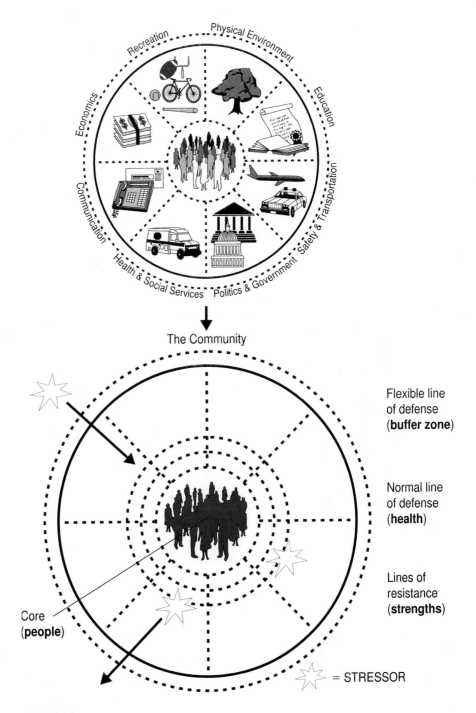

The Community

Flexible line
of defense
(**buffer zone**)

Normal line
of defense
(**health**)

Lines of
resistance
(**strengths**)

Core
(**people**)

= STRESSOR

FIGURE 6-3
The community assessment wheel, featuring lines of resistance and defense within the community structure.

divisions both define the major subsystems of a community and provide the community health nurse with a framework for assessment.

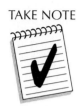

TAKE NOTE   *Take a moment to examine the selection of subsystems that have been identi-fied. Can you think of any that have been omitted? Think of the community where you live—what examples of each susbystem can you identify?*

Within the community are *lines of resistance,* internal mechanisms that act to defend against stressors. An evening recreational program for young people implemented to decrease vandalism and a free-standing, no-fee health clinic to diagnose and treat sexually transmitted diseases are examples of lines of resistance. Lines of resistance exist throughout each of the subsystems and represent the community's *strengths.*

Stressors are tension-producing stimuli that have the *potential* of causing disequilibrium in the system. They may originate outside of the community (for example, air pollution from a nearby industry) or inside the community (the closing of a clinic). Stressors penetrate the flexible and normal lines of defense, resulting in disruption of the community. Inadequate, inaccessible, or unaffordable services are stressors on the health of the community.

The *degree of reaction* is the amount of disequilibrium or disruption that results from stressors impinging on the community's lines of defense. The degree of reaction may be reflected in mortality and mor-bidity rates, unemployment, or crime statistics, to name a few examples.

TAKE NOTE   *The outcome of a stressor impinging on a community is not always negative. Often it is positive. For example, in the face of a crisis, people may band together and develop a community group to deal with the crisis. This group may continue to function after the crisis is over—strengthening the community and continuing to contribute to its "health."*

Assessment

The community's core and subsystems, its lines of defense and resis-tance, its stressors, and its degree of reaction comprise assessment para-meters for the community worker who views the *community as partner.* Analyzing data on these parameters *with the community* leads to the *community nursing diagnosis.* Note the similarities and differences between a nursing diagnosis of an individual and a community nursing diagnosis depicted in Table 6-2.

TAKE NOTE

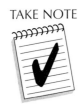

The term community health diagnosis *is preferred over community* nursing *diagnosis for three reasons: It is holistic and does not imply that only a nurse can address the identified problem, it underscores that work in the community is* by nature *inter- and intradisciplinary (not even confined to* health *professions but incorporating many others), and it places the emphasis once again on the* community, *which is the focus of our practice.*

Diagnosis and Planning

The community health diagnosis gives *direction* to both nursing's goals and its interventions. The goal is derived from the stressors and may include the elimination or alleviation of the stressor or strengthening of the community's resistance through strengthening the lines of defense. By stating the degree of reaction, the nurse can plan interventions to strengthen the lines of resistance through one of the prevention modes.

TABLE 6-2   Nursing Diagnosis: Comparison of Individual and Community Focus

Response	System/ Function	Source of Situation	Manifestation of Problem
Individual			
Patient behavior	Biopsychosocial-spiritual	Etiology	Symptoms from head-to-toe assessment
Example: Alteration in status	Oral integrity	Loose-fitting dentures	Oral pain; redness in mucosa; 10-cm open sore, and so on
Community			
Degree of reaction	Community subsystem	Stressor	Systems assessment (for example, rates)
Example: Increased	Respiratory disease	Air pollution	Increased hospital admissions for respiratory problems; higher rate of chronic obstructive pulmonary disease readmissions

Intervention

Primary prevention is the nursing intervention that aims at strengthening the lines of defense so that stressors cannot penetrate to cause a reaction or at interfering with a stressor by taking action against it. An example of primary prevention is the immunization of preschoolers to increase the percentage of immunized children in the community. *Secondary prevention* is applied after a stressor has penetrated the community. Interventions support the lines of defense and resistance to minimize the degree of reaction to the stressor. Conducting a breast cancer screening (breast self-exam and mammography) and referral program is an example of secondary prevention. Such a program is aimed at early *case finding* to reduce the degree of reaction (such as the severity of the cancer when found). *Tertiary prevention* is applied after the stressor penetrates and a degree of reaction has taken place. There has been system disequilibrium, and tertiary prevention is aimed at preventing additional disequilibrium and promoting equilibrium. For example, a school fire has occurred, and a large number of children are suffering from shock (physical and emotional). Teams of specialists (including community health nurses) are brought in to provide appropriate therapies and long-term follow-up as needed to reestablish equilibrium in the community and prevent additional problems in the children.

TAKE NOTE

In the school fire example, both tertiary and primary prevention are illustrated—tertiary, by providing appropriate therapy to prevent further trauma to the children due to this fire, and primary, by strengthening the children's coping mechanisms should another traumatic event occur in the future.

Evaluation

Feedback from the community provides the basis for evaluation of the community health nurses's interventions just as involvement of community persons in all steps of the nursing process ensures relevance to the community. Often the parameters that were used for assessment are also used for evaluation. For example, after the immunization program, did the percentage of immunized preschoolers increase? How many persons with breast lumps were identified and referred for medical care? What was the long-term effect of the school fire? Were the children reassimilated into their classes? Were fire codes investigated? Were additional precautions (increased fire drills, replacement of flammable materials) instituted in the schools? Such is the process of working with the community as partner. Interconnections, overlap, and interdisciplinary considerations are the rule rather than the exception.

Summary of the Model and Its Use

Consider the community-as-partner model (Figure 6-2) once more. The *goal* represented by the model is system equilibrium, a healthy community, and includes the preservation and promotion of community health.

TAKE NOTE

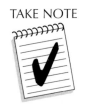

Health may not be a primary goal of the community (although it may be that of the community health nurse). It is, however, an important resource for the community to meet its goals. Realizing that we do not always share the same goals is important for anyone working in the community and must at least be considered (if not reconciled) as we plan, implement, and evaluate programs aimed at improving health.

The model's *target* (patient, in individual-focused practice) is the total community, the aggregate, and as such includes individuals and families. The nurse's *role* is to assist the community to attain, regain, maintain, and promote health; that is, to act as a facilitator, catalyst, and advocate for health so that the community is empowered to regulate and control its responses to stressors that are the source of difficulty. The *intervention focus* is the actual or potential disequilibrium or an inability of the community to function. The *intervention mode* is comprised of the three levels of prevention: primary, secondary, and tertiary. The *consequences intended* in this model include a strengthened normal line of defense, increased resistance to stressors, and a diminished degree of reaction to stressors by the community. Congruent with the principles of primary health care, it is the *community's competence* to deal with its own problems, strengthen its own lines of defense, and resist stressors that dictates the inverventions. Let us now begin the process.

BIBLIOGRAPHY

Neuman, B.N. (1972). A model for teaching total person approach to patient problems. *Nursing Research, 21*(3), 264–269.

SUGGESTED READINGS

Barnum, B.J.S. (1994). *Nursing theory: Analysis, application, evaluation*. Philadelphia: J. B. Lippincott.

Chinn, P.K. & Kramer, M.K. (1991) *Theory and nursing: A systematic approach*. St. Louis: C. V. Mosby.

Hawkins, J.W., Thibodeau, J.A., Utley-Smith, Q.E., Igou, J.F., & Johnson, E.E. (1993). Using a conceptual model for practice in a nursing wellness centre for seniors. *Perspectives, 17*(4), 11–16.

Nicoll, L.H. (1992). *Perspectives on nursing theory*. Philadelphia: J. B. Lippincott.

7

Community Assessment

Objectives

Preceding chapters have focused on foundational concepts such as primary health care, epidemiology, ecology, culture, and ethics. A community-focused model was introduced in Chapter 6 to guide you in the nursing process. This chapter and the four that follow focus on the *application* of the nursing process to the community. Consequently, the objectives are practice oriented. After studying this chapter, you will be able to complete a community health assessment using a nursing model.

Introduction

Assessment is the act of becoming acquainted with a community. To direct the assessment process, the community-as-partner model is used (see Figure 6-2). Recall that a system is a whole that functions because of the interdependence of its parts. A community, too, is a whole entity that functions because of the interdependence of its parts, or *subsystems*. The community assessment wheel (Figure 7-1) identifies the eight community subsystems and the community core. The community of Rosemont will be used to illustrate the use of the model in conducting a community assessment (and subsequent analysis, diagnosis, planning, intervention, and evaluation). Although we have chosen an urban community defined by census tracts (CT), the assessment wheel can be used

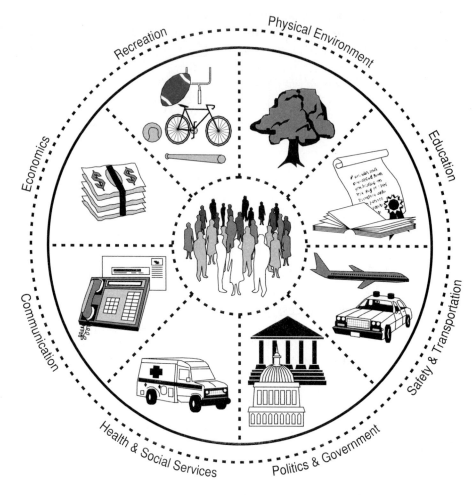

FIGURE 7-1
The community assessment wheel, the assessment segment of the commmunity-as-partner model.

as a guide to assess any community regardless of size, location, resources, or population characteristics. It can also be used to assess a "community within a community" (for example, a specific school, industry, or business); this will be illustrated in Part III, where we provide a variety of examples of the community-as-partner concept. The *process* of assessment, regardless of where it is applied, always remains the same.

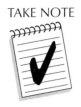

TAKE NOTE

Community assessments are not done in a vacuum. You are probably already familiar with some aspects of the community by virtue of your involvement in caring for people who reside there, perhaps in a clinic or a nearby hospital. In addition, this is not a solo job; many people will contribute to the assessment, so try not to get discouraged by the seeming enormousness of the task. Tackle it in increments.

Community Assessments

Looking to our community assessment wheel for guidance, we find eight subsystems surrounding the community core; therefore, we will first assess the core and then proceed to assess each subsystem. To facilitate the work of data collection, a "guide table" has been presented with each subsystem. Some information on these tables may not be available in your community, may not apply, or may be redundant. You may decide to include other information, omitted from the areas suggested in the tables, for your community. This is to be expected, for every community is a unique and special entity. It is this uniqueness that we seek to record.

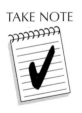

TAKE NOTE

It may be that in your community health nursing course, time limitations will not permit each student to complete an entire community assessment. Therefore, teams of students may be assigned to assess one or two community subsystems. At the end of the course, each team will present its assessment, and the total community assessment is thus completed. A similar situation frequently arises in agencies when health care providers, who are frequently from a variety of disciplines, are assigned one aspect (one subsystem) of a community to assess; later, all the subsystems are assembled, and the assessment is completed.

Assessment is a skill that is refined through practice. Everyone feels awkward and unsure as they begin (remember the first time you took a blood pressure?); this is normal. The first step is always the most difficult. It is time to take the first step.

Community Core

The definition of *core* is "that which is essential, basic, and enduring." The core of a community is its people—their history, characteristics, values, and beliefs. The first stage of assessing a community, then, is to learn about its people. Table 7-1 is a guide that lists the major components of the community core along with locations and sources of information about each component. Because every community is different, information sources available to one community may not be available to another. The text that follows presents core information about Rosemont.

TABLE 7-1   Community Core Data

Components	Sources of Information
History	Library, Historical Society
Demographics	Census of Population and Housing
Age and sex	Planning board (local, city, county, state)
characteristics	Chamber of commerce
Racial distribution	City Hall, City Secretary archives
Ethnic distribution	
Household types by	
Family	
Nonfamily	
Group	
Marital status by	
Single	
Separated	
Widowed	
Divorces	
Vital statistics	State Department of Health (Information
Births	distributed through city and county
Deaths by	health department)
Age	
Leading causes	
Values/beliefs/religion	Personal contact
	Windshield survey (To protect against
	stereotyping, avoid the library for this
	portion of the assessment)

The History of Rosemont

Rosemont includes CT 402 and CT 403. The Rosemont property was originally deeded to a Miss Ima Smith, who received a land grant of 3370 acres in 1827. For almost 100 years, the area remained as prairie, dotted with cattle ranches and small farms. In 1920, John Walker and William Bell formed a land corporation and began developing the Smith property. The first area that was improved and deed restricted was named Rosemont after a legendary town in Scotland. Following development, Rosemont prospered and attracted newcomers to the area. Numerous prominent families made their homes in Rosemont, including a state governor, a Nobel laureate, and a president of the United States. However, during the economic depression of the 1930s and the years before and during World War II, a drastic decrease in building activities occurred. Many stately homes deteriorated and either became multifamily dwellings or were left to decay. Eventually economic forces succeeded in breaking deed restrictions, and residential areas were forced to accept the introduction of industry and small businesses. As a result, property values plummeted, leaving quaint boutiques and antique shops to exist alongside an increasing number of night clubs and nude-modeling studios.

From 1950 to 1970, Rosemont witnessed the influx of a large population of young adults, commonly referred to as "hippies," who used the large, spacious homes for group living. This practice was also taken up by drug addicts and runaways. Rosemont gradually assumed the reputation of tolerating nontraditional lifestyles—a factor that precipitated the more recent influx of a large population of male homosexuals.

Because of lower property values and affordable rent during the mid to late 1970s, large groups of Vietnamese and Mexicans settled in Rosemont. Simultaneously, established families and single professionals, weary of the lengthy commute from suburbia to the inner city, began returning to Rosemont—a trend that still continues today. Today, older homes are being refurbished, businesses are being revitalized, and pride, once lost, is being reclaimed.

Demographics—The People of Rosemont

Tables 7-2 and 7-3 set forth age, sex, race, and ethnicity data for CT 402 and CT 403 as well as for the nearest city and county. (The census lists only numbers of persons; you must calculate percentages.) Tables 7-4 and 7-5 list data on family types and marital status.

TABLE 7-2   Population Age and Sex Characteristics for CT 402, CT 403, Hampton, and Jefferson County

AGE (YEARS)	CT 402			CT 403			Hampton		Jefferson County	
	MALES	FEMALES	TOTAL %	MALES	FEMALES	TOTAL %	NUMBER	TOTAL %	NUMBER	TOTAL %
Under 5 yr	370	362	10.6	29	11	0.6	123,150	7.8	189,246	8.4
5–19	1,200	991	31.9	241	195	6.5	377,345	23.9	569,991	25.3
30–34	395	437	12.2	1,965	911	42.6	514,705	32.6	716,431	31.8
35–54	837	970	26.2	1,758	721	36.7	339,453	21.5	484,380	21.5
55–64	222	370	8.6	221	181	5.9	116,835	7.4	157,705	7
65 and over	270	450	10.5	175	349	7.7	107,361	6.8	135,176	6
Total	3,294	3,580	100	4,389	2,368	100	1,578,849	100	2,252,929	100

(Data from Census of Population and Housing, Selected Characteristics.)

TAKE NOTE

During the next step of the nursing process (in other words, analysis), you will need city and county population data; therefore, collect all needed data now.

TABLE 7-3   Population Race and Ethnic Distribution for CT 402, CT 403, City of Hampton, and Jefferson County

	CT 402		CT 403		Hampton		Jefferson County	
	NUMBER	TOTAL %	NUMBER	TOTAL %	NUMBER	TOTAL %	NUMBER	TOTAL %
White	852	12.4	5,871	88.5	970,489	61.5	1,562,091	69.4
Black	3,732	54.3	305	4.6	434,014	27.5	467,177	20.7
Asian/Pacific Islander	1,312	19.1	54	0.7	32,335	2.1	45,432	2
Hispanic	625	9.1	321	4.7	131,763	8.3	163,774	7.3
American Indian	242	3.5	38	0.6	3,203	0.2	4,923	0.2
Other	111	1.6	58	0.9	7,045	0.4	9,532	0.4
Total	6,874	100	6,757	100	1,578,849	100	2,252,929	100

(Data from Census of Population and Housing, Selected Characteristics.)

TABLE 7-4   Population by Family Types, CT 402 and CT 403

	CT 402		CT 403	
	NUMBER	TOTAL %	NUMBER	TOTAL %
Family	5706	83	2443	36.2
Nonfamily	1168	17	4103	60.7
Female-headed household	721		994	
Male-headed household	447		2189	
Group quarters			211	3.1
Total	6874	100	6757	100

(Data from Census of Population and Housing, Selected Characteristics.)

Vital Statistics

Table 7-6 lists birth and death vital statistics for CT 402 and CT 403 as well as for the city and county. Using a similar format, Table 7-7 lists the leading causes of death.

Values, Beliefs, and Religion

Part of the community core is the values, beliefs, and religious practices of the people. All ethnic and racial groups have values and beliefs that

TABLE 7-5   Persons 15 and Over by Sex and Marital Status, CT 402 and CT 403

MARITAL STATUS	CT 402			CT 403		
	MALE	FEMALE	TOTAL %	MALE	FEMALE	TOTAL %
Single	348	408	15.2	2418	1016	53.5
Married	1510	1498	60.1	796	768	24.4
Separated	120	245	7.2	113	72	2.8
Widowed	52	119	3.4	68	198	4.3
Divorced	294	407	14.1	572	397	15
Total	2324	2677	100	3967	2451	100

(Data from Census of Population and Housing, Selected Characteristics.)

TABLE 7-6   Selected Birth and Death Vital Statistics for CT 402, CT 403, Hampton, and Jefferson County

	CT 402	CT 403	Hampton	Jefferson County
Births	*210*	*117*	*30,726*	*56,865*
Deaths				
Infant deaths	7	2	372	698
Neonatal deaths	5	2	245	471
Fetal deaths	16	1	387	870
Total deaths	72	42	9,533	16,440

(Data from State Vital Statistics, Department of Health.)

interact with each community system to influence the people's health. Review the chapter on cultural competence for methods to help you understand these cultural elements of the community.

To validate the demographic data, a windshield survey (Table 7-8) is needed to establish the presence and geographic location of different racial and ethnic groups. It is during this phase—assessment of the physical system—that we step into the community to learn and experience the values, beliefs, and religious practices of the community.

Notice that Table 7-1 cautions against the use of the library for information about values, beliefs, and religious practices—the reason being that books and articles frequently offer broad generalizations to describe the practices of ethnic and racial groups (for example, the lifestyles of urban blacks) or discuss one practice of one ethnic group (like breast-feeding practices of Mexican-born hispanics). Each community is unique, with values, beliefs, and religious practices that are rooted in tradition and continue to evolve and exist because they meet the community's needs.

Physical Environment

Just as the physical examination is a critical component of assessing an individual patient, so it is in the assessment of a community. And just as the five senses of the clinician are called into play in the physical exam

TABLE 7-7   *Deaths by Selected Causes for CT 402, CT 403, Hampton, and Jefferson County*

CAUSE OF DEATH	CT 402		CT 403		Hampton		Jefferson County	
	NUMBER	TOTAL %	NUMBER	TOTAL %	NUMBER	TOTAL %	NUMBER	TOTAL %
Heart disease	16	22.2	10	23.8	3,186	33.4	5,932	36
Malignant neoplasms	17	23.6	11	26.1	2,078	21.8	3,972	24.2
Cerebrovascular	6	8.3	2	4.7	690	7.3	1,213	7.4
Accidents	4	5.6	4	9.5	585	6.2	932	5.7
Emphysema, asthma, bronchitis	0	0	0	0	79	0.8	115	0.7
Diseases of early infancy	7	9.7	1	2.4	248	2.6	501	3
Homicides	6	8.3	1	2.4	592	6.2	831	5.1
Cirrhosis of liver	0	0	1	2.4	163	1.7	253	1.5
Pneumonia	2	2.8	1	2.4	210	2.2	365	2.2
Suicides	3	4.2	1	2.4	195	2	234	1.4
Diabetes mellitus	0	0	2	4.8	139	1.4	305	1.8
Congenital anomalies	0	0	2	4.8	99	1	245	1.5
Nephritis and nephrosis	0	0	0	0	13	0.1	26	0.2
Tuberculosis	1	1.4	0	0	17	0.2	28	0.2
All other causes	10	13.9	6	14.3	1,239	13	1,488	9.1
Total deaths, all causes	72	100	42	100	9,533	100	16,440	100

(Data from Hampton Vital Statistics, City of Hampton Health Department.)

of a patient, so, too, are they needed at the community level. Table 7-9 provides the components of the physical examination, both of an individual and a community, and compares tools and sources of data for each.

Our partner, the Rosemont community, is located within the city of Hampton and is in Hampton's central business district. It is bounded by Way Drive on the west, Buff's Bayou on the north, Live Oak Boulevard on the south, and Hampton Street on the east. Figure 7-2 is a map of the

TABLE 7-8   *Windshield Survey Components*

Element	Description
Housing and zoning	What is the age of the houses? What is their architecture and of what materials are they constructed? Are all the neighborhood houses similar in age and architecture? How would you characterize the differences? Are they detached from or connected to others? Do they have space in front and behind? What is their general condition? Are there signs of disrepair—broken doors or windows, leaks, or missing locks? Is there central heating, modern plumbing, and air conditioning?
Open space	How much open space is there? What is the quality of the space—green parks or rubble-filled lots? What is the lot size of the houses? Are there lawns and flower boxes? Do you see trees on the pavements or a green island in the center of the street? Is the open space public or private? Used by whom?
Boundaries	What signs are there of where this neighborhood begins and ends? Are the boundaries natural—a river or a different terrain? physical—a highway or railroad? economic—difference in real estate or presence of industrial, commercial units along with residential units? Does the neighborhood have an identity, a name? Do you see it displayed? Are there unofficial names?
"Commons"	What are the neighborhood hangouts (e.g., schoolyard, candy store, bar, restaurant, park, or 24-hour drugstore)? For what groups, at what hours? Does the "commons" have a sense of "territoriality," or is it open to the stranger?
Transportation	How do people get in and out of the neighborhood? Do they drive cars, take a bus, bike, walk, and so on? Are the street and roads conducive to good transportation and also to community life? Is there a major highway near the neighborhood? Whom does it serve? How frequently is public transportation available?
Service centers	Do you see social agencies, clinics, recreation centers, and signs of activity at the schools? Are there offices of doctors and dentists? Palmists, spiritualists, and the like? Parks? Are they in use?
Stores	Where do residents shop? At shopping centers, or neighborhood stores? How do they travel to shop?
Street people	If you are traveling during the day, whom do you see on the street? An occasional housewife or a mother with a baby? Do you see anyone you would not expect? Teenagers? Unemployed males? Can you spot a welfare worker, an insurance collector, or a door-to-door salesman? Is the dress of those you see representative or unexpected? Along with people, what animals do you see? Stray cats, dogs, pedigreed pets, or "watchdogs"?
Signs of decay	Is this neighborhood on the way up or down? Is it "alive"? How would you decide? Do you see trash, abandoned cars, political posters, neighborhood meeting posters, real estate signs, abandoned houses, or mixed zoning usage?
Race	Are the residents all of the same race, or is the area integrated?
Ethnicity	Are there indices of ethnicity—food stores, churches, private schools, and information in a language other than English?
Religion	Of what religion are the residents? Do you see evidence of heterogeneity or homogeneity? What denomination are the churches? Do you see evidence of their use other than on Sunday mornings?
Health and morbidity	Do you see evidence of acute or of chronic diseases or conditions? Of accidents, communicable diseases, alcoholism, drug addiction, mental illness, and so on? How far is it to the nearest hospital? Clinic?
Politics	Do you see any political campaign posters? Is there a present headquarters? Do you see any evidence of a predominant party affiliation?
Media	Do you see outdoor TV antennas? What magazines and newspapers do residents read? Do you see *Forward Times, Hampton Post, Enquirer,* and *Readers' Digest* in the stores? What media seem most important to the residents? Radio or TV?

(Adapted from Terry Mizrahi Madison: School of Social Work, Virginia Commonwealth University.)

| | **Sources of Data** | |
COMPONENTS	*INDIVIDUAL*	*COMMUNITY*
Inspection	All senses	All senses
	Otoscope	Windshield survey
	Ophthalmoscope	Walk through community
Auscultation	Stethoscope	Listen to community sounds/residents
Vital signs	Thermometer	Observe climate, terrain, natural boundaries,
	Sphygmomanometer	and resources
		"Life" signs such as notices of community
		meetings; density
Systems review	Head-to-toe	Observe social systems, including housing,
		businesses, churches, and hangouts
Laboratory studies	Blood tests	Almanac; census data
	X-rays	Chamber of commerce planning studies and
	Scans, other tests	surveys

TABLE 7-9   Physical Examination Components and Sources of Data

Rosemont community. Using the windshield survey (see Table 7-8) as a guide, we step into the community.

Inspection

Rosemont Boulevard bisects the community and serves as a major north–south thoroughfare for residents traveling to or through the community. It is tree-lined and divided by a grassy median in sections. Many businesses, especially restaurants, are located along Rosemont Boulevard. Many of the restaurants are of the "specialty" type that serve quiche, sprout sandwiches, and herbal teas. Other businesses situated along the boulevard are gas stations, office buildings, art-supply stores, a veterinarian, small art galleries, a nursery, one Mexican *barbacoa* stand in a grocery store, florists, a bank, a pharmacy, and various shops specializing in leather goods, books, and handcrafted items. (See the Economics section of this chapter for a summary of business units.

The major east–west thoroughfare through Rosemont, Pecan Drive, is also lined with businesses and, with fewer trees, presents a more urban face. At the east end can be seen nude modeling studios, small restaurants specializing in various ethnic foods (Greek, Pakistani, Mexican, Vietnamese, and Indian, to name a few), and numerous small art shops. The Rosemont Health Center, which is discussed later in this

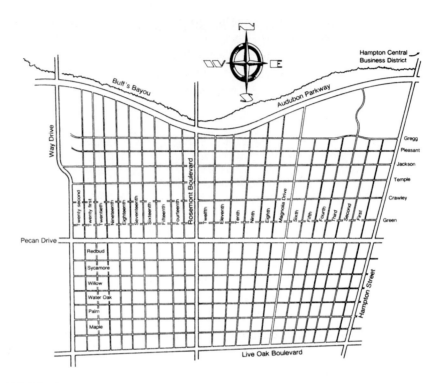

FIGURE 7-2
Rosemont Community.

chapter, is located in this area. Further west on this street is a large theater that attracts many first-run productions. There are a couple of "adult"
movie houses and the ubiquitous specialty restaurants (in this area they
are of the type that caters to the business or professional crowds—quiet
tea rooms that play classical music). Along this street, too, are many large
old houses, many of which have been converted into antique shops,
flower shops, and other small stores. There is no large industry in
Rosemont. Behind the two business-filled thoroughfares that divide the
community, Rosemont can give one the feeling of having entered a different world. The streets are narrower, and some are cobbled; old oaks
and pecan trees are abundant, and in many areas, the branches of the
trees meet over the streets to form protective canopies of green.

The streets (except the thoroughfares) are narrow, and most of
them have sidewalks, as is typical of older neighborhoods in Hampton.

In general, the streets and sidewalks are in good repair and free from debris; however, because there is little off-street parking, many residents park on the streets, so there is traffic congestion at the times when most residents are home (primarily nights and weekends).

Vital Signs

The climate of Rosemont (and the Hampton Standard Metropolitan Statistical Area [SMSA]) is mild and moderated by sea winds. Summers are hot (the temperature is 90°F or higher, approximately 87 days a year) and humid (averaging 62%), but evenings are cool, and there is rarely a hard freeze in the winter. Flora, both temperate and tropical, abounds—live oaks, hibiscus, and pines may grow in one block, for example.

The terrain is generally flat, with little variation in grade. It is 20 feet above sea level. The only naturally occurring water in the area is Buff's Bayou, a concrete-lined "river" that serves to carry off excess rain and drainage to reduce chances of flooding in Hampton. The bayou ends in the Hampton Channel, which leads to the sea.

Rosemont is the third most densely populated area in Hampton, with 14.4 persons per acre. An area in CT 402 that contains the subsidized housing complex is the most densely populated in all of Hampton, with 221 persons per acre (1980 Census).

The variety of local stores reflects the diversity of interests in Rosemont. Posters advertising a meeting of the Gay Political Caucus share bulletin-board space with senior citizens' meetings, church announcements, educational programs at the community college's "Sundry School," Vietnamese relocation services, the community's STD (sexually transmitted diseases) Clinic, and a musical show by "El Barrio" from the Mexican-American area. Rosemont is a community of rich diversity, a microcosm of Hampton.

The churches of Rosemont also reflect its diversity—virtually all denominations are represented. From the large Methodist and Presbyterian churches on its borders to the small storefront churches for refugees, Rosemont contains resources for all major religious groups.

Systems

Most of Rosemont is developed; there is little space not in use. Four small neighborhood parks, a narrow strip along the bayou, and the land

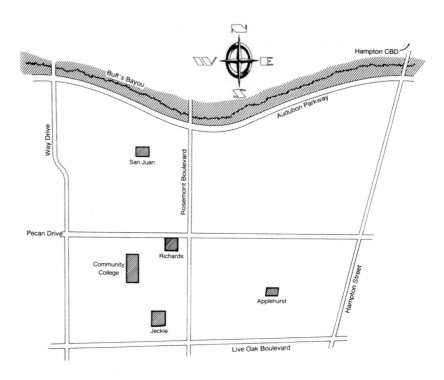

FIGURE 7-3
Rosemont Community Greens and Parks.

around the Community College are the "greens" available to the community (see Figure 7-3), although most houses have well-kept lawns with trees and shrubs. Table 7-10 presents land use data for Rosemont.

The majority of houses in Rosemont are old, reflecting the early development of the area. Within certain sections, the houses resemble each other (for example, all one-story, wood frame houses with porches); however, there may also be great heterogeneity from one block to the next. In the northeast quadrant is a large subsidized housing area comprised of run-down apartments with broken windows and poorly kept streets, whereas in the southwest quadrant are houses that have been well maintained and remodeled. Also in the northeast is an area covering several blocks of what are called "shotgun houses" (the story is told that one can shoot a shotgun from the front door, and the shot will go out the back door); placed side by side, they are tiny and poorly maintained. See Table 7-11 for housing information.

TABLE 7-10   Rosemont Land Use

	CT 402		CT 403	
LAND USE	**NUMBER OF ACRES**	**TOTAL %**	**NUMBER OF ACRES**	**TOTAL %**
Single family dwellings	161.2	28.03	95.4	31.78
Multifamily dwellings	46.4	8.06	46.5	15.49
Commercial	210.2	36.55	61.2	20.39
Industrial	44.9	7.8	0.2	0.06
Public	6.8	1.18	11.1	3.69
Open	52.9	9.2	53.2	17.72
Water	6.3	1.09	4.7	1.56
Undeveloped	46.3	8.05	14.6	4.86
Right-of-way	0	0	13.2	4.39
Total acres	575	100	300.1	100

(Data Book, Rosemont Community Development, City of Hampton. Planning Department.)

During the day, most of the people seen on the streets move quickly and purposefully as though on business or an errand. Those who could be described as "strolling" are elderly persons or young men, usually alone. Few children are seen during the day except in the school-yards, which are not on the main thoroughfares. Dogs are heard to bark as one walks through the neighborhoods, and cats sun themselves in windows; however, few pets run loose in the area.

At night, Rosemont assumes a different flavor along Pecan Drive: All the restaurants are open, and many have outdoor patios for serving. Smells of fajitas, curry, exotic spices, and charbroiling fill the air. "The

TABLE 7-11   Average Value of Housing and Rent for Years 1980 and 1990

	CT 403		CT 402		Hampton	
	1980	**1990**	**1980**	**1990**	**1980**	**1990**
Average value of housing	$58,432	$62,400	$25,777	$43,300	$49,630	$61,900
Average rent	$259/mo	$346/mo	$243/mo	$284/mo	$244/mo	$337/mo

(Data from Census of Population and Housing, Bureau of Census.)

Strip," as Pecan Drive is called, comes alive with sounds of disco, punk, and rock'n'roll, along with the stroking of a sitar or quiet strumming of a guitar.

Most of the clients in these restaurants and nude modeling "studios," according to residents, come from outside of Rosemont. Many are attracted by the food and some by the free-wheeling sex that is reputed to be available in the area.

Many of the residents express disdain for the Strip, calling it a "tourist attraction," and they feel that it is contributing to the deterioration of Rosemont. They state that "outsiders" and "cowboys" exploit and prey on unsuspecting tourists and that the unsavory reputation of the area is not the fault of the people who live there. An absence of zoning laws has facilitated the establishment of some of the less-than-desirable businesses in the area.

The physical examination of Rosemont reveals it to be a community of contrasts: churches and nude modeling studios, subsidized city housing units and restored homes from a more affluent time, old people and young, white and black (and all shades between), quiet tree-lined streets and busy thoroughfares, sedate tea rooms and garish adult movie theaters, families and singles, and the rich and poor.

Health and Social Services

One method of classifying health and social services is to differentiate between facilities located outside the community (*extracommunity*) versus those within the community (*intracommunity*). Once the health and social service facilities are identified, group them into categories, perhaps by type of service offered (for example, hospitals, clinics, extended care), by size, or by public versus private usage. Table 7-12 suggests a classification system as well as possible major components of each facility requiring assessment.

Extracommunity Health Facilities

Hospitals

Jefferson County has 50 hospitals with a total of 12,321 beds, of which 4,321 are in the Hampton Medical Center—a complex that includes all medical subspecialties as well as sophisticated diagnostic and treatment

TABLE 7-12   Health and Social Services

Component	Sources of Information
Health Services	
Extracommunity or intracommunity facilities. Once identified, group into categories (e.g., hospitals and clinics, home health care, extended care facilities, public health services, emergency care).	Chamber of commerce Planning board (county, city) Phone directory Talk to residents
For each facility, collect data on	Interview administrator or someone on the staff
1. Services (fees, hours, and new services planned and those discontinued)	Facility annual report
2. Resources (personnel, space, budget, and record system)	
3. Characteristics of users (geographic distribution, demographic profile and transportation source)	
4. Statistics (number of persons served daily, weekly, and monthly)	
5. Adequacy, accessibility, and acceptability of facility according to users and providers	
Social Services	
Extracommunity or intracommunity facilities. Once identified, group into categories (e.g., counseling and support, clothing, food, shelter, and special needs).	Chamber of commerce United Way directory Phone directory
For each facility, collect data on areas 1–5 listed above.	

services. The Medical Center is located seven miles from Rosemont. All patients admitted to the Medical Center must be referred by a physician; self-referral is not permitted. (*Self-referral* allows the individual independently to choose and acquire medical care.) Although existence of the Medical Center is common knowledge among Rosemont residents, few persons know anyone who has sought or received care there. Numerous private hospitals are located in Jefferson County, most being in Hampton. All private hospitals require third-party reimbursement for services rendered. (*Third-party reimbursement* means payment for services by an entity other than the patient. For example, Medicare, Medicaid, insurance, and workmen's compensation are third-party reimbursers.) In addition to private hospitals, most communities use tax revenues to support at least one hospital for the general public—in Jefferson County, the public hospital is Jefferson Memorial.

Jefferson Memorial is a full-service facility located five miles south of Rosemont. Care units and clinics at Memorial include medical, surgical, pediatrics, maternity, gynecology, trauma and burns, psychiatry, and emergency rooms. Persons can self-refer to Jefferson Memorial. According to the director of the emergency room (ER), 290 persons are seen daily in the ER (approximately 100,000 persons annually). Of these, some 40% are admitted. Follow-up care is provided by Memorial's outpatient clinics. Memorial is supported by city and county taxes as well as by fees collected for services. The base charge for an ER visit classified as minor is $85.20; a visit deemed major costs $274.40. Health care provider fees, as well as treatments and diagnostic services are in addition to the base fee. All fees are on a sliding scale according to income and family size. Rosemont residents use Memorial but complain of lengthy waits of up to eight hours and of having to undergo repeated assessments as they are moved from one health care provider to another. Hospital personnel recognize the lengthy waiting period and fragmentation of care, but they cite budget constraints and high staff turnover as major obstacles to improving care. No services have been discontinued at Memorial, and no new services or staff positions are budgeted for the next two years.

Private Care Providers, Group Practices, and Specialty Clinics

A full selection of general medical and specialty care is available in Jefferson County through private practitioners, group practices, and specialty clinics. Payment is usually third-party reimbursement. Two health maintenance organizations (HMOs) are located in Jefferson County. Rosemont residents with adequate finances use a variety of private practitioners and specialty clinics. The residents usually self-refer themselves following a favorable recommendation from a neighbor, friend, or work colleague.

Public Health Services: The Health Department

To monitor, maintain, and promote the public's health, each state has a state health department and accompanying regional, county, and sometimes city health departments. National, state, and local tax revenues are used to support public health services. There exists a Hampton Health Department as well as a Jefferson County Health Department. Because Rosemont is within the city limits of Hampton, the services of the Hampton Health Department are assessed.

   The Hampton Health Department offers all medical outpatient services through its seven satellite clinics. The Sunvalley Clinic, located six miles from Rosemont and closest to the area, provides the following services:

- Immunizations
- Well and ill infant, child, adolescent, and adult care
- Antepartum/postpartum care
- Family planning
- Nutrition counseling
- Screening and testing for genetic and acquired conditions such as sickle-cell anemia, diabetes, and phenylketonuria (PKU)
- Dental assessment, cleaning, and restoration
- Mental health counseling and referral
- Health education
- Maternal and infant home visitation following early hospital discharge (defined as earlier than 48 hours after dlivery)
- Child abuse, battered spouse, and abandoned person counseling and referral
- STD screening and follow-up (including HIV testing)

Additional services include a pharmacy, laboratory, and radiation department. Payment for most services is on a sliding scale; remaining services are free to all city residents. Free services include immunizations as well as screening and treatment for STDs. The majority of Rosemont residents who use the health department attend antepartum or postpartum clinics. The staff nurse in the maternity clinic estimates that of the 75 women seen in the prenatal clinic each week, 20 to 25 are Rosemont residents.

The major service-delivery problem cited by nurses in the maternity clinics is the long waiting period (frequently 8 to 10 weeks) between a woman's initial request for an appointment and the scheduled appointment date. Because many women wait until they are six or seven months pregnant to request antepartum care, the first available appointment time may be after the woman's expected delivery date. Consequently, a large number of women from Rosemont deliver at Jefferson Memorial having received no antepartum care. The administrator of the Sunvalley Clinic felt a top service priority to be additional education, support, and monitoring services for pregnant women and new mothers.

No services have been discontinued in the recent past. With regard to the question of services that are needed, the elderly were identified as a target group. Plans were underway to establish a nursing clinic for the elderly as well as a wellness program to be offered at day care for the elderly and at senior centers. There are presently more than 10 such facilities for seniors within the city of Hampton.

Numerous Rosemont residents use the health department services, especially the Sunvalley Clinic. Problems cited include lack of a direct bus connection to the clinic (presently, three bus transfers are required) and "impersonal" service. Because patients are not assigned to a primary care provider, it is customary for them to see a different health care provider at each visit. Maternity patients have an additional concern. Each woman must make her own delivery arrangements, and frequently women who qualify for antepartum care at Sunvalley Clinic do not meet eligibility requirements for delivery at Jefferson Memorial. Consequently, women must search for a facility that will admit them for labor and delivery. All too often, they are forced to deliver at home, a situation documented by Sunvalley nurses and confirmed by several Rosemont residents.

Home Health Agencies

The Visiting Nurses Association (VNA) of Hampton is the largest home health agency in Jefferson County. Services of the VNA include home health care by registered nurses, physical and occupational therapists, speech therapists, social workers, and home health aides. The VNA accepts paying clients and third-party reimbursements. Paying clients are charged on a sliding scale according to income and family size. Patients who are unable to pay a fee can request financial assistance from several community social service agencies such as the United Way.

Numerous other home health agencies are located in Hampton and Jefferson County. Although more limited in scope of service, all offer home health services and require fees or third-party reimbursement for payment.

Long-Term, Extended-Care, and Continuing-Care Facilities

There are two long-term facilities within eight miles of Rosemont: the Pinewoods Rest Center and the Windsail Nursing Home. Each facility is classified as an intermediate-care facility and is licensed by the State Department of Health. A profile of the services, resources, and characteristics of the residents for each facility is presented in Table 7-13. In addition, several hospitals offer extended-care services.

Emergency Services

The Poison Control Center provides information to individuals and health care providers on harmful substances and methods of assessment and treatment. The center provides educational materials and programs

TABLE 7-13   Services, Resources, and Resident Characteristics at Pinewoods Rest Center and Windsail Nursing Home During the Preceding Year

	Pinewoods Rest Center	Windsail Nursing Home
Services	Convalescent nursing care; physical, occupational, and speech therapy	Convalescent nursing care
Full-time personnel	Six RNs, four licensed visiting nurses (LVNs), three nurse aids, one administrator	Three RNs, two LVNs, one nurse aide, one administrator
Licensed bed capacity	96	38
Patient days	33,524	12,965
Occupancy rate	0.96	0.93
Certified bed capacity[*]	96	38
Median age of residents	79	76
Average duration of stay	Four years	Six years

[*]Recommended occupancy rate for nursing home beds is 90%.

(Jefferson County Planning Council, Pinewoods Rest Center, and Windsail Nursing record books.)

for schools and interested groups. Their easy-to-remember number is 1-POISON.

Medical Emergency Ambulance Service (MEAS) is financed by Hampton city taxes, public donations, Jefferson County contributions, and organized fund-raisers. The MEAS first-aid services are free and available 24 hours a day to all residents of Rosemont. (The MEAS operates in conjunction with the local fire stations. See the Safety and Transportation section of this chapter for a description of fire protection services.)

The MEAS closest to Rosemont has two ambulances; one is used daily, and the other serves as a backup. The MEAS averages 90 to 110 calls a month, with a response time of less than eight minutes. (Table 7-14 presents specific reasons for ambulance service to persons in Rosemont during the last three-month period.) Calls are received through the central fire department and dispatched by radio to the nearest MEAS team. Each MEAS team consists of 26 persons: 3 paramedics having completed 100 hours of classwork and 200 hours of hospital experience and 22 emergency medical technicians (EMTs) with basic paramedic training

TABLE 7-14   Reasons for MEAS to Persons in Rosemont During the Preceding Three-Month Period

Reason	Total %
Cardiac-related problems and cerebrovascular accidents	25
Falls and household accidents	19
Respiratory problems	12
Dizziness and weakness	12
Lacerations	11
Fractures and dislocations	9
Abdominal pain	7
Mental-psychiatric disorders	5

(MEAS paramedics records.)

and additional experience in intravenous therapy and intubation. Both paramedics and EMTs are certified. In addition to emergency service, the MEAS team offers CPR and first-aid classes to community groups.

Special Services

Frequently, special facilities exist to serve specific groups such as the handicapped or retarded. After surveying the immediate extracommunity area, no such facilities were located within a 10-mile radius of Rosemont.

Intracommunity Health Facilities

According to the Health Systems Agency (HSA) of Jefferson County, CT 402 is a medically underserved area; CT 403 is not.

The type and number of practitioners offering health services in Rosemont are listed in Table 7-15. A need for gynecological and obstetric services was frequently expressed by female residents. Numerous persons cited the need for family practitioners as well as bilingual health care providers. (One of the nurse practitioners listed in Table 7-15 speaks Spanish, but none speaks Vietnamese.) Rosemont residents with financial resources tend to select from extracommunity medical services; indigent residents rely on medical services within the community. All private practitioners require payment when services are rendered or third-party reimbursement; the nurse practitioners use a sliding scale to calculate fees. In addition to private practitioners, two clinics—the Third Street Clinic and the Rosemont Health Center—are located in Rosemont.

TABLE 7-15   *Practitioners in Rosemont*

Type	Number
Dentist	6
General medical	1
Optometrist	2
Orthodontist	1
Osteopath	2
Podiatrist	1
Chiropractor	3
Nurse Practitioner	2

(Windshield survey, chamber of commerce, and phone directory.)

Third Street Clinic.   The Third Street Clinic was founded in 1968 by concerned citizens and church leaders in Rosemont. The clinic, located in the center of CT 402, was initially financed by public donations and church-sponsored fund-raisers. All professional time and supplies were donated. Today the Third Street Clinic serves 30% to 40% of Rosemont residents and has an annual operating budget of $750,000, a reduction of $220,000 from two years ago. The majority of funds are from federal and state grants as well as from client fees and Medicare and Medicaid reimbursements. Although patients are charged according to a sliding scale, no one is denied care. Services provided at Third Street Clinic are summarized in Table 7-16. The clinic provides no acute or trauma care services. One part-time physician, two part-time nurses, one social worker, one administrator, and a clerk form the clinic's staff. Both nurses speak Spanish, but none of the staff speaks Vietnamese. Optometry students and supervising faculty provide services one day a week and one nurse midwife provides antepartum care two mornings a week. The clinic is open Monday through Friday, 8 A.M. to 5 P.M. On average, 125 people are seen weekly. Medical professionals and citizens form the board of directors. According to the clinic's director, immediate medical needs for the residents of CT 402 include the following:

- Ill infant, child, adolescent, and adult assessment, treatment, and follow-up
- Dental assessment and restoration

TABLE 7-16   Services and Number of People Served at Third Street Clinic

Service	Description	Patient Visits (Weekly Average)
Family planning	Physical exams, education, and prescriptions filled	24
Well child examinations	Physical assessment, referral for illness, immunizations, and screening	19
Antepartum and postpartum	Physical assessment and monitoring	42
Optometry	Eye exams and prescriptions filled	9
Podiatry	Assessment and treatment	6
Chronic disease counseling and treatment	Treatment and care instructions for hypertension, diabetes, and cardiovascular conditions	31

- Counseling, referral, and when possible, treatment for drug abuse and alcoholism
- Group health teaching, especially for pregnant women, parents of young children, and adolescents
- Wellness and self-care classes for all age groups
- Support groups for single parents and senior citizens

Presently there are no consistent health education or counseling services. Transportation services from area neighborhoods to the clinic, as well as dental and home nursing care, were discontinued two years ago following grant reductions. The major problem confronting the clinic is the recruitment of health care providers, especially nurses and physicians. Clinic services cannot be expanded (or maintained at the present level) unless additional health care providers are recruited and retained.

Most Rosemont residents are aware of the Third Street Clinic, and many use the clinic's services routinely. The major impediment to clinic use is the one- to two-mile walk to the clinic for many residents (there is no direct bus connection for most people). Rosemont residents feel welcomed at the clinic, and low staff turnover has fostered compliance with medical recommendations. Residents did, however, express a need for additional services at the clinic.

Rosemont Health Center. The Rosemont Health Center, centrally located in CT 403, is a nonprofit clinic devoted to the diagnosis and treatment of STDs (including HIV infection). The clinic is open Monday to Saturday, 6 P.M. to 10 P.M., and Sunday, 2 P.M. to 10 P.M. The center reports 20% of the syphilis cases and 60% of the gonorrhea cases in Jefferson County. Approximately 600 patient visits occur monthly (200 new cases, 200 repeat cases, and 200 follow-ups). All 75 professional staff members are volunteers and donate 4 to 10 hours of service a month. The director of the clinic is employed part-time. The state donates penicillin, tetanus cultures, and Venereal Disease Research Laboratory (VDRL) tests. Initially there were no fees for services—presently a fee of $10.00 per visit is assessed to defray costs of equipment, rent, and utilities. (However, no person is denied care.) Ninety percent of the patients are male homosexuals. Each patient is issued an identification number and card that is used with each visit. Persons in psychologic crisis are referred to the City Health Department for counseling. Most patients drive or walk to the clinic.

The director of the health center discussed the immediate need for expanded counseling and support groups, especially for persons who are HIV positive. A second need is for an orientation program and information update sessions for staff members, most of whom are former patients. The majority of patients are from the Rosemont area, although an increasing number of patients are commuting to the clinic from Hampton and surrounding Jefferson County. Patients surveyed in the waiting room rated the care as excellent; appointments are rarely cancelled by patients.

Observations at the clinic revealed a warm, caring atmosphere where people were treated with respect and were provided privacy when needed. In addition, however, were two open trash bags filled with syringes and attached needles and no visible emergency cart. There were no standard policy and procedure manuals and no posted protocol for an adverse treatment response (such as penicillin reaction) for the many volunteers who worked there.

Social Service Facilities

Because social service agencies are frequently located in office buildings, their location in the community may be difficult to determine during a windshield survey. It is preferable to use a directory such as the type compiled by the chamber of commerce or local planning board to begin identifying social service organizations relatively close to the community being assessed. If the community does not have a chamber of commerce, use the phone directory.

Extracommunity Social Service Facilities

Counseling and Support Services. The Hampton Comprehensive Counseling Center was founded in 1971 by concerned citizens of Hampton and Jefferson County for the purpose of providing counseling to adolescent drug users. Today the center offers a comprehensive mental health program for all residents of Hampton. The center is located two miles south of Rosemont. Although persons can self-refer to the center, most patients are referred from schools, clinics, and private practitioners. Fees are based on a sliding scale; third-party reimbursements are not accepted. Last year's operating budget was $200,000. The majority of revenues are from clients, although numerous churches and social service agencies sponsor individuals and families. The staff consists of six professionals and two clerks. Services are outlined in Table 7-17. An average of 300 patients are seen monthly. The director describes the patient population as white and middle to upper class, with more males than females. Most patients use private transportation to arrive at the

TABLE 7-17   Services Offered at the Hampton Comprehensive Counseling Center

Service	Description
Diagnosis	Screening procedure for the mentally handicapped; recommends services required for clients' needs
Information and referral	Liaison teams coordinate services with state schools for the mentally retarded and state hospitals for the mentally ill
Counseling and therapy	Group and play therapy provided
Alcohol and drug abuse services	Counseling services
Psychiatric evaluation and medical services	Psychiatric department provides evaluations and medications for clients
Emergency service	Handles crisis calls 24 hours/day, 7 days/week
Education and consultation	Center staff works with other community groups, including schools, police, and social service agencies, to solve local problems

(Hampton Comprehensive Counseling Center.)

clinic. No additional services are planned as the center staff feels they are adequately meeting the needs of the population. Rosemont residents queried were unaware of the existence of the counseling center, and no one knew of anyone having used the center, although all residents interviewed knew of several adolescent drug users.

The YMCA Youth Development Center borders Rosemont and offers a variety of educational and recreational programs. Adjacent to the "Y" is the YMCA Indo-Chinese Refugee Program, an agency that seeks to facilitate the resettlement of Asian immigrants. Major services include cultural orientation, job counseling and placement, and courses in English as a second language. The agency services have experienced a 200% increase in usage during the past three years. Presently, over 100 persons use the facility daily. Although all four staff members are bilingual, this is too small a staff to meet the needs of the Vietnamese community—a large proportion of which lives in Rosemont. The staff feels the immediate need is for counseling and therapy programs for alcohol and drug abuse as well as teaching basic survival skills (for example, finding a job, housing, and medical care). The staff estimates that 40% to 50% of the Asians using their services are from Rosemont. Asian residents in Rosemont agree that the "Y" is responsive to their needs, but when asked, they do acknowledge long waiting periods (sometimes weeks) for classes and counseling.

Clothing, Food, Shelter, and Basic Welfare Services.   Most churches and synagogues in the area have a food pantry, and many can arrange emergency shelter and provide clothing and essential transportation services. People are usually helped on a walk-in basis, but sometimes the church is referred to a family or individual in need. In Hampton a special organization, The Metropolitan Ministries, serves as an interfaith link between the religious communities of Hampton and community residents in need of social services. The Metropolitan Ministries acts to coordinate services, thereby avoiding duplication, and refers individuals to the program that can best meet their immediate needs.

TAKE NOTE

In most communities, churches must be contacted individually for a listing of services.

In addition to the churches and synagogues, numerous resale clothing shops are located in shopping areas close to Rosemont. Residents are very knowledgeable about available retail stores and actively promote preferred merchants.

The Jefferson County Welfare Department and the Hampton Welfare Department screen and process applicants for food stamps, housing subsidies, and financial aid checks. Each welfare department has a division of child protection that investigates reports of child abuse and neglect. The division provides casework services, foster home placement, and emergency shelter for women and children as well as parenting classes and child therapy groups. Welfare departments are financed by federal, state, and local tax revenues.

Special Services.   The United Way lists 42 private and public-supported social service agencies located in Hampton or Jefferson County. The United Way directory includes identifying information for each agency, plus services and fees. Agencies on the roster include the Society to Prevent Blindness, American Lung Association, March of Dimes, Woman's Center, Paralyzed Veterans Association, International Rescue Committee.

TAKE NOTE

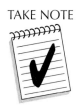

In your community assessment material, this would be an ideal location to append a list of social service agencies, along with identifying information (such as address, phone number, major services, and contact person). Brochures describing services, eligibility, and so on are useful to include as well.

Intracommunity

Two churches in Rosemont, South Main Methodist and Westpark Episcopal, have extensive social outreach programs including preschool and day care services; benevolence funds for food, clothing, and shelter; and numerous support groups (for example, parents without partners, singles, and solitaires). Westpark has a seniors center open 8 A.M. to 6 P.M. daily. The seniors enjoy a variety of recreational and educational programs and a hot noon meal. In addition, volunteers are enlisted to assist with shopping and errands, minor home repairs, light housekeeping, and meals for fellow seniors who are permanently or temporarily incapacitated. Noticeably absent from Westpark were any support groups or programs directed at the large male homosexual population. When asked about this, staff members responded that "that problem does not exist in this community." South Main does offer a coffee klatch on Friday night and plans to offer additional services to the male homosexual population, although there is strong resistance from the older parishioners.

On the north side of CT 403 is Lambda Alcoholics Anonymous (AA), a program specifically for homosexuals, a group originally not allowed to join Alcoholic Anonymous. Lambda AA in CT 403 is an active group, with the present participation exceeding 200. All socioeconomic groups are represented in the meetings, and members take turns leading the support groups.

Economics

The economic subsystem includes the "wealth" of Rosemont; that is, the goods and services available to the community as well as the costs and benefits of improving patterns of resource allocation. It should be evident that extracommunity factors such as the state of the U.S. and world economies affect in great measure the local economy. Nevertheless, intracommunity economic factors impinge upon all other subsystems, so they must be included in the assessment. Table 7-18 lists the suggested areas for studying a community's economy, along with sources of the data. The census data can be used to summarize most of these economic indicators.

Financial Characteristics of Households

The two census tracts that comprise the Rosemont community vary greatly in income characteristics. The census data show the median income for households in CT 402 to be $21,238, whereas in CT 403 it was $25,878. Table 7-19 lists the household income for the community and Hampton, comparing 1980 and 1990 figures.

Businesses

There are several high-rise office buildings located on the northern boundary of the area along the Audubon Parkway, including the National General Life Insurance complex of three towers, the new National Tower, the National Service Corporation, and the Second Mortgage Corporation's building. Way-on-the-Bayou, a new office complex, is also being constructed at the corner of Way Drive and Buff's Bayou. These buildings all feature spacious landscaped grounds, mod-

TABLE 7-18   Economic Indicators and Sources of Information

Indicators	Source
Financial Characteristics	
Households	
Median household income	
% households below poverty level	
% households receiving public assistance	Census records
% households headed by females	
Monthly costs for owner-occupied households and renter-occupied households	
Individuals	
Per capital income	
% of persons who live in poverty	Census records
Labor Force Characteristics	
Employment Status	
General population (age 18+)	
% employed	Chamber of commerce
% unemployed	Department of labor
% not participating in employment (retired)	Census records
Special groups	
% women with children under age 6 working	
Occupational Categories and Number (%) of Persons Employed	
Managerial	
Technical	
Service	
Farming	Census records
Production	
Operator/laborer	
Union Activity and Membership	*Local unions(s) office*

ern architecture, and covered parking. Some of the residents of the area are employed in these offices; most employees, according to local residents, live in other areas of Hampton.

Other major area businesses include the Rose Milk Company factory at the northern edge of the area on Way Drive, the Sheet Metal Workers Union Local No. 54 at the corner of Way Drive and Jackson, and American Life Insurance Company on Green.

All of the main thoroughfares in the area are lined with locally owned businesses such as grocery stores, craft stores, antique shops,

TABLE 7-19   Income Indices for the Years 1980 and 1990 for CT 402, CT 403, and Hampton

INCOME INDICES	CT 402		CT 403		Hampton	
	1980	1990	1980	1990	1980	1990
Median household income	$4,776	$21,238	$16,019	$25,878	$15,321	$29,378
% of all families with incomes below poverty level	53.7	18.3	5.4	13.3	7.1	14.2
% of female-headed households	49.2	NA	11.1	NA	15.4	12.7

NA = not available

(Data from 1980 Census, Selected Characteristics; 1990 Census, Selected Characteristics.)

cleaners, and small restaurants (see the Physical Description section). In addition, these kinds of businesses are also dispersed throughout the area within the residential districts. The Hampton Lighting and Power Service Center is located near the northern edge of the area. Hampton's Vehicle Maintenance Department and its Street Repair Department are also located on West Pleasant in the northern part of the Rosemont area. There are also a considerable number of printing houses (probably the largest concentration in Hampton) on the northern edge of the area, as well as the broadcast studios of Channel 11 (KHAM-TV).

According to local residents, the economic impact of these businesses on the Rosemont area is minimal because most residents are employed outside of Rosemont, and although they do patronize neighborhood convenience stores, they tend to shop for major purchases in other areas of the city. The residents also indicated that the vast majority of the businesses do not directly participate in the life of the community. Selected industries of the area are listed in Table 7-20.

When there are major businesses within a community that employ a substantial number of community residents, a thorough assessment is required. An excellent guide for assessing an occupational setting is included in Appendix A at the end of this book. This guide may be used by either the community nurse who needs more information about a major economic factor in the community or by the occupational health

TABLE 7-20   Selected Industries in Rosemont

	CT 402		CT 403	
	NUMBER	TOTAL %	NUMBER	TOTAL %
Manufacturing	92	10	430	15
Wholesale and retail trade	450	48	1084	37
Professional and related services	387	42	1423	48
Total	929	100	2937	100

(Data from Census, Selected Characteristics.)

nurse employed by the business. A completed industry assessment using the guide is also presented in Appendix B.

Labor Force

Employment Status

The labor force of a community is comprised of persons 16 years of age and over. Table 7-21 summarizes key data relating to the workforce of the Rosemont community. The majority of workers are categorized under "private wage and salary," as shown in Table 7-22.

Occupation

General occupational categories are included in the census. Table 7-23 lists the occupations of the citizens of Rosemont.

TABLE 7-21   Rosemont Labor Force, 1980

	CT 402	CT 403	Hampton
Persons 16 and over	4,580	6,470	1,189,136
Labor force	1,825	5,472	850,389
Percent of persons 16 and over	39.8	85.4	71.5

(Data from Census of Population and Housing.)

TABLE 7-22 *Class of Worker, Rosemont*

	CT 402		CT 403	
	NUMBER	*TOTAL %*	*NUMBER*	*TOTAL %*
Private wage and salary	1219	67	4168	76
Government	326	18	664	12
Local government	238	13	307	6
Self-employed	42	2	333	6
Total	1825	100	5472	100

(Data from Census of Population and Housing.)

TAKE NOTE

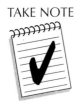

Census occupational categories are quite general. To determine more precisely what sort of work is incorporated in a category, it is necessary to ask those who do the job or to look up the category in the Department of Labor publications.

Differences between the two census tracts that comprise Rosemont are clearly seen in the occupational makeup of the community. Whereas almost half of the workers in CT 402 are categorized under "service," a similar percentage of workers in CT 403 are classified under "managerial and professional specialty."

TABLE 7-23 *Occupations, Rosemont*

	CT 402		CT 403	
	NUMBER	*TOTAL %*	*NUMBER*	*TOTAL %*
Managerial and professional specialty	117	7.1	2238	42.1
Technical, sales, administrative support	198	12.1	1813	34.1
Service	724	44.2	560	10.5
Farming	28	1.7	11	0.2
Precision production	186	11.3	463	8.7
Operators, fabricators, laborers	387	23.6	230	4.3
Total	1640	100	5315	100

(Data from Census of Population and Housing.)

Safety and Transportation

Table 7-24 lists the major components of safety and transportation that affect the community.

Protection Services

Fire, police, and sanitation services are provided by the city of Hampton. Rosemont residents pay for these services through their city taxes. Therefore, these services are extracommunity, located outside the community of Rosemont.

TABLE 7-24   Safety and Transportation

	Sources of Information
Safety	
Protection services	Planning office (city, county, and state)
Fire	Fire department (local)
Police	Police Department (city and county)
Sanitation	
Waste sources and treatment	Waste and water treatment plants
Solid waste	
Air quality	Air control board (state, regional, and local offices)
Transportation	
Private	
Transportation sources	
Number of persons with a	Census data: Population and Housing
transportation disability	Characteristics
Public	
Bus service (routes, schedules, and fares)	Local and city transportation authorities
Roads (number and condition;	
primary, secondary and farm-to-	
market roads	State Highway Department
Interstate highways	
Freeway system	
Air service (private and public-owned	Local airports (Note: Local airports are frequently owned and operated by city government.)
Rail service	In the United States, Amtrak is the primary source of intercity rail transportation

Fire Protection

The fire department and MEAS are combined in Hampton. (For a description of the MEAS, see the Health and Social Services section.)

The fire station serving Rosemont maintains two fire trucks, one air boat (for evacuations during flooding), and 20 personnel. Firemen must complete 335 hours of basic certification courses. The fire captain reports a response time of less than 10 minutes. During the 90 days prior to the assessment, the station responded to 45 fires. This compares to 39 responses during the same period of the previous year. Forty responses were to homes—the major culprit being grease fires that started in the kitchen. Other leading causes of fires include children playing with matches and lighted cigarettes. In addition to responding to fires, personnel perform safety checks of homes; teach fire prevention classes to school and community groups; and distribute window stickers that specify the location of children, elderly citizens; and pets for emergency alert during a fire.

Police Protection

The police department serving Rosemont has a staff of 27 full-time employees, including 21 police officers and 6 civilians (4 dispatchers and 2 record clerks). Equipment includes five marked and four unmarked patrol cars, two motorcycles, and a complete computerized data storage and retrieval system. This station has one holding cell where persons are detained until they can be transported to the Hampton Jail.

According to the dispatcher, response time to Rosemont is four to six minutes. Crime statistics for CT 402 and CT 403 are presented in Table 7-25.

The most frequent crimes are burglaries and thefts, which the police captain feels are committed mainly by nonresidents of Rosemont. Speeding and driving while intoxicated (DWI) are also frequent crimes in Rosemont, although following the addition of two motorcycle police officers two years ago, the number of traffic accidents has decreased by 38%. The police department offers the following services to Rosemont residents:

- Housewatch—When residents are out of town, the police will check their house three times a day for up to 30 days.
- Identification—The police department loans an engraver to citizens who wish to engrave personal belongings. The department

TABLE 7-25   Crime Statistics for CT 402 and CT 403

	1990		1991		1992		1993	
	CT 402	CT 403	CT 402	CT 403	CT 402	CT 403	CT 402	CT 403
Murder	5	3	7	7	8	6	10	3
Rape	24	19	22	18	27	11	34	17
Robbery	196	100	204	104	252	165	328	186
Aggravated assault	40	17	47	27	58	27	94	29
Burglary	263	288	274	279	295	321	345	339
Theft	403	462	423	371	397	384	384	363
Vehicle theft	103	144	113	214	112	232	109	327
Total	1034	1033	1090	1020	1149	1146	1304	1264

(Data from City of Hampton Police Department.)

also provides household possessions registration and pamphlets on how to protect one's home from burglary.

- Fingerprinting—Fingerprinting is done, and a record of the prints is provided to the person for personal identification as well as for immigration requirements. The police department is presently pursuing a special project, a citywide campaign to fingerprint all children and adolescents. A copy of the fingerprint record is given to parents, and the original remains with the police. Following several weeks of radio and TV announcements, police personnel are now present at local shopping centers every weekend to explain and complete the fingerprinting process. This special project is in response to citizen concern and requests for police assistance in locating an increasing number of missing children.
- Animal Protection Officer—The city of Hampton has a leash and fence law for dogs. The animal protection officer picks up stray animals and detains them in the city kennel until the owner or an adopter can be found.
- Public Education—Crime prevention programs are offered to community and school groups.

Residents of Rosemont repeatedly voiced concern about their personal safety. Elderly citizens expressed fear of being mugged and related stories of friends who have been harassed and robbed during the day as they walked to and from local stores. (One area grocery store owner reported that he has stopped cashing social security checks because so many patrons had been mugged after leaving his store.) The feeling of being a prisoner in one's own home was repeatedly expressed, as were questions regarding what people could do to protect themselves.

Homosexual males described experiences of perceived harassment by police as well as incidences of marked delay (up to 30 minutes) in police response time to requests for help. Residents reported that brawls, quarrels, and physical violence are becoming commonplace in Rosemont. The citizens are concerned for themselves and others; they want a safe place to live.

Sanitation

Water Sources and Treatment.   The terrain of Rosemont is flat with minimal changes in elevation. Stagnant pools of water are common—a situation that promotes mosquito populations during the warm months. Drainage is toward the northeast and into Buff's Bayou, the only open stream in Rosemont. All storm water and sewage is gathered into Hampton's sewage system. There is no separate system for storm water disposal. As a result, raw sewage backs up during heavy rains and residents complain of the smell and problems associated with toilets that cannot be flushed.

Sewage from Rosemont is treated at the 5th Street Plant. Presently a sewage moratorium exists for Rosemont owing to overcapacity at the 5th Street Plant. Consequently, only single- family dwellings can be built on plotted lots. Builders requesting permits for multifamily dwellings are given the option of delaying building indefinitely *or* being assessed a fee based on projected occupancy of their building and the associated gallons of sewage that will be produced. The assessed fee is used to increase the capacity of the treatment plant. However, even if the assessed fee option is chosen, it may be three to four years before the permit is issued.

Potable (drinking) water for Rosemont comes from Lake Hampton, located 20 miles north of the city. Residents are concerned about possible contamination of the drinking water with lead and other heavy metals. Presently there is no routine testing of the drinking water except to meet state health department requirements for chlorine content. Fluoride is not added to the Rosemont's drinking water, and it is not present naturally.

Solid Waste.   Garbage is collected twice weekly; residents state that the service and frequency are adequate. The major complaint is that illegal dumping of large items, such as refrigerators, stoves, and so forth, has increased, and despite numerous calls to proper authorities, the trash is not cleaned up with any regularity. Parents are concerned that children attracted by abandoned machinery and appliances may be hurt as they explore. In addition, inoperable automobiles are abandoned in parking spaces on the streets, and months can pass before the cars are removed by the city.

Air Quality

The Federal Air Quality Act of 1967 provided for the establishment of air-quality control regions. Regional offices maintain an inventory of air-pollution sources and monitor air status. In similar fashion, individual states formed advisory boards that developed air-quality standards and long-range air-quality programs. Local air-monitoring stations sample and record information levels on such pollutants as ozone, carbon monoxide, sulfur dioxide, and nitrogen dioxide. In addition, some 30 to 40 suspended particles in the air (solids) are measured and recorded, as are certain gaseous substances (for example, ammonia).

To assess the air quality of Rosemont, the Air Control Board was contacted; its recent reports document a rise in air pollution, which is attributed to an increase in industrial growth and a high population density. Some 25 miles east of Rosemont is a large industrial complex, and although the daily emissions from the industries are within acceptable limits, certain wind and temperature patterns act to compound emissions. This causes a visible yellow haze to form that shrouds Rosemont and surrounding communities many days of the year. Area residents complain of eye irritation and increased frequency of respiratory conditions. The chemical reactions that lead to the haze and the contribution of automotive and industrial emissions, as well as potential health effects associated with the haze, are unknowns presently being researched.

TAKE NOTE

Air pollution is a frequently used term; it means the presence of one or more contaminants in such concentration and of such duration that they may adversely affect human health, animal life, vegetation, or property.

Despite the pollution increase and industrial growth, there has been no significant increase in the amount of pollutants introduced into the atmosphere surrounding Rosemont. This is attributed to compliance of industries with the Air Control Board regulations and the permit system for new industries. Citizens can contest industry construction permits and through this process provide a forum for public opinion and objections that regulation boards take into consideration during the permit decision-making process. Citizens are also entitled to complain to the board regarding a specific industry's emissions; the board will then investigate and file a report.

During the past year, Rosemont has experienced three air stagnation advisories. Because the pollution concentration is greater than usual, persons with respiratory conditions such as bronchitis and emphysema are advised to remain indoors and limit outside activities until the air stagnation clears.

TAKE NOTE   *Air stagnation occurs when a layer of cool air is trapped by a layer of warmer air above it; the bottom air cannot rise, and pollutants cannot be dispersed.*

The board feels citizens are ill informed regarding the meaning of and the appropriate actions that should be taken during air stagnation advisories as well as each citizen's responsibility in minimizing pollution. For example, citizens seem unaware that transportation sources (such as automobiles and buses), not industry, are the major contributors of air-pollution problems and that a citizen who burns leaves or trash is releasing tiny particles of matter into the air that can the irritate the eyes, nose, and lungs. To promote public awareness and understanding, the local office makes presentations to organizations, schools, and citizen groups. Numerous public television and radio programs were planned for the year following the assessment.

Transportation

Private

The primary means of transportation in Rosemont include walking, bicycle riding, automobiles, Hampton city buses, Hampton city vans (special transportation for the elderly and handicapped), and school buses.

The major source of private transportation is the automobile. Table 7-26 presents the types of transportation used to commute to work, and

TABLE 7-26   Transportation Sources to Work That Are Used by Residents of CT 402 and CT 403

	CT 402		CT 403	
	NUMBER	TOTAL %	NUMBER	TOTAL %
Drive alone	1351	42.8	3279	63.8
Carpool	749	23.7	808	15.7
Public transportation	721	22.8	567	11
Walk	231	7.3	300	5.8
Other means	79	2.5	130	2.5
Work at home	27	0.9	58	1.2
Total	3158	100	5142	100

(Data from Census of Population and Housing.)

Table 7-27 indicates the number of persons 16 years of age or older that have a transportation disability. According to the census data, mean travel time to work for Rosemont residents is 17.7 minutes as compared to 26.6 minutes for Hampton residents.

Public

The major source of public transportation within Rosemont and surrounding communities is the Hampton bus system. The city provides

TABLE 7-27   Noninstitutionalized Persons 16 Years of Age or Older by Transportation Disability Status for CT 402 and CT 403

	With Disability		Without Disability		Total	
	NUMBER	TOTAL %	NUMBER	TOTAL %	NUMBER	TOTAL %
Age 16–64						
CT 402	221	5.9	3495	94.1	3716	100
CT 403	15	0.3	5908	99.7	5923	100
Age 65 and Over						
CT 402	197	21.3	728	78.7	925	100
CT 403	55	10.5	469	89.5	524	100

(Data from Census of Population and Housing.)

east–west bus service at half-hour intervals during the day on Pecan Drive and Live Oak Boulevard. The same service is provided on north–south routes for Way Drive, Rosemont Boulevard, and Hampton Street. For persons that qualify (such as the elderly and/or handicapped), the bus company provides door-to-door service from the individual's home to essential services such as food shopping or medical-care visits. The cost of this service varies from $0.50 to $1.00 per trip according to geographic area. Although all users agree the service is reliable, it is only available Monday through Friday, 8:30 A.M. to 5:00 P.M., and reservations are required several days in advance—a requirement that is impossible to meet in situations such as during acute illnesses.

Roads

Jefferson County (of which Rosemont is a part) has adequate primary, secondary, and farm-to-market roads. In addition, several miles of a freeway system circle Hampton. Two major interstate highways transect Hampton, and the State Highway Department has budgeted $2 billion for highway construction and maintenance for Jefferson County over the next 20 years. Recently, the residents of Jefferson County voted for an additional tax devoted entirely to improving intracounty transportation. Rosemont residents complain of congested freeways and damaged roads that go without repair for months. The need was expressed for a road system that efficiently handles local traffic.

Air Service

Jefferson County has four small, privately owned airports. The city of Hampton owns and operates two airports; both provide national and international service.

Rail Service

Amtrak connects Hampton to other major cities in the state as well as to other states. There are no private or public commuter rail services within Jefferson County or Hampton.

Politics and Government

Rosemont falls within the city limits of Hampton, which has a mayor–council form of government. There are 14 council members (5 at-large), one of whom represents Rosemont and nearby communities. Each serves a two-year term. The city council meets at City Hall on the first Tuesday of each month. The meetings are open to the public, and Rosemont residents often attend.

The city council and mayor comprise the policy-making body as well as the administrative head of Hampton. Their duties include the following: maintaining competent staff to operate all city services (the health department and police, for instance), passing ordinances, and appropriating funds to carry out policies.

The councilman for District Three, which includes Rosemont, is James Browning. Councilman Browning was elected by a wide margin of votes and has been popular with the Rosemont community because he has spearheaded the fight against sexually oriented businesses (the "SOB Fight," as it is popularly called). This issue has not been settled, and the citizens are supporting Councilman Browning's reelection so that he may continue the fight.

The active participation in the Hampton council of Councilman Browning is only one indicator of Rosemont's politics. There are several politically oriented organizations and civic clubs in the area, all of which seek to improve the quality of life in Rosemont and help to support inter-community activities.

A brief synopsis of several organizations that are politically active in Rosemont is presented in Table 7-28. (Contact person, address, and phone number should be included in such lists but have been omitted from this description.)

Several other groups in the community are less visible and active unless an issue of particular interest becomes "hot." For instance, many voluntary agencies such as the American Lung Association–Hampton Chapter are located in the community and can be called upon to assist specific campaigns (for example, smoking-prevention programs in the schools or antipollution campaigns aimed toward extracommunity sources). The Community Services Directory lists all such organizations both by interest (heart, lung, crime, and so on) and general area (Rosemont groups can usually be found under "Southwest, near downtown").

Political activism is evident throughout Rosemont: During election years there are campaign posters everywhere; talk at gathering places (barbershops, grocery stores, bars) inevitably turns to politics; and numerous rallies are held in support of candidates or issues. In Rosemont there appear to be two major political factions. Voting records show CT 403 residents to be more liberal than residents in CT 402. This

TABLE 7-28 *Organizations Politically Active in Rosemont*	
	Description
Neartown Business Alliance (Founded 1949)	Owners of businesses in the area meet monthly and work to promote the area and its businesses. The alliance contributes to campaigns of supporters of Rosemont.
Gay Political Caucus (Founded 1964)	This is a very active and visible group. It works to influence elections through voter registration, campaign work, and education. It has been credited with the election or defeat of certain candidates. Membership is open to all interested in community improvement. It meets on third Tuesday, 7:00 P.M.
Rosemont Firehouse (Founded 1973)	This is a coordination and referral group; it operates a 24-hour crisis hotline. It is sponsored by donations from most of the area's churches as well as the civic groups, and most of the workers are community volunteers.
Rosemont Watch (Founded 1978)	The Watch works to prevent crime in the area through education and visible activities such as "Block Awareness Week." It coordinates activities with the Hampton City Police. All citizens are encouraged to become involved. It meets monthly.
Seniors for a Safe Community (Founded 1980)	Comprised primarily of retired persons (but open to all interested residents), this group was formed to address the problem of the mugging or robbing of senior citizens, especially on the days in which social security checks arrived. The original small group has expanded, as have their goals, so that now they are actively involved in promoting a better quality of life for all in the community (with a special emphasis on the elderly). This group is active in the "SOB Fight" and also works closely with Rosemont Watch.

may reflect the fact that CT 403 is comprised of more affluent, younger, and professional residents than is CT 402.

Communication

Communication may be formal or informal. Formal communication usually originates outside the community (extracommunity) as opposed to informal communication, which almost always originates and is disseminated within the community. Salient components of formal and informal communication, as well as sources of data, are presented in Table 7-29.

Formal Communication

Hampton has one major newspaper, *The Hampton Herald*. Additional daily newspapers include a business journal, *Current Issues;* a black-oriented paper, *Progress;* one Spanish-language paper, *La Prensa;* and a Vietnamese tabloid. Hampton has 12 AM stations and 10 FM stations, six commercial TV stations and one educational network. Cable television is available to Rosemont residents on a monthly subscription basis. Residents receive home mail delivery.

Informal Communication

Bulletin boards and posters dot community and municipal buildings in Rosemont. Posters are placed on trees and tacked to buildings throughout the community, and a rainbow of fliers can be seen tucked into fence and door crevices. Radio and television announcements herald forthcoming events and offer open forums on community issues. The

TABLE 7-29   Communications

Components	Sources of Information
Formal	**Chamber of commerce**
Newspaper (number, circulation, frequency, and scope of news)	Newspaper office
	Telephone company
Radio and television (number of stations, commercial versus educational, and audience)	Yellow pages
	Telephone book
Postal service	Census data on phone use
Telephone status (number of residents with service)	
Informal	
Sources: bulletin boards; posters; hand-delivered fliers; and church, civic, and school newsletters	Windshield survey
	Talking to residents
	Survey
Dissemination (How do people receive information?)	
Word of mouth	
Mail	
Radio, television	

Rosemont Civic Association publishes a bimonthly four-page newsletter to notify residents of upcoming meetings and social activities. Polls and surveys are a regular feature of the newsletter, which is distributed free to all residents.

Key informants within Rosemont include the civic association secretary, local ministers, and fire and police personnel as well as community civic board members. People can be seen "chatting" throughout Rosemont, and when asked how information is received, they mention all of the above formal and informal sources.

Education

The general educational status of a community can be summarized using census data. Census information lists the number of residents attending schools, years of schooling completed, and percentage of residents who speak English. To supplement this broad assessment, information is needed about major educational sources (for example, schools, colleges, and libraries) located inside the community. Table 7-30 is a suggested guide for assessing a community's educational sources.

TABLE 7-30   *Education*

Components	Sources of Information
Educational Status	
Years of school completed	Census data—Social characteristics section
School enrollment by type of school	Census data—Social characteristics section
Language spoken	Census data—Social characteristics section
Educational Sources	
Intracommunity or extracommunity (collect data for each facility)	Local board of education
Services (educational, recreational, communication, and health)	School administrator (such as the principal or director) and school nurse
Resources (personnel, space, budget, and record system)	School administrator
Characteristics of users (geographic distribution and demographic profile)	Teachers and staff
Adequacy, accessibility, and acceptability of education to students and staff	Students and staff

TABLE 7-31   Years of School Completed for CT 402, CT 403, and Hampton

	CT 402	CT 403	Hampton
Persons 25 years and over	3,459	4,948	888,269
Elementary			
0 to 4 years	611	26	41,695
5 to 7 years	665	164	66,775
8 years	409	101	37,373
High School			
1 to 3 years	800	278	136,179
4 years	661	914	240,320
College			
1 to 3 years	181	1,173	160,999
4 or more years	132	2,292	204,928
% High school graduates	28.2	88.5	68.3

TAKE NOTE

It is sometimes difficult to decide which educational sources to include in the assessment. Community usage is probably the single most important indicator. Primary and secondary schools attended by the majority of youngsters in a community, regardless of intra- or extracommunity location, are major educational sources and require a thorough assessment, whereas schools composed primarily of students from outside the community do not require such an extensive appraisal.

Educational Status

Table 7-31 presents the years of schooling completed by adults in CT 402 and CT 403. In a similar format, Table 7-32 lists school enrollment by type of school, and Table 7-33 presents the number and percentage of community residents who speak English.

Educational Sources

Intracommunity—Temple Elementary School

Temple Elementary School is located on the corner of Pecan Drive and Magnolia Drive, close to the center of CT 402. Asphalt lots bound three sides of Temple; two are used for vehicle parking, and one is for play. A

TABLE 7-32   School Enrollment and Type of School for CT 402, CT 403, and Hampton

	CT 402	CT 403	Hampton
Type of School			
Public nursery school	94	44	20,735
Private nursery school	77	44	15,427
Public kindergarten	194	14	21,863
Private kindergarten	25	14	4,833
Public elementary (1 to 8 yr)	1,258	186	198,367
Private elementary (1 to 8 yr)	10	136	18,440
Public high school (1 to 4 yr)	482	92	94,099
Private high school (1 to 4 yr)	12	25	7,154
College	92	922	78,472
Total enrolled in schools (age 3 years and over)	2,120	1,258	413,536

(Data from Census of Population and Housing.)

small patch of grass persists on the remaining side, a fenced-in area that contains several large trees, a swing set, and three teeter-totters. Several broken windows were seen, and no graffiti was noted.

Temple is in its 64th year of continuous operation teaching grades kindergarten to eighth. Present enrollment is 924; 42% of the students are black, 33% are Asian, 18% are hispanic, and 5% are white. Most of the children live in Rosemont and either walk to school or ride the school bus (provided for children living further than two miles from Temple).

TABLE 7-33   Ability to Speak English for CT 402, CT 403, and Hampton

	Percentage Who Speak English Poorly or Not at All	
	AGE 5–17	*AGE 18 YEARS AND OVER*
CT 402	75.9	73.8
CT 403	11	19.3
Hampton	21.4	26.2

(Data from Census of Population and Housing.)

As part of the Hampton School District (HSD), Temple receives funding from the district revenues obtained from local property taxes, state coffers, and the federal budget. State monies to HSD are based upon average daily attendance of students at each school. Most policies affecting Temple are formed and enforced by the HSD Board. The board is composed of eight nonsalaried persons, each elected from one of eight regions in the school district. Each term of office is four years. Board member Jane Roberts represents Rosemont; at the time of assessment, she was in the second year of her four-year term. Responsibilities of the HSD board include prescribing qualifications of employees, establishing salary schedules, setting goals and objectives for the district, establishing the policies to implement the goals and objectives, and evaluating the performance of the district in relationship to adopted goals and objectives. The General Superintendent is the administrative head of the board and is salaried and recruited by the Board.

Principal.   Temple's principal cited truancy and the related problem of academic failure as the school's major problems. According to office records, some 6% to 8% of the student body is absent each day, and most of those absent are not ill. Compounding the problem is the fact that many parents do not have phones. As a result, it is not uncommon for a youngster to be absent for two or three days before parental contact is made. (In most cases it is found that the parent assumed the child was in school.) The principal believed that truancy is most common among seventh and eighth graders, especially among hispanic boys.

Regarding bilingual education for non-English-speaking students, the principal felt that all classes should be in English and that the presence of bilingual education at Temple only slows the progress of the children who are learning English. Presently, there are two bilingual teachers at Temple; they reported that they have a list of over 100 youngsters who have requested and have been assessed as needing the bilingual program.

Teachers.   Teachers repeatedly stated the need for improved communication with parents. They felt that parents need to have current information about their child's learning needs and school performance as well as a knowledge of specific techniques for fostering academic achievement. (Presently, school policy allows for two, 20-minute, parent–teacher conferences yearly—a time allotment that was rated as extremely inadequate by the teachers.) The teachers reported that 22% of the student body at Temple failed last year. Major impediments to learning were listed as poor English-speaking skills and understanding of English, stressful home environments, and inadequate adult supervision at home. Teachers felt overwhelmed and frustrated; the average employment stay at Temple is two years.

School Nurse. The school nurse at Temple is present two days a week; she is at West Hampton High the remaining three days. A review of the daily clinic register for the preceding six weeks noted a clinic attendance of 141; the majority (72%) of those visting suffered from stomachache or headache. Although none of the stomach ailments required early dismissal, 60% of the headaches were associated with fever and necessitated early dismissal from school. Remaining complaints were sore throats and minor cuts or falls. All children were screened biannually for vision and hearing problems. The nurse recognized the need for yearly screening but said she lacked the necessary time. She stated that if school policy would permit the recruitment and training of a parent volunteer(s), then yearly screening would be feasible. In addition to vision and hearing testing, all children are screened for head lice twice a year; children found to be infected are dismissed from school and are not readmitted until they have been successfully treated. Some 62% of the youngsters participate in the free lunch program. The nurse expressed concern that several children who appear undernourished (displaying, for example, low weight for height and small arm circumference for age) do not qualify for the lunch program, whereas others who appear to be well nourished do qualify. Eligibility is based on family size and income.

Major health problems as described by the nurse include lack of hygiene (children frequently come to school dirty and inadequately clothed for cold weather); dental caries; high (30%–40%) annual incidence of youngsters with head lice, especially in primary grades (kindergarten, first grade, and second garde); incomplete immunization status (92% of the youngsters have up-to-date immunizations); and lack of parent follow-through for needed medical care and treatment during illnesses. To assess dental status, the nurse performed oral assessment of children who came to the clinic during one four-week period. She found 62% of the children to have discolored areas or cavitations in the pits of their teeth or between teeth. Most of the youngsters stated they had never been to a dentist, and many reported frequent tooth pain and difficulty chewing.

The nurse does not do any health teaching in the classroom because school policy mandates that the nurse be present in the clinic at all times. The ruling causes considerable frustration as the nurse's participation in the teaching and promotion of health habits is restricted to one-to-one clinic encounters (a time when the child is ill and not receptive to learning). When asked about staff and teacher usage of the clinic, the nurse discussed at length the need for health information expressed by both teachers and staff. Questions regarding exercise, stress, and diet modifications are common. The nurse would like to assess and identify specific health needs of staff and teachers.

Community Service.   As a community service, Temple sponsors scout troops and basketball and softball teams and provides a meeting place for several newly formed church and community action groups. In addition, Monday through Thursday nights, Temple houses extension courses from Hampton Community College. A full range of subjects is offered, including academic, vocational, and enrichment courses. Present enrollment exceeds 1200, an increase of 22% from the previous year.

All Rosemont residents were familiar with Temple Elementary; most had children who attended Temple, or else they themselves had attended Temple as youngsters. Residents felt that Temple was a community landmark and symbol of unity that links one generation to the next. The primary complaint, repeated by several families, was a perceived insensitivity of Temple's staff and teachers to ethnic and racial differences and needs. For example, all school notices are written in English, and all programs offered by the Parent Teachers Organization (PTO) are presented in English. Both Asian and hispanic parents have brought specific concerns and needs to the staff and teachers at Temple but have repeatedly been told that all parental requests must come from appropriate PTO committees—an organization that seems alien to many Asian and hispanic parents.

Day Care.   One day care center is located in CT 402—the Busybee Nursery. There are no day care facilities in CT 403. Housed in a renovated building, the Busybee accepts children aged two to five years. Some 60 youngsters are cared for by five staff members, and 43 children (primarily toddlers) are on the waiting list. The center is licensed by the state. Rosemont residents repeatedly lamented the lack of day care facilities. Many parents felt forced to leave their young children with other mothers or teenagers who have dropped out of school. Several mothers reported leaving their children daily with a babysitter who cares for from 8 to 10 youngsters.

Library. The Rosemont library is conveniently located adjacent to the main shopping district and offers a variety of adult, teen, and youth book programs, films, and special educational activities. Notices of all programs are published in the Rosemont civic association newsletter and posted on local bulletin boards.

Extracommunity

High school students from Rosemont attend Central Hampton High, a complex that houses 4800 students and is located eight miles from Rosemont. Concerned about truancy and grade failure, Central Hampton began a "Failproof" program two years ago. Some 82% of students and their parents have participated. As a result, school scores on state and national proficiency tests have improved, and truancy has decreased. The principal described numerous community outreach services offered by the school, including recreational programs in the evening and on the weekends, as well as a full complement of adult education courses.

The nurse at Central Hampton is present five days a week. The majority of visits to the clinic (an average of 30 daily) involve allergy-related complaints, gastrointestinal upsets, and minor sprains or strains that occur during physical exercise class. Because of HSD policies, the high school nurse is also prohibited from offering health education in the classroom.

The nurse's major concern is the increased number of teenage pregnancies and the HSD Board's decision of two years ago not to permit sex education information in the classroom. Classes in sexuality, sexually transmitted disease, contraception, and decision-making in the area of sexual activity had been offered at all high schools in Hampton prior to the new ruling. The nurse does not know the sequence of events that resulted in the sex education decision. A second major concern is the increased use of alcohol among students. A drug awareness curriculum was prepared by the State Board of Education and will be implemented during the next semester as part of the biology courses' content.

Numerous private preschool and grade schools are available in Hampton, and some are used by the residents of Rosemont, especially by persons in CT 403. Some 20 colleges and universities are located in

Hampton and Jefferson County; most offer a variety of general education and specialty training programs. One unique aspect of the area's educational resources is Hampton Community College, a junior college that provides classes in 21 public schools in Hampton and Jefferson County. (Temple Elementary is one of these campuses.) Numerous residents state that they prefer Hampton Community College to other area resources because of its convenient locations, low tuition, and employment-oriented approach to education.

Recreation

The recreation facilities within and adjacent to Rosemont are listed in Table 7-34 and pictured in Figure 7-3 on page 190. With the exception of the schoolyards, there is very little recreational area for children and almost none for adults and teenagers. Although there are funds in the budget of the Hampton Parks and Recreation Department for the acquisition of property, there are no plans for any development in the Rosemont area. However, the city has recently begun an improvement program along the banks of Buff's Bayou in order to create a "River Walk" similar to those in other cities with rivers. It will be several years before the project is completed.

TABLE 7-34   *Recreational Facilities in Rosemont and Adjacent Areas*

	Acreage	Location	Facilities
San Juan	2.6	1650 Pleasant	Shelter building, playground equipment, softball field, and baseball field
Richards	1	1414 Redbud	Shelter building, playground equipment, picnic area, and basketball court (swimming pool recently filled in)
Applehurst	1.9	600 Water Oak	Recreation center, rest room, playground equipment, picnic area, tennis, basketball, and volleyball courts
Jeckle Park	0.08	1500 Maple	None
Buff's Bayou	?	"Greens" along the bayou	Park benches and jogging/bicycle trail

(City of Hampton, Parks and Recreation Department, interview with JB, (Director), May 1994.)

The Rosemont Sports Association, according to its president, provides "quality organized recreation opportunities" for the local community. Programs consist of teams for winter bowling, spring bowling, summer bowling, softball, flag football, tennis, and so forth. The Rosemont Sports Association, however, is open only to members who pay a fee of $20 per year.

Churches of Rosemont (two were visited—see the Social Services section) offer a wide variety of activities for all ages. Exercise classes, craft classes, Mother's Day Out, preschool classes, senior citizens' groups, and many other programs are available to church members. Although other community residents are welcome to take advantage of these activities, the persons interviewed at the churches reported that their participants are almost all church members.

Several residents spoke of an area along the northern bank of Buff's Bayou (just east of Way Drive) that is used as a gathering place by residents who live nearby. Families take their children there on summer evenings so that parents can visit while the children play. The only facilities at this area are benches that have been placed along the grassy area.

A bicycle/jogging trail follows the bayou for several miles and is popular with the health-conscious residents who use it frequently, especially in the early morning and late evening hours. Some people have expressed fear of being mugged while using this trail, but there have been no official reports of crime in this area over the past year. The trail and all the land along the bayou are maintained by the city of Hampton.

The area residents of the east side tend to congregate for recreation on sidewalks and in neighborhood bars. The one playground in the area, other than the one at Temple Elementary, is located adjacent to the Audubon Parkway Village (the low-rent housing complex), but it is used exclusively by the residents of that complex. The playground equipment is in very poor repair, and there is virtually no grass left in the area. The Parks and Recreation Department has no plans to upgrade or replace the equipment or to replant the grass.

There is one movie theater and one theater for stage production in Rosemont, but movie theaters are accessible and near almost all areas surrounding the community. Other forms of evening entertainment are reflected in the numerous bars and restaurants that feature live music (as was mentioned in the physical examination of the community).

Extracommunity recreational facilities abound. A large city park that includes museums, a zoo, a bandshell, and picnic areas is less than a mile to the south of Rosemont. Another city park in downtown Hampton, called Serenity Park, is less than a mile to the northeast.

Virtually every major league sport has a team in Hampton. The sports arenas are some distance from the area, but there is adequate bus service to them.

An abundance of music and theater is available to those who can afford it. Hampton has a symphony orchestra, a ballet, both grand and light opera, and a legitimate stage company, to name a few options.

In addition, water activities such as boating and fishing are as close as 30 miles away. According to several residents of Audubon Parkway Village, a special day out includes crabbing along the bay—which is often a successful endeavor to fill the dinner pot as well as provide fun for the whole family.

Summary

The community assessment is complete. A description of each community subsystem has been recorded. Note that at every step of the assessment, *people* in the community were included. Not only did we interview the "professionals" (for example, school nurses, principal, police chief, and so on), but clients of the subsystems were also included (parents, shoppers, patients, and people on the street). The assessment, like all steps in the process, is carried out in *partnership* with the community. The next step is *analysis,* a process that synthesizes the assessment information and derives from it diagnoses specific to the community.

Crucial to community assessment is a model, or map, to direct and guide that process. The model shown in Figure 7-1 was used to guide the assessment of Rosemont. In the Suggested Readings list, several other approaches to community assessment are presented. Consider these sources as you continue your practice of community health assessment.

SUGGESTED READINGS

*American Indian Health Care Association. (1990). *Promoting healthy traditions workbook: A guide to the Healthy People 2000 campaign.* St. Paul, MN: Author.

Barton, J.A., Smith, M.C., Brown, N.J., Supples, J.M. (1993). Methodological issues in a team approach to community health needs assessment. *Nursing Outlook, 41*(6), 253–261.

Bennett, E.J. (1993). Health needs assessment of a rural county: Impact evaluation of a student project. *Family & Community Health, 16*(1), 28–35.

Gregor, S., & Galazka, S.S. (1990). The use of key informant networks in assessment of community health. *Family Medicine, 22*(2), 118–121.

Kretzman, J.P., & McKnight, J.L. (1993). *Building communities from the inside out: A path toward finding and mobilizing a community's assets.* Chicago: ACTA Publications.

Martin, A. (1988). Community assessment: The cornerstone of effective marketing. *Pediatric Nursing, 14*(1), 50–53.

Muir, K., Wilson, O., Rooney, F., O'Connor, T., & Murphy, T. (1992). Student corner-community assessment. *Nursing Praxis in New Zealand, 7*(2), 25–29.

Nettle, C., Laboon, P., Jones, N., Pavelich, J., Pifer, P., & Beltz, C. (1989). Community nursing diagnosis. *Journal of Community Health Nursing, 6*(3), 135–145.

Palfrey, J.S. (1994). *Community child health: An action plan for today.* Westport, CT: Praeger.

Ruth, J., Eliason, K., Schultz, P.R. (1992). Community assessment: A process of learning. *Journal of Nursing Education, 31*(4), 181–183.

Schultz, P.R., & Magilvy, J.K. (1988). Assessing community health needs of elderly populations: Comparisons of three strategies. *Journal of Advanced Nursing, 13,* 193–202.

Urrutia-Rojas, X., & Aday, L.A. (1991). A framework for community assessment: Designing and conducting a survey in a Hispanic immigrant and refugee community. *Public Health Nursing, 8,* (1), 20–26.

*Walker, M., & Breuer, S. (1992). Community assessment, health care and you. Austin, TX: Health Care Options for Rural Communities (P.O. Box 15587, Austin, TX 78761-5587; Fax [512] 465–1090.)

White, J.E., & Valentine, V.L. (1993). Computer assisted video instruction & community assessment. *Nursing and Health Care, 14*(7), 349–353.

*Women's Environment & Development Organization. (Not dated). *Women for a healthy planet—Community report card.* Available from the author at 845 Third Avenue, 15th Floor, New York, NY 10022; Fax (212) 759-8647. (Also available in Spanish.)

---

*Documents that can be used throughout the planning process.

8

Community Analysis and Nursing Diagnosis

Objectives

This chapter is focused on the second phase of the nursing process, *analysis,* and the associated task of forming community nursing diagnoses. After studying the chapter, you will be able to

- Critically analyze community assessment data
- Formulate community nursing diagnoses

Introduction

Analysis is the study and examination of data. Analysis is necessary to determine community health needs and community strengths as well as to identify patterns of health responses and trends in health care use. During analysis, any need for further data collection is revealed as gaps and incongruencies in community assessment data surface. The end product of analysis is the community nursing diagnosis.

Community Analysis

Analysis, like so many procedures we carry out, may be viewed as a process with multiple steps. The phases we will use to help in the analysis are categorization, summarization, comparison, and inference elaboration. Each is described and illustrated below.

Categorize

To analyze community assessment data, it is helpful to first *categorize the data.* Data can be categorized in a variety of ways. Traditional categories of community assessment data include the following:

1. Demographic characteristics (family size, age, sex, and ethnic and racial groupings)
2. Geographic characteristics (area boundaries; number and size of neighborhoods, public spaces, and roads)
3. Socioeconomic characteristics (occupation and income categories, educational attainment, and rental or home ownership patterns)
4. Health resources and services (hospitals, clinics, mental health centers, and so forth)

However, models are being used increasingly in the organization and analysis of community health data because they provide a framework for data collection and a map to guide analysis. Because the community assessment wheel (see Figure 7-1) was used to direct the community assessment process in the Rosemont sample study, that same model can be used to guide analysis. Each of the community subsystems will be analyzed, and components within each subsystem specify the categories to be evaluated.

Summarize

Once a categorization method has been selected, the next task is to *summarize the data* within each category. Both summary statements and summary measures such as rates, charts, and graphs are required.

TAKE NOTE

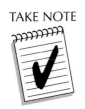

Many health care agencies and educational institutions have access to computerized information systems—a system through which formatted data can be retrieved in a variety of forms—including summary health statistics. For example, data entered into a computer system as census figures can be configured into population pyramids, and census and vital statistics information can be programmed to calculate birth, death, and fertility rates. Calculations that previously required hours to complete are now computed in seconds. In your practice, make it a point to inquire as to the availability of computer systems and, if possible, use computer processes to complete quantitative data analysis.

In addition, your local health department may be able to furnish the rates for you, for instance, the infant mortality rate. Note, however, that the denominator used may not be your community as you have defined it.

Compare

Additional tasks of data analysis include the *identification of data gaps, incongruencies,* and *omissions.* Frequently, comparative data are needed to determine if a pattern or trend exists or if data do not seem correct and the need for revalidation of original information is required. Data gaps are inevitable, as are mistakes in recording data; the important task is to analyze data critically and be aware of the potential for gaps and omissions. To have professional colleagues review the analysis is helpful. Every person has a unique perspective; it is only through the sharing of views that a whole and comprehensive picture of community assessment data can evolve.

Using the data from your community, compare it with other similar data. For instance, you calculate (or discover) an infant mortality rate of 12 per 1000 live births—how does this compare with the city? the state? the nation? Is it for the *entire* infant population of your community? Is the IMR different based on race? NOTE: This is a good time to review Chapter 2 to assist you with epidemiologic reasoning as you try to make sense of your data.

Other resources for comparison are the documents dealing with objectives—for the nation and for individual states. *Healthy People 2000* (U.S. Department of Health and Human Services, 1990) presents national figures, such as incidence and prevalence when available, for our major health problems and proposes goals and objectives for each. *Healthy People 2000*—along with state and, if available, local health planning documents—can be invaluable to you both as you analyze your data and as you develop a plan based on those data.

Draw Inference

Having categorized, summarized, and compared the data you have collected, the final phase is to draw logical conclusions from the evidence; that is, to draw inferences that will lead to the statement of a community nursing diagnosis.

Rosemont Sample Community Analysis

Following the analysis examples given below, information on how to form community nursing diagnoses is presented (see the Community Nursing Diagnosis section later in this chapter). The analysis of the Rosemont assessment data, as in the assessment process, begins with the community core, for it is the core (the *people* and their health) that is of interest to the community health nurse. Recall that the core is affected by (and affects) all of the subsystems depicted in the model surrounding it. Some subsystems will influence certain problems more than others, but *it is important to assess the subsystems because of their contribution to the causes and alleviation of problems in the core.*

Community Core

An analysis of Rosemont's core is presented in Table 8-1. Community core data include many demographic measures, a type of data that is especially amenable to graphs and charts. The adage One picture is worth a thousand words is particularly meaningful for demographic characteristics.

Perhaps the most representative illustration of the age and sex composition of a population is the *population pyramid.* Population pyramids for census tracts (CTs) 402 and 403 appear in Figure 8-1.

TAKE NOTE

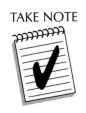

The population pyramid is formed of bars; each bar represents an age group. Usually 5- or 10-year age groups are used, although adaptations can be made for smaller or larger age ranges. Bars are stacked horizontally, one on another, with bars for males on the left of a central axis and those for females on the right. The percentage of males and females in a particular age group is indicated by the length of the bars, as measured from the central axis. All age groups in a pyramid should be the same interval.

To construct a population pyramid, use Table 8-2 to calculate the percentage contribution of each age and sex class and Table 8-3 for actual pyramid construction. Note that parts of the population pyramids in Figure 8-1, those depicting people younger than 20 years and older than 65, are shaded; this was done to denote the dependent portions of the population.

(*Text continues on page 242*)

TABLE 8-1   Analysis of Rosemont's Core

Categories of Data	Summary Statements/Measures	Inferences
History		
	Cultural and ethnic diversity	
	Renovation of businesses and homes	Community revitalization
	Pride and concern evident	Community pride
Demographics		
Age		
CT 402	42.5% of population $\leq$19 years	Large % of children and adolescents
	53% of population $\leq$19 years or $\geq$65 years	High dependency ratio[*]
	10% of population $\geq$65 years	Large % of elderly compared to Hampton and Jefferson County

Data gap: Need prior census data to determine if demographics are consistent or changing.

CT 403	7.5% of population $\leq$19 years	Small % of children and adolescents
	15.2% of population $\leq$19 years or $\geq$65 years	Low dependency ratio
	7.7% of population $\geq$65 years	

Data gap: Need census data on 5-year increments to construct population pyramids.

Sex		
CT 402	48% of population is male.	Equal % of males and females
	45% of population aged 20–64 is male.	
CT 403	65% of population is male.	High % of males
	69% of population aged 20–64 is male.	

Data gap: Need prior census data to determine if demographics are consistent or changing.

Racial/ethnic		
CT 402	Diversity: black 54%, Asian 19%, white 12%, hispanic 9%	Racial and ethnic diversity
CT 403	Homogeneity: white 89%	Racial and ethnic homogeneity

Data gap: Need census data from 1970 to determine if demographics are consistent or changing.

Household types		
CT 402	83% of households are family.	Family households dominate.
CT 403	36% of households are family.	Nonfamily households dominate.
Marital status		
CT 402	15% single, 60% married, 14% divorced	Small % of single adults
		Majority of adults married
CT 403	53% single, 24% married, 15% divorced	Large % of single adults
		Small % married

Data gap: Need prior census data to determine if demographics are consistent or changing.

TABLE 8-1   (continued)

Categories of Data	Summary Statements/Measures	Inferences

Vital Statistics
(Refer to Chapter 2 for rate calculation)

		(When Compared to Hampton and Jefferson County)
Births	Rate per 1000	
CT 402	30.5	A higher birth rate
CT 403	17.3	A lower birth rate
Hampton	19.4	
Jefferson County	25.2	

Data gap: Need general fertility rate and age-specific birth rate.

		(When Compared to Hampton and Jefferson County Data)
Deaths	Rate per 1000	
CT 402		
Infant	33.3	A higher death rate for all ages
Neonatal	23.8	
Fetal	76.2	
Crude	10.4	
CT 403		
Infant	17.1	A higher infant and neonatal
Neonatal	17.1	rate
Fetal	8.5	
Crude	6.2	

Data gap: Need vital statistics from previous 3 to 5 years to determine if rates are consistent or changing.

Hampton		
Infant	12.1	
Neonatal	7.9	
Fetal	12.6	
Crude	6.0	
Jefferson County		
Infant	12.3	
Neonatal	8.3	
Fetal	15.3	
Crude	7.3	

		(When Compared to Hampton and Jefferson County Data)
Causes of Death	Rate per 1000	A much higher % of deaths
CT 402	Heart disease 22.2%; malignant neoplasms 23.6%; cerebrovascular 8.3%; accidents 5.6%; diseases of early infancy 9.7%; homicides 8.3%; pneumonia 2.8%; suicides 4.2%; tuberculosis 1.4%; all other causes 13.9%	due to Diseases of infancy Homicides Suicides Tuberculosis A higher % of deaths due to cerebrovascular disease A lower % of deaths due to heart disease

(continued)

237

TABLE 8-1   (continued)

Categories of Data	Summary Statements/Measures	Inferences
		(When Compared to Hampton and Jefferson County Data)

Causes of Death
CT 403
	Rate per 1000
	Heart disease 23.8%; malignant neoplasms 26.1%; cerebrovascular 4.7%; accidents 9.5%; diseases of early infancy 2.4%; homicides 2.4%; cirrhosis of liver 2.4%; pneumonia 2.4%; suicides 2.4%; diabetes mellitus 4.8%; congenital anomalies 4.8%; all other causes 14.3%
		A higher % of deaths due to
		    Accidents
		    Diabetes mellitus
		    Congenital anomalies
		A lower % of deaths due to
		    heart disease

Data gap: Need comparative data for past 3 to 5 years.		
Hampton	Disease of heart 33.4%; malignant neoplasms 21.8%; cerebrovascular 7.3%; accidents 6.2%; emphysema, asthma, bronchitis 0.8%; diseases of early infancy 2.6%; homicides 6.2%; cirrhosis of liver 1.7%; pneumonia 2.2%; suicides 2%; diabetes mellitus 1.4%; congenital anomalies 1%; nephritis and nephrosis 0.1%; tuberculosis 0.2%; all other causes 13%	
Jefferson County	Disease of heart 36%; malignant neoplasms 24.2%; cerebrovascular 7.4%; accidents 5.7%; emphysema, asthma, bronchitis 0.7%; diseases of early infancy 3%; homicides 1.5%; pneumonia 2.2%; suicides 1.4%; diabetes mellitus 1.8%; congenital anomalies 1.5%; nephritis and nephrosis 0.2%; tuberculosis 0.2%; all other causes 9.1%	

Dependency ratio describes the potentially self-supporting portion of the population and the dependent portions at the extremes of age. The dependency ratio is usually computed as follows:

$$\frac{\text{population under 20 + population 65 and over}}{\text{population 20 to 64 years of age}} \times 100$$

The dependency ratio for CT 402 is 91, meaning for every 100 persons aged 20 to 65 (supposedly self-supporting because of age) there are 91 persons under age 20 or over age 65 needing support (because of age). In contrast, the dependency ratio for CT 403 is 19.

TABLE 8-2 *Calculations for a Population Pyramid*

COMMUNITY NAME, CENSUS TRACT,
OR GEOGRAPHIC BOUNDARIES: _____

TOTAL POPULATION: _____

	Males		Females	
AGES (YEARS)	*NUMBER*	*% OF TOTAL POPULATION*	*NUMBER*	*% OF TOTAL POPULATION*
Total				
Younger than 5				
5–9				
10–14				
15–19				
20–24				
25–29				
30–34				
35–39				
40–44				
45–49				
50–54				
55–59				
60–64				
65–69				
70–74				
75 and over				

TABLE 8-3   *Constructing a Population Pyramid*

POPULATION PYRAMID FOR _____ : 19 _____

Males														Females
						75 & Over								
						70–74								
						65–69								
						60–64								
						55–59								
						50–54								
						45–49								
						40–45								
						35–39								
						30–35								
						25–29								
						20–24								
						15–19								
						10–14								
						5–9								
						Younger than 5								

8   6   4   2   0   2   4   6   8

Percentage of Population

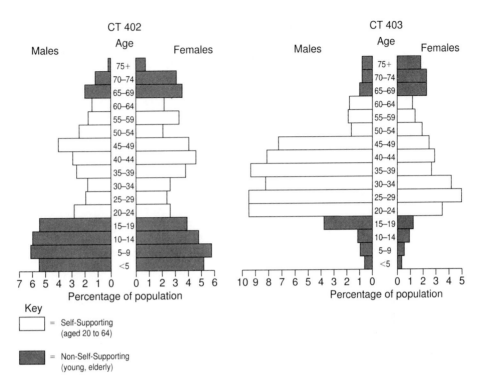

FIGURE 8-1
Population Pyramid: Age and sex structure of CT 402 and CT 403.

Studying the population pyramids for CT 402 and CT 403 reveals striking age and sex differences, and this illustrates an important lesson. If the demographics of Rosemont had been presented as one population pyramid (Figure 8-2), important age and sex differences might have been minimized or have gone unrecognized, and their associated age- and sex-related health needs would be left unmet. This hazard in data analysis is referred to as *aggregating* or *pooling the data*. It is important to divide data along all possibly meaningful lines so that important information is not overlooked. Be alert to this problem as you proceed with your analysis.

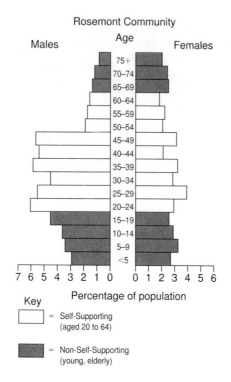

FIGURE 8-2
Population Pyramid of Rosemont Community: Age and sex structure.

Studying the inferences presented in Table 8-1, in conjunction with the population pyramids, Figures 8-1 and 8-2, the following statements can be made about Rosemont's core. In CT 402 there exists the following:

- A large percentage (42.5%) of children and adolescents
- A high dependency ratio
- An equal percentage of adult men and women aged 20 to 64 years
- A larger percentage (10%) of elderly than Hampton or Jefferson County
- A small percentage (15.2%) of single adults
- A moderate percentage (60.7%) of married adults
- A predominance (83%) of family households

- A mixed racial/ethnic composition with 54% black, 19% Asian, 12% white, and 9% hispanic
- An extremely high infant and fetal death rate:
  —Infant mortality rate (33 per 1000 live births)
  —Neonatal mortality rate (24 per 1000 live births)
  —Fetal mortality rate (76 per 1000 live births)
- A higher birth rate (31 per 1000 population) than Hampton (19 per 1000 population) or Jefferson County (25 per 1000 population)
- A higher crude death rate (10 per 1000 population) than Hampton (6 per 1000 population) or Jefferson County (7 per 1000 population)
- A much higher percentage of deaths owing to diseases of early infancy, homicides, suicides, and tuberculosis than Hampton or Jefferson County
- A slightly higher percentage of deaths owing to cerebrovascular disorders than Hampton or Jefferson County

In contrast, it can be seen that CT 403 has the following factors:

- A small percentage (7.5%) of children and adolescents
- A low dependency ratio
- A larger percentage (7.7%) of elderly than Hampton or Jefferson County
- A high percentage (69%) of adult males aged 20 to 64 years
- Racial and ethnic homogeneity, with 89% of the population white
- A predominance (64%) of nonfamily households
- A large percentage (53%) of single adults
- A small percentage (24%) of married adults
- A lower birth rate (17 per 1000 population) than Hampton or Jefferson County
- A higher infant mortality (17 per 1000 live births) and a higher neonatal mortality (17 per 1000 live births) than Hampton or Jefferson County
- A lower crude death rate (6.2 per 1000 population) than Hampton or Jefferson County
- A higher percentage of deaths owing to accidents, diabetes mellitus, and congenital anomalies than Hampton or Jefferson County
- A lower percentage of deaths due to heart disease than Hampton or Jefferson County

Having analyzed the core characteristics of Rosemont, it is evident that major differences exist between CT 402 and CT 403, although both are part of Rosemont. In the following sections, this finding will be given more detail as each subsystem in our community assessment wheel model is analyzed.

Physical Environment

To study the physical components of Rosemont, data were collected that began with community inspection (that is, the windshield survey) and concluded with a systems review and laboratory studies (in other words, census and chamber of commerce data). Table 8-4 presents an analysis of the *physical examination data.*

Studying the inferences in Table 8-4, the following statements about Rosemont's physical components can be made:

- Rosemont is a community of contrasts and diversity.
- Densely populated residential areas, composed mainly of older homes, abut businesses of various types.
- Industry is minimal and is concentrated entirely in CT 402.
- Housing values increased greatly in CT 402; in both CT 402 and CT 403, only rents rose at the same rate.

Health and Social Services

An analysis of the health and social services in Rosemont is presented in Table 8-5. Because the data were categorized initially as extra- and intra-community health and social services, the same format has been used in the analysis. Notice that statements from health care providers have been reported separately from those of health care recipients. This is because health care providers frequently have a different concept of the adequacy, accessibility, and acceptability of health services than that held by health care recipients. Be sure to collect and analyze data from both perspectives.

After reviewing Table 8-5, the following statements can be deduced about Rosemont's health services:

TABLE 8-4   *Analysis of Rosemont's Physical Examination Data*

Categories of Data	Summary Statements/Measures	Inferences
Inspection Windshield survey	A community of contrast; bustling business areas and quiet neighborhoods Ethnic diversity evident in foods	Ethnic and business diversity Congested streets lined with homes or businesses Minimal industry Little "open" space
Vital Signs	Flat terrain and mild climate Densely populated (14 persons per acre) Posters abound, sharing information and heralding forthcoming events.	Mild climate, abundant flora Densely populated (14 persons per acre) Note: In CT 402 there are 221 persons per acre at one housing development.
Systems Review *Land Usage* CT 402 CT 403	37% of land in commercial usage, 28% single family, 8% multifamily, and 9% open 20% of land in commercial usage, 32% single family, 15% multifamily, and 18% open	CT 402 has almost twice the commercial usage of land (37%) compared to CT 403 (20%). CT 403 has twice the percentage of open space (18%) compared to CT 402 (9%)
Housing Values CT 402 CT 403	From 1980 to 1990, average home values increased 68% and average rents increased 16.9%. From 1980 to 1990, average home values increased 6.8% and average rents increased 16.9%.	Sharp contrast between average home values; in CT 402 average home value is $43,300 compared to $62,400 in CT 403. Average rent is similar for both census tracts and comparable to Hampton.

(Note: No data gaps identified; data for this area are complete.)

- A variety of private hospitals, home health care agencies, and continuing-care facilities are located outside Rosemont; however, most require fee-for-service or third-party reimbursement.
- There is only one full-service public hospital in the area, Jefferson Memorial, which is located five miles from Rosemont; users of Jefferson Memorial complain of lengthy waits for outpatient care and fragmented service.

TABLE 8-5   Analysis of Health and Social Services in Rosemont

Categories of Data	Summary Statements/ Measures	Inferences
Health Facilities		
Extracommunity		
Hospitals	Most are referral or private. One public hospital, Jefferson Memorial, has problems of Long waits (≥8 hr) Fragmented care Inaccessibility	Only one public hospital; users complain of lengthy waits and fragmented care.
Private care	Numerous options, including HMOs	Variety of private care options
Health department (Sunvalley Clinic)	Health providers feel Sunvalley Clinic has Inadequate antepartal services; women wait 8–10 weeks for an initial appointment that is often after their expected data of confinement (EDC) Inadequate nursing services to meet elderly's needs Rosemont residents feel the clinic is Inaccessible (no direct bus connection) Impersonal (no primary care providers)	Inadequate antepartal services Many women deliver at Jefferson Memorial with no antepartal care. Many women are forced to self-deliver at home because they do not meet eligibility requirements at Jefferson Memorial. Inaccessibility and unacceptability of Sunvalley services.

Data gap:
   Number of Rosemont residents using
      Well and ill infant, child, adolescent, adult services
      Mental health counseling and referral services
   User's perception of adequacy, accessibility, and acceptability of the above services

Home health	One large Visiting Nurse Association (VNA) Numerous home health agencies; most require fee-for-service or third-party reimbursement.	Numerous options for home health care

Data gap: Frequency and type of VNA services used by Rosemont residents

Continuing care	Two long-term licensed facilities close (eight miles) from Rosemont	Two long-term licensed facilities

Data gap: Adequacy of facilities as perceived by health administrators, staff, and patients

Emergency services: Medical emergency ambulance service (MEAS)	Cardiac and CVA are major reasons for MEAS visits to Rosemont.	Cardiac and CVA are major reasons for MEAS visits, followed by accidents and home falls.

Data gap: Number of persons using MEAS and their age, sex, race, and ethnic characteristics

TABLE 8-5   (continued)

Categories of Data	Summary Statements/ Measures	Inferences
Intracommunity Health Services		

Health care practitioners	Rosemont has no
	  Obstetric, gynecologic, or
	  family practitioners
	  Bilingual health practitioners
		Lack of ob/gyn and family
		  practitioners
		No bilingual health practitioners

Clinics		

Third Street Clinic	Health care providers feel immediate
	  health needs include
	    Ill infant, child, adolescent,
	    and adult assessment,
	    treatment, and follow-up
	    Dental assessment and
	    restoration
	    Counseling, referral, and
	    treatment for substance abuse
	    Group health teaching
	    Support groups for single
	    parents and senior citizens
	  Additional needs of the clinic
	  include recruitment and
	  retainment of health care providers.
		Inadequate health services for
		  Ill persons (all ages)
		  Dental assessment and
		  restoration
		  Counseling and treatment
		  for substance abuse
		  Health education
		  Self-help/support groups

	Many Rosemont residents use the
	  clinic routinely; people feel
	  welcomed and comply with
	  medical care.
	Residents agree that additional
	  services are needed.
		Rosemont residents state that care
		  at Third Street Clinic is
		  acceptable and accessible.

Data gap:
  Number of persons requesting services that health care providers feel are needed
  Characteristics of persons requesting medical care services

Rosemont Health
  Center
	Director of clinic feels immediate
	  needs are
	    Formation of counseling and
	    support groups
	    Orientation program and
	    inservice for staff (all are
	    volunteers
		Highly acceptable, accessible
		  and affordable care for STD
		Inadequate counseling and
		  support groups
		Lack of orientation and inservice
		  for the staff
		Lack of procedure manuals and
		  posted protocols for
		  emergency care
		Lack of safety procedures
		  including visible emergency
		  cart and proper syringe
		  disposal

Data gap: What do staff perceive as needs?

(continued)

TABLE 8-5 *(continued)*

Categories of Data	Summary Statements/ Measures	Inferences
Social Facilities		
Extracommunity		
Hampton Community Counseling Center (HCCC)	HCCC offers counseling to adolescent drug users. Most patients are middle- or upper-class males; all are white. Staff feels that they are meeting community needs. Rosemont residents are not aware that the center exists.	HCCC is close to Rosemont and offers needed counseling for substance abuse, yet HCCC is not used by Rosemont residents.

YMCA Indo-Chinese Refugee Program	Cultural-orientation programs for Asian immigrants; staff perceive immediate needs are for programs on the following:
	    Substance abuse
	    Basic life survival skills (for example, employment, self-health care)
	Many Rosemont residents use the YMCA services; all agree the programs are excellent but state the waiting period for classes is long and frustrating.
		Insufficient number of cultural programs resulting in long waiting periods and frustration

Intracommunity		
Churches		
South Main	Extensive social service programs; social program for homosexual males despite resistance from older members	Social outreach programs offered by both churches Only South Main offers program for homosexual males although older members of South Main resent the program.
Westpark	Extensive social service program No social programs for homosexual males	
Lambda Alcoholic Anonymous (AA)	Active AA program for homosexual males; membership exceeds 120.	Active chapter of Lambda AA

- The Sunvalley Clinic, operated by the city health department, has inadequate antepartum services for Rosemont women; this results in
  —Many women delivering at Jefferson Memorial with no antepartum care
  —Women forced to self-deliver at home because they do not meet eligibility requirements at Jefferson Memorial
- There are no practicing private obstetric, gynecologic, or family practitioners in Rosemont.
- The Third Street Clinic has inadequate health services, specifically a lack of
  —Assessment and treatment of persons who are ill
  —Dental assessment and restoration
  —Counseling and treatment programs for substance abuse
  —Health education programs responsive to residents' needs
  —Support and self-help groups as needed and requested by residents
- The Rosemont Health Center offers acceptable, accessible, and affordable services for sexually transmitted diseases (STD); however, there is a lack of
  —Orientation and education for the staff
  —Procedure manuals and posted protocols for emergency care
  —Safe disposal methods for syringes
  —A visible emergency cart

The following deductions can be made about Rosemont's social services:

- Hampton Community Counseling Center (HCCC) is located close to Rosemont but is not used by Rosemont residents, although residents repeatedly expressed a wish for substance-abuse counseling programs.
- The YMCA Indo-Chinese Refugee Program is heavily used by Asians in Rosemont; however, present programs of cultural orientation are inadequate to meet the demand. Both the YMCA staff and Rosemont residents see a need for additional programs.
- South Main and Westpark churches offer numerous social service programs; however, only South Main offers a social program especially for the male homosexual population—a program that is resisted by older parishioners.
- An active chapter of Lambda AA is located in Rosemont.

Economics

An analysis of the economic and financial characteristics of Rosemont is presented in Table 8-6. The analysis begins with individual wealth indices (such as income), proceeds to indicators of business and industrial wealth, and concludes with employment status of community residents. As with other subsystems, the categories for data assessment have become categories for data analysis.

After studying Table 8-6, the following statements can be made about the economic status of Rosemont. Striking differences exist in the financial characteristics between households in CT 402 and CT 403.

In CT 402 it was found that

- The median household income of $10,693 is only 34% of the median income in CT 403 and Hampton

TABLE 8-6   Analysis of the Economic Indicators of Rosemont

Categories of Data	Summary Statements/ Measures	Inferences
Financial Characteristics of Households		
Median household income (1990)		
CT 402	$10,693	Median household income in
CT 403	$31,273	CT 403 is considerably higher
Hampton	$30,483	than in CT 402.
% of families with incomes below poverty level (1990)		
CT 402	53.7%	In CT 402, over half of all
CT 403	5.4%	families have incomes
Hampton	7.1%	below the poverty level.
% of families on public assistance/welfare		
CT 402	36.4%	In CT 402, 36.4% of all families
CT 403	4.3%	are on public assistance/
Hampton	3.4%	welfare compared to 4.3% in CT 403 and 3.4% in Hampton.
% of female head of households (1990)		
CT 402	49.2%	In CT 402, half of the
CT 403	11.1%	households are headed by
Hampton	15.4%	females.

TABLE 8-6   (continued)

Categories of Data	Summary Statements/ Measures	Inferences
Financial Characteristics of Households		
Business/industry		
characteristics (1990)		
CT 402	Nearly equal percentage of wholesale/retail (48%) and professional (42%)	In CT 402, equal percentage of wholesale and professional businesses
CT 403	Predominance of professional (48%) over wholesale/retail (37%)	In CT 403, predominance of professional businesses
Labor force characteristics (1990):		
age (% of persons ≥16 years)		
CT 402	39.8%	Only 40% of persons in CT 402
CT 403	85.4%	are of employable age
Hampton	71.5%	(≥16) compared to 85% in CT 403 and 71% in Hampton.
Wage class: % Private, % government,		
% self-employed		
CT 402	67%, 18%, 2%	Wage class data similar for CT
CT 403	76%, 12%, 6%	402 and CT 403, with the majority of all wages derived from private businesses
Occupational groups		
Managerial/professional		
CT 402	7.1%	Striking differences between
CT 403	42.1%	occupational categories
Technical/sales		
CT 402	12.1%	In CT 402, 67% of workers are
CT 403	34.1%	in service or operator occupations, compared to 14.8% in CT 403.
Service		
CT 402	44.2%	In CT 403, 76% of workers are
CT 403	10.5%	in managerial or technical occupations, compared to 19% in CT 402.
Operators/laborers		
CT 402	23.6%	
CT 403	4.3%	

(Note: No data gaps identified; data in this area are complete.)

        —The majority of families (53.7%) have incomes below the poverty level
        —Half of all households are headed by females
        —One third of all families receive public assistance/welfare
- In CT 403 the following factors exist:
        —The median household income of $31,273 is much greater than that of CT 402, as well as that of Hampton.
        —Only 5.4% of families have incomes below the poverty line.
        —Only 11.1% of all households are headed by females.
        —Only 4.3% of families receive public assistance/welfare.

Striking differences also exist between the labor force characteristics of CT 402 and CT 403.

- In CT 402 it was found that
        —Only 39.8% of the population is of employable age (16 years or older)
        —Most people (67.8%) work in service or operator/labor occupations
- CT 403 presented a contrasting picture:
        —Of the population, 85.4% is of employable age (16 years or older).
        —Most people (76.2%) work in managerial or professional positions.

Safety and Transportation

An analysis of the safety and transportation services in Rosemont are set forth in Table 8-7.

Reviewing the data, the following statements can be made about Rosemont's safety (protection) services and associated concerns:

- Grease fires are the major cause of house fires.
- Thefts and burglaries are the major reported crimes, followed by robbery and vehicle theft; elderly persons and male homosexuals feel especially victimized. Both groups related numerous stories of harassment and violence.

TABLE 8-7 Analysis of Safety and Transportation Services in Rosemont

Categories of Data	Summary Statements/ Measures	Inferences
Safety		
Protection Services		
Fire	45 fires during past 90 days; of these, 40 occurred in homes (usually a grease fire).	Major cause of fires within last 90 days was grease.

Data gap:
    Obtain additional data (12 months) and determine if grease fires are major cause.
    Document age, sex, and racial characteristics, as well as time of day and associated circumstances.

Police	Crime statistics for past four years show thefts as the leading crime, followed by burglary. Frequency of occurrence is high for both census tracts. Robbery is twice as prevalent in CT 402 compared to CT 403, and vehicle theft is three times more common in CT 403. Residents expressed fear and related stories of muggings and violence directed especially toward the elderly and male homosexual population.	Thefts and burglaries are the major crimes; the elderly and male homosexuals feel especially victimized.

Data gap:
    Assess residents' knowledge about self-protection measures against crime.
    Assess residents' interest and past participation in crime prevention programs.
    Assess available crime prevention programs.

Sanitation		
Sewage	Sewage moratorium exists owing to overcapacity of present facility.	Inadequate sewage treatment facilities resulting in building restrictions.
Potable water	No fluoride in drinking water No routine testing of drinking water for arsenic or heavy metals (elements that residents believe may be contaminating the water)	Lack of fluoride in drinking water No routine tests of drinking water for arsenic or heavy metals

Data gap:
    Assess history of fluoride issue. Has fluoride been proposed, voted on? What is the present position of the health department, city council, civic associations, and the general public?
    Regarding arsenic and heavy metals: Is Lake Hampton tested for arsenic or heavy metals? What is the position and plan of the health department, city council, and civic associations?

(*continued*)

TABLE 8-7   *(continued)*

Categories of Data	Summary Statements/ Measures	Inferences
Sanitation		
Solid waste	Increased illegal dumping of machinery and appliances; unoperable autos are parked on the streets for months before removal by the city of Hampton	Potential for accidents (with consequences such as trauma and suffocation) as persons explore abandoned objects and automobiles

Data gap:
   Document laws and fees for illegal dumping. Are signs posted to notify persons of law and associated fines? What actions have been taken by residents, civic associations, businesses?

Air	Rise in air pollution attributed to increase in industrial growth and population density. Residents complain of eye irritation and increased number of respiratory conditions.	Increased air pollution
	Air Board feels citizens are inadequately informed regarding actions needed during an air stagnation advisory and individual responsibility to decrease pollution.	Citizens may be inadequately informed regarding personal actions needed during an air stagnation advisory to decrease air pollution.

Data Gap:
   Assess if public awareness programs have occurred. If so, when, and what was the response? What do residents understand about air pollution, air advisories, and their role in decreasing air pollution? Do residents desire more information about air pollution?

Transportation		
Private (To Work)		
CT 402	43% of people drive alone; 24% carpool, and 23% use public transportation.	Almost half (43%) drive alone to work, with equal percentages (24%) carpooling or using public transportation.
CT 403	64% of people drive alone; 16% carpool, and 11% use public transportation.	Most people (64%) drive alone to work, some carpool (16%), and only a few use public transportation (11%).

| | Summary Statements/ | |
Categories of Data	Measures	Inferences
Transportation		
Transportation Disability		
CT 402	6% of persons aged 16 to 64 and 21% of over age 65 have a disability.	When compared to CT 403, a large percentage of residents in CT 402 have a transportation disability, especially those over age 65.
CT 403	0.3% of persons aged 16 to 64 and 11% of those over age 65 have a disability.	

TABLE 8-7   (continued)

- There is no fluoride in Rosemont's drinking water, and neither is there routine testing for arsenic or heavy metals, substances that residents fear are contaminating the water.
- Owing to abandoned vehicles and dumping of machinery and appliances, residents, especially children, are at increased risk of accidental injury.
- Air pollution has increased; the Air Control Board feels citizens are inadequately informed about air pollution advisories as well as personal actions that can be taken to decrease pollution.

Regarding Rosemont's transportation services, the following deductions are made:

- A large percentage of residents in CT 403 drive to work alone (64%) compared to those in CT 402 (43%); however, 48% of the residents in CT 402 use carpools or public transportation to get to work, compared to 26% in CT 403.
- When compared to CT 403, a substantially larger percentage of the population in CT 402 have a transportation disability, especially among those over age 65.

Politics and Government

A rich diversity of political organizations exists in Rosemont. However, at this point in the nursing process—analysis—it is sufficient to describe the organizations and identify key persons. Consider your information about the political system and form of government to be reference material that will be useful at the next stage of the nursing process—program planning with the community.

Communication

Ample formal and informal communication sources exist in Rosemont. No analysis is required of the data. Consider the communication data to be reference material that will be useful at the next stage of the nursing process—program planning with the community.

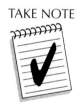

TAKE NOTE

If sufficient information is collected regarding a community's communication system (refer to Table 7-29 in Chapter 7 for components to assess), then there is no need to analyze the data.

Education

An analysis of Rosemont's *general educational status* (characteristics of school enrollment, years of schooling completed, and language spoken) and *specific educational sources* (for example, public and private schools both intra and extracommunity) is presented in Table 8-8.

Major differences exist between the general educational status of CT 402 and CT 403. The status in CT 402 is as follows:

- A small percentage of residents are high school graduates (28%), with the majority of persons enrolled in school attending elementary grades. Some 75% of the population has poor English proficiency.

In contrast, the CT 403 data show that

TABLE 8-8   *Analysis of Educational Sources in Rosemont*

Categories of Data	Summary Statements/ Measures	Inferences
Educational Status		
Years of schooling completed: % high school graduates		In CT 402, only 28% of persons over age 25 are high school graduates, compared to 89% in CT 403 and 68% in Hampton.
CT 402 28%		
CT 403 89%		
Hampton 68%		
School enrollment: % elementary, % high school, % college		The majority of persons attending school in CT 402 are elementary grade students; in CT 403, the majority of those attending school are in college.
CT 402 59%, 23%, 4%		
CT 403 15%, 7%, 73%		
Hampton 48%, 23%, 19%		
Language spoken: % of population with poor English proficiency		In CT 402 some 75% of the population has poor English proficiency, compared to small percentages in CT 403.
Age 5–17 Age 18+		
CT 402 76% 74%		
CT 403 11% 19%		
Hampton 21% 26%		
Educational Sources		
Intracommunity		
Temple Elementary	Grades K to eighth Enrollment 924 Ethnicity 42% black 33% Asian 18% hispanic 5% white	Mixed ethnicity, predominance of black children
	Principal feels major problems are Truancy Academic failure Principal wants to stop bilingual classes.	According to staff, major problems are Truancy Academic failure (22%) Inadequate parent– teacher relationships English insufficiencies Stressed home environments with inadequate adult supervision

Data gap:
  Explore the principal's statement about bilingual education. Why the opposition? What is the
  position and policy on bilingual education in HISD?
  What is the principal's perception of parental concerns?

(continued)

TABLE 8-8 (continued)		

Categories of Data	Summary Statements/ Measures	Inferences
Educational Sources		
	Teachers feel major impediments to student learning are: Inadequate parent–teacher communication Poor English proficiency Stressed home environment Inadequate adult supervision	Same as above

Data gap:
  Explore teachers' perceptions of bilingual education.
  What are teachers' perceptions of parental concerns?

| Temple Elementary | *Nurse feels* major health problems of youngsters are Poor hygiene Dental caries Prevalence of head lice Incomplete immunizations Lack of parent follow-through for needed medical care | Major student health problems are Inadequate Hygiene Control of dental caries Control of head lice Parent follow-through with needed medical care Health education |

Data gap:
  Document age, sex, ethnicity, and racial characteristics of children with specific health problems.

| | *Nurse feels* more health teaching and screening would be possible with parent volunteers. Present policy restricts nurse to clinic, permitting no classroom teaching. | Same as above |

Data gap:
  Document school policy regarding
    Recruitment and training of parent volunteers
    The nurse's presence and role in the clinic
  Explore nurse's attitude toward health education.
    Discuss options for health programs for students, staff, and parents.

TABLE 8-8   *(continued)*

Categories of Data	Summary Statements/ Measures	Inferences
Educational Sources Temple Elementary	*Parents feel* Temple is a community strength *but* the present staff members are insensitive to ethnic and racial needs; attempts to discuss these concerns with Temple's staff have been frustrating.	Parental concern and involvement are evident; however, attempts to discuss concerns with staff have been frustrating.

Data gap:
   Identify officers and key people (committee chairs) of Temple's PTO. Are these officers/key people aware of ethnic and racial needs?
   Identify students' perceptions of their school. What activities do they enjoy? Are there afterschool activities? Who participates? What activities are needed?

Busybee Day Care	One day care center in CT 402; no facility in CT 403	Inadequate day care facilities Parents leave children in crowded homes
Extracommunity Central Hampton High	Truancy and grade failure reversed with "Failproof" program Increased number of teenage pregnancies Decision by school board not to permit sex education classes Increased use of alcohol	Increased number of teenage pregnancies Increased use of alcohol among high school students Sex education classes not permitted in high school

Data gap:
   Number of pregnancies last 3 to 5 years (for comparison) and age, grade level, racial, and ethnic characteristics of girls.
   History and reason for Hampton Independent School District (HISD) Board decision to stop sex education
   Document scope of alcohol use and characteristics of users.

- A large percentage of residents are high school graduates (89%), and the majority of the persons who attend school are in college. Only 19% of the residents have poor English proficiency.

With regard to specific educational sources, Temple Elementary is the primary educational resource in Rosemont. Temple has an enrollment of 924 youngsters. The principal, teachers, nurse, and parents were interviewed during the assessment process. To summarize the situation at Temple, it has been concluded that

- Probems of truancy exist, especially among hispanic boys. There are large numbers of academic failures (22% of students last year).
- Large numbers of students have English-skills insufficiencies, further documented by general educational data.
- Inadequate working relationships exist between parents and teachers, compounded by the language barrier.
- Student health problems consist of
  —Dental caries (62% of youngsters)
  —Head lice, especially in grades kindergarten to second
  —Incomplete immunizations
  —Poor hygiene
  —Inadequate parent follow-through of needed medical care
  —Inadequate health education program
- There is parental concern and involvement and a desire to communicate needs to staff.

One day care facility exists in Rosemont—the Busybee. This facility is extremely inadequate. As a result, parents are forced to leave children in conditions that may be crowded and undersupervised.

The major extracommunity educational facility is Central Hampton High. The major problems of Central Hampton High, according to the school nurse, include

- Increased number of teenage pregnancies
- Lack of sex education classes
- Increased use of alcohol

Central Hampton has succeeded in reducing truancy and grade failure through a program called "Failproof."

Recreation

Recreational space and facilities are minimal. A sum of 5.6 acres of public recreational space is available for a population of 13,631 (combined populations of CT 402 and CT 403). The organized sports and recreational programs that are available through churches and associations require membership and usually charge a fee. There are no public recreational programs, and the few pieces of public recreational equipment that exist are in need of repair.

Community Nursing Diagnosis

In the preceding pages, each subsystem of the Rosemont sample has been analyzed in relation to its effect on the core (the people), and inferences have been drawn. The final task of analysis is the synthesis of the inference statements into community nursing diagnoses.

A *diagnosis* is a statement that synthesizes assessment data. A diagnosis is a label that both *describes a situation* (or state) and *implies an etiology* (reason).

A *nursing diagnosis* limits the diagnostic process to those diagnoses that represent *human responses to actual or potential health problems that nurses are licensed to treat.* This stipulation is based on the American Nurses' Association (ANA) Social Policy Statement (see the Suggested Readings list). Although no standard format exists, most nursing diagnoses have three parts:

- A *description* of the problem, response, or state
- Identification of factors *etiologically* related to the problem
- *Signs and symptoms* that are characteristic of the problem

A *community nursing diagnosis* focuses the diagnosis on a *community*—usually defined as *a group, population, or cluster of people with at least one common characteristic* (such as geographic location, occupation, ethnicity, or housing condition). To derive a community nursing diagnosis, community assessment data are analyzed, and inferences are presented. Inference statements shape nursing diagnoses. Some inference statements form the descriptive part of the nursing diagnosis— that is, they testify to a potential or actual community health problem or concern, for example

- High infant mortality rate in Rosemont
- High prevalence of dental caries among youngsters at Temple Elementary School in Rosemont

Other inference statements are etiologic and document the possible reasons for the health problem or concern. Etiologic statements are linked to the descriptive statements with a "related to" clause, for example

- High infant mortality in Rosemont is *related to*
    —Inadequate resources at the Health Department's Sunvalley Clinic to meet antepartum care needs
    —Inaccessibility and unacceptability of present antepartum services at the Sunvalley Clinic
    —Lack of obstetric and family practitioners in Rosemont
- High prevalence of dental caries among youngsters at Temple Elementary School in Rosemont is *related to*
    —Lack of dental assessment and treatment at the Third Street Clinic
    —Lack of fluoride in Rosemont's drinking water
    —Low median household income in CT 402 and associated limited economic resources for purchasing dental care
    —No dental hygiene education offered at Temple Elementary

Finally, the *signs and symptoms* of the community nursing diagnosis are the inference statements that *document the duration or magnitude of the problem.* Examples of documentation include record accounts, census reports, and vital statistics. This final piece of the community nursing diagnosis is linked to the first two parts with an "as manifested by" clause, for example

- High infant mortality rate in Rosemont is related to
    —Inadequate resources at the Health Department's Sunvalley Clinic to meet antepartum care needs
    —Inaccessibility and unacceptability of present antepartum services at the Sunvalley Clinic
    —Lack of obstetric and family practitioners in Rosemont
    As manifested by many Rosemont women who deliver at Jefferson Memorial with *no* antepartum care, many Rosemont

women who self-deliver at home, and an IMR of 17 per 1000 live births
- High prevalence of dental caries among youngsters at Temple Elementary School in Rosemont is related to
  —Lack of dental assessment and treatment at the Third Street Clinic
  —Lack of fluoride in Rosemont's drinking water
  —Low median household income in CT 402 and associated limited economic resources for purchasing dental care
  —No dental hygiene education offered at Temple Elementary *As manifested by* 62% of youngsters at Temple Elementary who have dental caries on inspection

Although a single problem is stated, the etiology(ies) and signs and symptoms may be multiple. Also notice that although the health problem inference is drawn from the analysis of one subsystem (such as the health and social services subsystem or the educational subsystem), the etiologies may be, and usually are, drawn from several subsystems. For example, regarding the health problem of dental caries among youngsters at Temple Elementary, etiologic inferences were derived from four subsystems—educational, health and social services, safety and transportation, and economic. This example sums up the most important lesson of community health nursing: *All community factors (subsystems) join to determine the health status of a community.* No one subsystem is more important or crucial than any other in determining a community's health.

The process of deriving community nursing diagnoses always remains the same—*first,* assessment data are categorized and studied for inferences that are descriptive of potential or actual health problems amenable to nursing interventions; *next,* associated inferences are identified that explain the derivation or continuation of the problem; and *last,* documentation is presented. Additional community nursing diagnoses for Rosemont are presented in Table 8-9. There is no particular order to the list, and neither is the list conclusive. Determining the order of priority among community nursing diagnoses is part of program planning and is dependent on existing community goals and resources this important skill is discussed in the next chapter.

Deriving community nursing diagnoses requires critical decision making and astute study; it is a challenging and vital task. The completeness and validity of the diagnoses that have been derived will be tested during the next stage of the nursing process and will form the

TABLE 8-9   Community Nursing Diagnoses

Community Response/ Concern/Problem (Actual or Potential)	Etiology Related to...	Documentation Signs and Symptoms as Manifested by...
Stress and anxiety of being criminally victimized	Increased episodes of thefts and burglaries Inadequate knowledge on the part of residents regarding self-protection measures	Police crime statistics of past four years Personal testimony of residents, especially homosexual males and the elderly
Potential for accidents (such as trauma and suffocation) as children and adults explore abandoned goods	Illegal dumping of machinery and appliances Abandonment of automobiles Nonenforcement of city ordinances	Parental concern for safety Observation of persons exploring abandoned goods
Potential for health problems associated with air pollution (such as initiation and exacerbation of respiratory conditions)	Increased air pollution Lack of knowledge regarding personal action required during an air stagnation advisory to decrease air pollution	Air Board reports of current air pollution levels Residents' complaints of eye irritation and increased number of respiratory conditions
Truancy and academic failure at Temple Elementary	Large number of students with poor English proficiency Stressed home environment in CT 402, where 50% of homes are headed by females and 54% of families are below poverty level Inadequate communication links between parents and school personnel	Records at Temple Elementary
Stress within Rosemont between the homosexual and nonhomosexual populations	Differing lifestyles of homosexual males Lack of acceptance of homosexual male lifestyle	Lack of social programs for homosexual males in Westpark Church Resistance of older church members in South Main to existing program for homosexual males Large percentage of single males in CT 403
Potential for inadequate coping of single parents, the elderly, and persons with STDs	Lack of support groups and programs for single parents, the elderly, and persons with STDs Inadequate resources at Third Street Clinic to offer programs although the need is recognized Inadequate resources at Hampton Health Center to offer programs although the need is recognized	Health providers' perceptions of the Third Street Clinic Health providers' perceptions of the Rosemont Health Center High percentage of deaths owing to homicides and suicides in CT 402

TABLE 8-9 *(continued)*

Community Response/ Concern/Problem (Actual or Potential)	Etiology Related to. . .	Documentation Signs and Symptoms as Manifested by. . .
Unsafe working environment at Rosemont Health Center	Lack of orientation and inservice programs for staff Lack of procedure manuals and posted protocols for emergency care Lack of safety procedures	Visual assessment Perceptions of administration Perception of volunteer nurse
Potential for inadequate cultural assimilation of Asian immigrants	Lack of programs to meet present needs Lack of staff at Indo-Chinese Refugee Program Increased need for programs Large Asian population in CT 402 (19%) Large percentage of population in CT 402 (75%) with poor English proficiency	Perceived needs of Asians in Rosemont
Incomplete immunization status of children at Temple Elementary	Inadequate communication between parents and school's staff Inaccessibility and unacceptability of Health Department's Sunvalley Clinic Inadequate income in CT 402 to purchase immunizations	School health records at Temple Elementary
High infant, neonatal, and fetal mortality rate	Inadequate antepartum care at Sunvalley Clinic Lack of obstetric and family practitioners in Rosemont Lack of bilingual practitioners in Rosemont Inadequate income in CT 402 to purchase essential medical care	Vital statistics
Potential for boredom and associated consequences (violence, vandalism)	Lack of public, no-fee recreational programs. Minimal public recreational areas and equipment	A total of 5.6 acres of public recreational space in Rosemont Visual inspection of available land and equipment
High prevalence of capitis pediculosis among children at Temple Elementary	Crowded living conditions Knowledge deficit regarding transmission and treatment	Cases reported by school nurse at Temple Elementary

tested during the next stage of the nursing process and will form the foundation of that stage—the planning of a health program.

TAKE NOTE

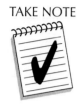

This is an excellent time to share your assessment data with colleagues and persons in the community to solicit their analysis. Because we all have opinions and values that color our perceptions, group critiquing and analysis of assessment data are ways to foster objectivity.

Summary

Critical analyses of the Rosemont community have been completed using the community assessment wheel as a guide. Subsequently, community nursing diagnoses were formulated, based on the inferences of the analyses. Although community nursing diagnoses are new to practice, community health nurses have, since the profession's inception, derived inferences from assessment data and have acted on those data. However, the terminology and format that has surrounded these informally produced inferences (diagnoses) have been inconsistent. There is considerable discussion, and some controversy, regarding the structure and terminology that would be optimal for community-focused nursing diagnoses. In your practice, you will be exposed to various formats for making community nursing diagnoses; evaluate and test the usefulness of each. It is only through collaboration and vigorous testing that a standard format will evolve. In the Suggested Readings list, there are sources that trace the development of community nursing diagnoses as well as suggested frameworks for deriving diagnoses.

SUGGESTED READINGS

Allor, M.T. (1983). The "community profile." *Journal of Nursing Education, 22,* 12–16.

American Nurses' Association. (1980). *Nursing: A Social Policy Statement.* Kansas City, MO: Author.

Anderson, E.T. (1990, Fall). Community diagnosis: A guide for planning. *Visions* (A publication of Population-Focused Community Health Nursing Edcuation at Pacific Lutheran University, Tacoma, WA), 8–10.

Bjaras, G. (1993). The potential of community diagnosis as a tool in planning an intervention programme aimed at preventing injuries. *Accident Analysis & Prevention 25,* 3–10.

Stoner, M.H. Magilvy, J.K., & Schultz, P.R. (1992). Community analysis in community health nursing practice: The GENESIS Model. *Public Health Nursing, 9,* 223–227.

U.S. Department of Health and Human Services. Public Health Service. (1990). *Healthy People 2000: National Health Promotion and Disease Prevention Objectives.* Washington, D.C: U.S. Government Printing Office.

9

Planning a Community Health Program

Objectives

This chapter covers the planning of nursing actions to promote the health of a community. After studying this chapter, you should be able to

- Validate your community nursing diagnoses with your community
- Use principles of change theory to direct the planning process
- In partnership with the community, plan a community-focused health program that includes
  — Measurable goals and behavioral objectives
  — A sequence of actions and a time schedule for achieving goals
  — Resources needed to accomplish the plan
  — Potential obstacles to planned actions and revised actions
  — Revisions to the plan as goals and objectives are achieved or changed
  — A recording of the plan in a concise, standardized, and retrievable form

Introduction

Once a community's health has been assessed, the data analyzed, and community nursing diagnoses derived, it is time to consider nursing interventions that will promote the community's health—to formulate a *community-focused plan*. Each of the three parts of the diagnosis statement—the descriptions of the actual or potential problem, its causes, and its signs and symptoms—directs planning efforts for the nurse. All three provide equally important information from which to plan. Figure 9-1 displays the process for deriving a community nursing diagnosis and summarizes how the parts of the diagnosis both describe the community assessment and give direction for program planning, intervention, and evaluation. Community-focused plans are based on the nursing diagnoses and contain specific goals and interventions for achieving desired outcomes. Planning, like assessment and analysis, is a systematic process completed in partnership with the community.

TAKE NOTE

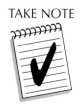

Before proceeding, let's stop and consider the word partnership *and its implications for community health nursing. Recall that a* community *is a social group determined by geographic boundaries and common values and interests. Community members function and interact within a particular social structure that both creates and exhibits behaviors and values. The normative behaviors and value systems of individuals, families, and the community that you have assessed may be very different from your own individual and family behaviors and values as well as the shared values of the community in which you reside. This creates a potential conflict. What may appear to you as a primary health problem of the community (for example, the incomplete immunization status at Temple Elementary in Rosemont) may not hold the same importance for the community's residents. They may be far more concerned about the possibility of being criminally victimized. Hence, there is a real need to* validate *community nursing diagnoses with the community. There is one question to ask: Are the community nursing diagnoses of importance to community residents? Methods of validating community nursing diagnoses will be presented in this chapter.*

Validating your community nursing diagnoses with the community residents is an important step for establishing and maintaining the partnership. Equally important is the right of community leaders, organizations, and residents to confidentiality of privileged information and their right to choose *not to participate* in health planning. Communities have the right to identify their own health needs and to negotiate with the community health nurse with regard to interventions and specific programs. In turn, the community health nurse has the responsibility to provide or assist with the development of information needed for this process. The American Nurses' Association's *Code for Nurses with Interpretive Standards* (1985) provides a guide for the many human rights issues that the community health nurse encounters.

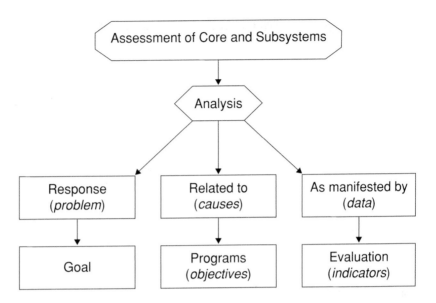

FIGURE 9-1
Using a community nursing diagnosis to plan.

In addition to forming a partnership with the community, the community health nurse must consider the influences of social, economic, ecological, and political issues. Many (if not all) community health issues are directly and profoundly affected by larger policy issues. The high prevalence of dental caries among youngsters at Temple Elementary is related as much to the lack of fluoride in Rosemont's drinking water as it is to the lack of dental hygiene education at the school. In turn, each etiologic antecedent is influenced by city, county, state, and national legislative actions and policies. None of the nursing diagnoses for Rosemont can be considered to be separate from the remaining diagnoses; all diagnoses document the health status of Rosemont and must be considered as a whole during the community-focused planning.

Additional considerations of the nurse who is involved in community-focused health planning are the health needs of populations at risk. Special at-risk groups reside in all communities—the homeless, the poor, persons who are infected with HIV, pregnant women, infants, children, and the elderly are groups at increased risk for decreased health status.

The health needs of at-risk groups must be considered as part of all community health plans.

Lastly, community-focused planning involves an awareness and application of planned change—a process of well-thought-out actions to make something happen. Planned change is discussed in detail later in this chapter.

Validating Community Nursing Diagnoses

In reviewing the community nursing diagnoses for Rosemont (see Table 8-9), it can be seen that several diagnoses focus on the health status of

---

Community Nursing Diagnosis for Rosemont by Population Group

Children
- Potential for accidents (for example, trauma or suffocation as children explore abandoned machinery)

Specific to children at Temple Elementary:
- Truancy and academic failure
- Incomplete immunization status
- High prevalence of *capitis pediculosis*
- High prevalence of dental caries
- Lack of health promotion information including nutrition, exercise, and safety

Infants
- High infant, neonatal, and fetal mortality rate

Male Homosexuals
- Stress within Rosemont between the homosexual and heterosexual populations (especially the heterosexual elderly)
- Potential for inadequate coping of persons with sexually transmitted diseases (STDs)

All Rosemont Residents
- Stress and anxiety of being criminally victimized
- Potential for health problems associated with air pollution
- At Rosemont Health Center, unsafe working environment

---

children and others on the health of special groups such as the Asian and homosexual male populations. Many diagnoses seem to affect all residents, such as the stress and anxiety of being criminally victimized. It may be helpful to stop and review your community nursing diagnoses and categorize them according to the population most affected. A categorization of Rosemont's diagnoses appears in the displayed material, *Community Nursing Diagnoses for Rosemont by Population Group.*

Because several diagnoses focus on children and because the age and dependency status of children place them at increased risk of decreased health status, a decision was made to begin the planning process by validating the diagnoses that focused on children.

Planned Change

We all experience change. As you read these words, your knowledge level is changing. Yet *planned change* differs from *change* in that actions occur in a definite sequence, with each one serving as preparation for the next. Planned change is a well-thought-out effort designed to make something happen; all efforts are directed and targeted to produce change. (Many theorists have written about planned change; several works are listed at the end of this chapter.) Reinkemeyer's stages of planned change are presented in the displayed material. The stages are

Reinkemeyer's Stages of Planned Change

Stage 1   Development of a felt need and desire for the change
Stage 2   Development of a change relationship between the agent and the client system
Stage 3   Clarification or diagnosis of the client system's problem, need, or objective
Stage 4   Examination of alternative routes and tentative goals and intentions of actions
Stage 5   Transformation of intentions into actual change
Stage 6   Stabilization
Stage 7   Termination of the relationship between the change agent and the client system

Reinkemeyer, A. 1970. Nursing's need: Commitment to an ideology & change. Nursing Forum, 9(4), 340–355.

Lewin's Stages of Planned Change and Their Application to the Planning Process

Lewin's stages of planned change	Application to the Planning Process
>> ◆ Unfreezing	◆ Unfreezing
	● Identification of a need for change
>> >> ◆ Moving process	◆ Moving process
	● Presence of a change agent
	● Identification of problems
	● Consideration of alternatives
	● Adaptation of plan to circumstances
>> >> >> ◆ Refreezing	◆ Refreezing
	● Implementation of the plan
	● Stabilization of the situation

(Lewin, K. [1958]. Group decision and social change. In E. Maccoby (Ed.), Readings in social psychology *(3rd ed.). New York: Holt, Rinehart and Winston.*

like a recipe in that to produce the intended outcome, each step must be followed strictly and completely. One theorist, Kurt Lewin (1958), described three stages of planned change: *unfreezing, moving,* and *refreezing,* as shown in the displayed material on Lewin. It is during the unfreezing stage that the client system (in other words, the organization, community, or at-risk population) becomes aware of a problem and the need for change. Then the problem is diagnosed, and solutions to the problem are identified. From these alternative solutions one is chosen that seems most appropriate for the situation. In the moving stage, the change actually occurs. The problem is clarified, and the program for solving the problem is planned in detail and begun. Finally, the refreezing stage consists of the accomplished changes becoming integrated into the values of the client system. In this stage the idea is established and continues to be influential. Lewin also addressed forces that help or hinder change to occur, labeling them the *driving forces* and the *restraining forces,* respectively.

Theories of planned change are important because they can be used to guide and direct the planning process.

Applying Change Theory to Community Health Planning

To validate our nursing diagnoses and initiate the planning process, Reinkemeyer's stages of planned change have been chosen as a guide.

Stage 1: Development of a Felt Need and Desire for the Change

To initiate a felt need and desire for change within the Rosemont community, those organizations that reported actual or potential health concerns of youngsters were contacted, and a meeting was suggested in order to report the findings of the Rosemont community assessment. Meetings were arranged with the staffs of Temple Elementary, the Third Street Clinic, and the YMCA Indo-Chinese Refugee Program. During the meetings, input from all staff members was sought regarding their observations and perceptions of child health needs as well as their desire to become involved in a planned program of health promotion.

Temple Elementary requested that the assessment data be shared with representatives of the Parent Teacher Organization (PTO) as well as with the school's newly formed parent–teacher liaison group. Both the Third Street Clinic and the YMCA Indo-Chinese Refugee Program requested a presentation to their community advisory boards.

Stage 2: Development of a Change Relationship Between the Agent and the Client (Partner) System

Both Stages 1 and 2 were completed during the assessment presentations. All staff members were keenly aware of child health needs, and each organization desired to become involved in the planning process. To expedite planning, the *Rosemont Health Promotion Council* was formed. Each of the three organizations, Temple Elementary, the Third Street Clinic, and the YMCA Indo-Chinese Refugee Program, decided to send one staff member and one interested parent to the planning meetings. At this point the community health nurse functioned as a change agent to guide and facilitate but *not* to direct the planning process. The council elected a chairperson and agreed on meeting dates. The purpose of the council was to coordinate interagency planning for a community-focused health-promotion program.

Questionnaire to Validate Community Nursing Diagnosis

Dear Parent:

We are nursing students who are interested in learning more about what you think are the most important health needs of your family. Answering a few short questions will help us plan some information sessions for you about how to keep your family healthy. Please either place a √ in the appropriate box or fill in the line. Your participation is voluntary. All information is confidential, and you will not be identified in any way. If you have questions, please feel free to call us. Thank you.

Virginia Brown
Ricardo Guerrero
Ann Wang
Alice Washington

1. How many children do you have?
2. What are their ages?
3. If you have a baby, do you breast-feed? Yes[ ] No[ ]
4. If you have a baby, do you bottle-feed? Yes[ ] No[ ]
5. What other foods do you feed your baby?
6. What foods do you usually feed your children?
7. Would you like to know more about what to feed your baby and children to keep them healthy? Yes[ ] No[ ]
8. Would you like to know where you can take your children for health care, both when they are well and sick? Yes[ ] No[ ]
9. Check (√) the following common problems you would like to know more about.
   [ ] Vomiting
   [ ] Diarrhea
   [ ] Colds and allergies
   [ ] Skin rashes
   [ ] Cuts and falls
   [ ] Head lice
   [ ] Worms
   [ ] Fever
   [ ] Temper tantrums and angry behaviors
   [ ] Refusal to do homework or go to school
   [ ] Poor school grades

Questionnaire to Validate Community Nursing Diagnosis (continued)

10. Other concerns that you would like information about (this can include information for yourself, a friend, or a child):

    _____

    _____

11. Have you ever felt that you, a sibling, or another adult hurt your child when the child was punished? Yes[   ] No[   ]

12. Would you like to learn about ways to keep from hurting children when adults are angry? Yes[   ] No[   ]

13. Circle the best days and times for you to attend information sessions.

    Monday   am   pm
    Tuesday   am   pm
    Wednesday   am   pm
    Thursday   am   pm
    Friday   am   pm
    Saturday   am   pm
    Sunday   am   pm

14. Circle the best place for you to attend information sessions:
    Temple Elementary
    Third Street Clinic
    YMCA
    Other (specify where)

Stage 3: Clarification or Diagnosis of the Client System's Problem, Need, or Objective

Now the time had arrived to validate the community nursing diagnoses. At the conclusion of each presentation, the community health nurse proposed a survey questionnaire to assess the target population's perception of their health concerns. Revisions were solicited from staff and community groups, and the final, agreed-upon questionnaire is presented here. Notice that the questionnaire is directed to parents, yet the nursing diagnoses are focused on children. Why not ask the children? This suggestion was made by several council participants. Some members felt two questionnaires were necessary—one for the parents and one for the youngsters. What do you think? Because of the age of the youngsters (some had not learned how to read) and the associated time and costs of two questionnaires, it was decided to use one questionnaire directed at the parents.

Although the Rosemont questionnaire is focused on child health, the same format could be used to validate assessed health concerns of the elderly, well adults, teenagers, or pregnant women. The process of checking your assessed community data against the perceptions of the target population can be completed by a survey questionnaire (such as the one in the displayed material) that can be mailed or given as an interview. (An additional example of questions that may be used for validation is in the exemplar about rural Canada in Chapter 16.) Or you may choose to validate assessed data by interviewing community leaders and civic groups that are representative of the target population. The word *representative* is very important. For example, the Temple Elementary PTO would not be representative of parents in Rosemont because, as was noted during the assessment, most parents are not active in the organization.

Before we continue, a few words are needed about composing questionnaires. Everyone is confronted daily with people who are asking questions. Questionnaires arrive in the mail and people call on the phone. Frequently, the interviewees neither learn the purpose of the questionnaire nor how the information will be used. When you draft a questionnaire, begin with introductory information that states who you are and what the purpose of the questionnaire is. Emphasize that participation is voluntary and that the information given will be confidential. Sign your name and, if the questionnaire is to be mailed, include a phone number where you can be contacted. Write questions that can be answered quickly (the whole questionnaire should not take longer than 10 minutes to complete). Ideally, place all questions on one side of a standard 8½-inch by 11-inch piece of paper that, if it is to be mailed, can be refolded so that a return address shows. Before sharing the questionnaire with agencies or community residents, administer it informally to friends and family; any comments made (such as "What do you mean by . . .?" or "I don't understand . . .") signal the need for further rewriting and clarification.

Because Rosemont has a large population of Spanish- and Vietnamese-speaking residents, staff at Temple Elementary and the YMCA

Indo-Chinese Refugee Program volunteered to translate the questionnaire into these languages. The questionnaire was then ready for distribution.

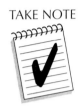

TAKE NOTE

How should the questionnaire be administered? Should the questionnaire be mailed to all households of children at Temple Elementary? Should the questionnaire be given to all adults who bring their children to the Third Street Clinic? Or should the questionnaire be used as an interview and given to a selected number of parents at Temple Elementary or to clients at the Third Street Clinic or to adults attending the YMCA Indo-Chinese Refugee Program? (Recall from research that persons who have been randomly selected can be considered representative of the total population.) What would you recommend? Before making a decision, list each option and consider the benefits and drawbacks of each. Here is some information for your decision making: Mailed questionnaires have about a 50% return rate that can be increased somewhat with a reminder postcard or telephone call, whereas questionnaires administered as an interview potentially have a 100% return rate. However, interviews require interviewers and about five minutes per person per page of questionnaire, whereas mailed questionnaires require less labor but have the financial cost of postage. Decisions . . . decisions . . .

Following several discussions of the Rosemont Health Promotion Council, it was decided to distribute the questionnaire from Temple Elementary by sending one form home with each child. The questionnaires were color-coded by language, and each child was given a questionnaire in the language that was spoken commonly at home.

Within two weeks, 410 of the 736 questionnaires had been returned. The results were tabulated and summarized by the community health nurse and the student nurses from the local university who were helping her. The summaries were then presented to the Rosemont Health Promotion Council. Examples of the summarized data are presented in Tables 9-1 through 9-4. Why do you think the information was presented by ethnicity? What differences do you notice between family composition and ethnicity, health information desired and ethnicity, and further concerns and ethnicity? Of what importance are these ethnic differences for community health planning?

TAKE NOTE

The Rosemont questionnaires were categorized by ethnicity (surmised from the language commonly spoken in the home). However, depending on the

TABLE 9-1   Family Composition by Ethnicity

NUMBER OF CHILDREN	Hispanic		Vietnamese		Other*	
	N	%	N	%	N	%
One only	82	57	44	61	31	16
Two children	12	8	3	4	112	58
Three children	24	17	10	14	34	18
Four or more children	26	18	15	21	17	8
Total	144	100	72	100	194	100

*Primarily white and black

community, responses may be categorized by urban versus rural residence, age of respondents, or other meaningful variables. Once summarized, no preferred day and time emerged for the classes. However, a definite preference was shown for location, with all Vietnamese-speaking families preferring the YMCA location and Spanish-speaking clients preferring the Third Street Clinic.

TABLE 9-2   Health Information Desired by Ethnicity

	Hispanic		Vietnamese		Other*	
	N	%	N	%	N	%
Vomiting	124	86	65	90	22	11
Diarrhea	134	93	71	98	34	18
Skin rashes	114	79	11	15	52	29
Cuts/falls	45	31	60	83	5	3
Colds/allergies	46	32	5	7	62	32
Head lice	24	17	10	14	74	38
Worms	85	59	70	97	10	5
Fever	132	92	69	96	93	48
Tantrums/angry behavior	10	7	4	5	175	90
School refusal	5	3	6	8	165	85
Poor grades	4	3	2	3	132	68
Total respondents	144		72		194	

*Primarily white and black

TABLE 9-3 Percentage of Respondents Noting Other Concerns by Ethnicity			
	HISPANIC (%)	VIETNAMESE (%)	OTHER (%)[*]
Legal issues (child support, custody rights)	32	15	64
Finances/budgeting	23	26	51
Child-care programs	82	12	75
Adult health (weight reduction, birth control)	75	11	68
Employment	82	95	75
Crime prevention, especially prevention of rape and child molestation	88	84	89

[*]Primarily white and black

Stage 4: Examination of Alternative Routes and Tentative Goals and Intention of Actions

Having validated the community nursing diagnoses, the Rosemont Health Promotion Council was anxious to establish a plan. Much discussion followed the presentation of the questionnaire results. Representatives from Temple Elementary focused on questions 9 and 10 and were anxious to present a series of effective parenting seminars on dis-

TABLE 9-4 Percentage of Respondents Answering Yes to Questions 11 and 12 by Ethnicity			
	Answered Yes		
	HISPANIC (%)	VIETNAMESE (%)	OTHER (%)[*]
Question 11: Have you ever felt that you, a sibling, or another adult hurt your child when the child was punished?	89	92	94
Question 12: Would you like to learn about ways to keep from hurting children when adults are angry?	94	95	98

[*]Primarily white and black

cipline. Temple also felt the high percentage of white and black families who requested information about school phobias and poor grades merited sessions on that topic. Temple's staff discussed how programs to meet the questionnaire needs were consistent with the school's goal of improved communication between teachers and parents as well as with the goals of their Failproof program. In addition, recent state programs developed to prevent child abuse were proposed for presentation.

The staff of the Third Street Clinic focused on the families with infants and the associated desire for information on nutrition and the care of common health conditions. The Third Street Clinic had recently initiated a Healthy Baby Program, consisting of evening and Saturday well child and prenatal clinics as well as a total service day on Friday when clients could drop in without appointments for immunizations and screening tests for blood pressure, vision, and hearing. Informal counseling was also offered on Friday. The goal for the next six months was to invite various service providers, such as optometry and dental hygiene students as well as Medicare and State Unemployment Commission representatives, to jointly use the clinic space for information sessions and services. After considering the results of the questionnaire, the staff began to discuss the possibility of offering health promotion classes on Fridays that would focus on weight reduction, exercise fitness, and information about common conditions. The idea of inviting the Police Department to make presentations on crime prevention and legal rights was proposed and agreed on by everyone.

Representatives from the YMCA Indo-Chinese Refugee Program felt that, because of cultural taboos against discussing topics such as birth control in public, the information would be best accepted if offered at the YMCA by a respected member of the Vietnamese community. The YMCA was beginning a day care service for mothers of preschoolers, and staff members felt that some of the information on child care could become part of the new program, as well as basic child health screening services of development, vision, and hearing. The YMCA representatives were equally concerned that Vietnamese refugees be culturally assimilated into the Rosemont community, and they wanted to plan interagency programs about crime prevention and legal rights that would bring the Vietnamese into more contact with other Rosemont residents. The suggestion was made that a program on crime prevention would bring not only residents of different cultures together but also residents of different lifestyles. Keenly aware of the tension and stress between the homosexual and heterosexual populations, a community awareness program on crime prevention was suggested that would involve all three agencies and all residents of Rosemont. The idea was agreed upon by all council members.

TAKE NOTE

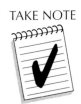

Notice that each agency is considering how information learned from the questionnaire can be assimilated into existing or planned programs. All agencies have budgets and a set number of staff members to deliver services. Agencies must be as cost-efficient as possible and will want to consider how to include new services (such as information desired by parents) into an existing program. Community health nurses can facilitate this process by becoming familiar with the organizational structure and purpose of each agency. When you establish a planned-change relationship with an agency, ask about their organizational structure (most agencies have an organizational chart with positions arranged according to authority). Decision making usually follows the organizational chart, with consent from all levels being required before major changes can be made or a new program can be begun. Learn the names of the staff members and their position on the organizational chart. (An organizational chart for the Third Street Clinic appears in Figure 9-2.) Ask for a statement of the agency's purpose and goals. Ask if you can attend a board meeting and pertinent committee meetings. Your purpose is to learn as much as possible about the services and decision-making process of the agency in order to facilitate the planned-change nursing interventions.

Community Health Goal

Now is the time to transform the ideas and proposals of each agency into a community-focused goal and concrete intentions of action. After validating the nursing diagnoses with the community, the community-focused goal was this: *to provide health-promotion programs on issues desired by the community residents, using methods acceptable to cultural norms and offered in an accessible location at a cost the community can afford.*

This is a very comprehensive statement and can be considered to be an umbrella goal for the Rosemont community under which each agency will have goals. Goals specific to Temple Elementary included

- Reduce truancy 20% by the end of one school year
- Reduce grade failures 20% by the end of one school year

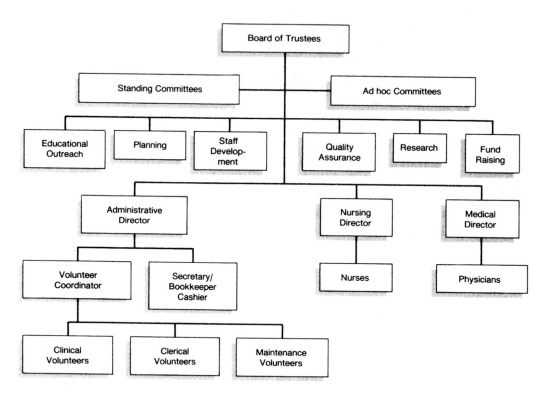

FIGURE 9-2
Organizational chart—Third Street Clinic.

- Increase immunization levels to 95% within one year
- Improve communication between parents and teachers
- Increase parental knowledge on how to protect children from molestation

Goals for the Third Street Clinic that were congruent with the community goal included

- Increased knowledge of community residents regarding crime prevention and legal rights
- Increased knowledge of parents regarding common health problems of children
- Increased knowledge and practice of effective parenting skills

- Increased percentage of adults who practice healthy lifestyle practices, including
  —Exercise fitness
  —Weight control
  —Stress management

Goals for the YMCA Indo-Chinese Refugee Program included

- 100% of children in the day care program screened for vision and hearing problems
- Increased knowledge and correct use of contraceptives
- Increased knowledge of parents regarding common health problems of children
- Increased rate of employed adults by 50%
- Increased rate of employed teenagers by 20%
- Increased knowledge of community residents regarding crime prevention and legal rights

Program Activities

After formulation of goals, the next step is specifying the program activities. *Program activities* map out the actions necessary to deliver the program and thereby reach the goal(s). For example, one goal of the Third Street Clinic was *increased knowledge of parents regarding health problems of children.* Program activities for the goal might include

- Third Street Clinic staff and the community health nurse will select topics that are congruent with the questionnaire results to be included in classes for parents on common health problems of children.
- Third Street Clinic staff and the community health nurse will select resources (such as audiovisual aids and pamphlets) for presentation on the selected topics.
- Third Street Clinic staff and the community health nurse will decide on a day, time, and presentation schedule that are congruent with the questionnaire results.

Each program activity deals with planning the program and is written as sequential steps, each step being required to reach the goal. In addition, each program activity needs a date of accomplishment (for example: "By June 15, the Third Street Clinic staff and the community health nurse will . . .").

Learning Objectives

Once program activities have been established, learning objectives are written. *Learning objectives* are derived from a goal and describe the precise behavior or changes that will be required to achieve the goal. Whereas program activities map out the actions necessary to deliver the program, learning objectives specify what changes in knowledge, behaviors, or attitudes are expected as a result of program activities.

Learning objectives focus on the learner and state what changes the learner can expect as a result of participating in the program. For example, one topic selected for presentation during the classes on common health problems of children was fever assessment and home management. The learning objectives were as follows:

- Following the class and practice session on fever assessment and management of the fever at home, each participant will be able to
  —Demonstrate how to take a rectal and axillary temperature
  —Discuss common causes and dangers of fever during childhood
  —State what constitutes a fever
  —Explain at least three methods to reduce a fever
  —Describe danger signs that require a medical assessment

Both program and learning objectives can be written in sequential steps that are required to reach the goal, or each objective may have different aspects that, when combined, achieve the goal. Goals and objectives need to be *measurable*. To make statements measurable, use precise words. Examples of precise terms and less precise terms appear below:

Less Precise Terms (many interpretations)
To know
To understand
To realize

To appreciate
To be aware
To lower

More Precise Terms (fewer interpretations)

To identify
To discuss
To list
To compare and contrast
To state
To decrease by 20%

In addition, strive for each goal and objective to include

- A time frame for attaining the change; for example, "By June 15th . . ."
- The direction and magnitude of the change; for example, "Increase immunization levels to 95%"
- The method of measuring the change; for example, "Following the session, each participant will demonstrate . . ."

Goals and subparts of the goals (objectives) help to clarify a program and establish the expected changes that will result from the program. Although much has been written on the mechanics of writing goals and objectives (several such texts are listed at the conclusion of this chapter), little information exists on the collaborative relationship that must exist between community health nurse and community agency(ies) before meaningful goals and objectives can result.

Collaboration

What is meant by a collaborative relationship? Recall from the initial community assessment data that the staff of Temple Elementary had voiced concerns about truancy and grade failure; these same concerns are their first two goals. However, when the nursing diagnoses were validated with the community, parents were more concerned about ways in which they could protect their children from molestation. Could the concerns of the parents and those of the Temple Elementary staff be addressed in the same program? If they could, what would be the program objective? the content objectives? This process is an example of *collaborative planning* and is the essence of community health nursing. You may be wondering how to establish collaborative planning and inform agencies about the usefulness of goals and objectives. Although you may be convinced of the value of planned change, how do you convince others to agree, especially since planned change is not commonly practiced in agencies? *Role modeling* is probably the best strategy. After reviewing the community nursing diagnoses and validating data with an agency, propose goals and objectives that are congruent with the agency's purpose and organizational structure. Solicit input from the group and continue to revise the goals and objectives until a group consensus is reached.

Resources, Constraints, and Revised Plans

Once goals and objectives are written, the next step is to identify available resources and any constraints to the plan. Lastly, revised plans are proposed to the planning group. *Resources* are all the available means for accomplishing a task, including staff and budget as well as physical space and equipment. For program planning, it is important to identify the *resources needed* as well as the *resources available. Constraints* are obstacles that restrict or limit actions and can include a lack of staff, budget, physical space, and equipment. Constraints may be thought of as the difference between needs and resources. *Revised plans* are actions that are proposed based on the knowledge of resources and constraints.

Following much discussion and self-examination, each agency of the Rosemont Health Promotion Council formed program goals and objectives. Then, alongside each goal and objective, necessary resources were listed. For example, at the Third Street Clinic, the following resources were identified as crucial to the goal.

GOAL

To increase the knowledge of parents regarding common health problems of children

Resources Needed

- Staff member to develop and assemble existing information on common health problems of children
- Staff member to present the information materials in English, Spanish, and Vietnamese
- Physical space and necessary equipment (thermometers, basins) to teach assessment and home care skills

Resources Available

- Staff members who speak English and Spanish
- Staff nurse with knowledge about the care of children
- Physical space and some necessary equipment
- Staff interest and desire to offer information requested by parents

Constraints

It may be helpful to consider constraints as the mismatch between resources needed and resources available. Constraints at the Third Street Clinic include

- No staff member who speaks Vietnamese
- Discomfort of staff because of inexperience in developing and adapting learning materials
- Time limitations
- Staff members' insecurity about their ability to perform group teaching (all previous teaching was one-on-one)
- Lack of resource material (for example, audio-visuals and brochures on care of common childhood problems)

TAKE NOTE

Universal constraints are staff and money—agencies never have enough. An additional constraint is resistance to change. All people are reluctant to change existing routines and patterns of behavior. Initially, change is uncomfortable, and until new roles are learned, there is anxiety. Making people aware of the natural discomfort associated with change can build rapport and establish a collaborative relationship.

When each agency had listed its program goals, activities, and objectives along with resources and constraints, several alternative actions became apparent. For example, a constraint of the Third Street

Clinic was lack of staff members who spoke Vietnamese. A similar constraint of the YMCA Indo-Chinese Refugee Program was lack of a staff with necessary knowledge to offer classes on contraception or the care of children with common health problems. Therefore, the following revised plan was proposed:

REVISED PLAN

A bilingual (English–Vietnamese) staff member from the YMCA would attend the classes offered in English at the Third Street Clinic and then offer the classes in Vietnamese at the YMCA.

Both the Third Street Clinic and the YMCA noted a lack of resource materials as a constraint to program implementation. However, further assessment of community health resources by the community health nurse revealed that the Sunvalley Clinic, as part of the Hampton Health Department, had access to various audiovisual aids and printed materials on the subjects; however, all materials were in English.

REVISED PLAN

One Spanish–English-speaking staff member from the Third Street Clinic and one Vietnamese–English-speaking staff member from the YMCA would translate the materials into Spanish and Vietnamese free of charge with the provision that they be given copies of all the translated materials.

An additional constraint to each agency was that their staffs felt unprepared to do group instruction.

REVISED PLAN

The community health nurse would provide instruction in basic principles of group teaching, including methods of presenting information. In addition, the community health nurse would participate in the development and adaptation of materials and the teaching of classes.

For each constraint, a revised plan was proposed, discussed, and adopted. This is a period of intense collaboration between the community health nurse and community agencies, and only at the completion of this stage is the community ready for Stage 5 of planned change—transformation of intentions into actual change behavior. This *transformation of intentions* is the actual program implementation (which is covered in the next chapter). However, before the plan is implemented, it must be recorded.

Recording

Community plans must be recorded in a standardized, systematic, and concise form that clearly communicates to others the purpose and actions of the plan as well as the rationale for revisions and deletions of actions. Discuss with each agency its present recording system and decide on a

Format for Recording a Community Health Plan

Agency: Third Street Clinic
Community Nursing Diagnoses Specific to Children
- Potential for decreased health status of children
- Incomplete immunization status of elementary-school-age children
- High prevalence of *capitus pediculosis* among elementary-school-age children

Validation Data
- Questionnaire sent to 736 families and returned by 410

Program Goal
- Increase knowledge of parents in regard to common health problems of children

Program Activities
- Third Street Clinic staff and the community health nurse will select topics to be included in classes that are congruent with questionnaire results.
- Third Street Clinic staff and the community health nurse will select resources (audiovisual aids, pamphlets) for presentation of the selected topics.
- Third Street Clinic staff and the community health nurse will decide on a day, time, and presentation schedule that is congruent with the questionnaire results.   *(continued)*

Format for Recording a Community Health Plan (continued)

Learning Objectives

Following the class and practice session on fever assessment and home management, each participant will be able to

- Demonstrate how to take a rectal and axillary temperature
- Discuss common causes and dangers of fever during childhood
- State what constitutes a fever
- Explain at least three methods to reduce a fever
- Describe danger signs that require a medical assessment

Resources

- Needed   Staff member to develop and assemble information on common health problems of children

  Staff member to present the information materials in English, Spanish, and Vietnamese

  Physical space and necessary equipment (thermometer, basins) to teach assessment and homecare skills

- Available   Staff members who speak English and Spanish

  Staff nurse with knowledge about the care of children

  Physical space and some necessary equipment

  Staff interest and desire to offer information requested by parents

- Constraints   No staff member who speaks Vietnamese

  Discomfort related to lack of experience in developing and adapting learning materials

  Time constraints

  Insecurities in staff's abilities to implement group teaching experience (all previous teaching was one-on-one)

  Lack of resource material (audiovisual aids, and brochures on care of common childhood problems)

Revised Plans

- A bilingual (English–Vietnamese) staff member from the Third Street Clinic and one Vietnamese–English-speaking staff member from the "Y" will translate needed materials into Spanish and Vietnamese free of charge, with the provision to have copies of all the translated materials.
- The community health nurse would provide instruction in basic principles of group teaching, including methods of presenting information. In addition, the community health nurse would participate in the development and adaptation of materials, as well as the teaching of the classes.

format and system for recording the plan. The format need not be elaborate, and a simple one such as that used at the Third Street Clinic would be adequate *if* agreed upon by the agency (see the displayed material).

Summary

Before concluding, let's review the learning objectives for this chapter and their application to community health nursing. The planning process begins with validation of the community nursing diagnoses—a process that establishes the community's perception and value of community health needs. Next, using theories of planned change, the community health nurse and the community form a collaborative partnership to establish program goals and objectives. Last, based on resources and constraints, plans are proposed, recorded, and adopted. Although only one example is offered here, the process of community health planning was the same for all eight programs that were developed by the Rosemont Health Promotion Council.

REFERENCES

American Nurses' Association. (1985). *Code for nurses with interpretive standards.* Kansas City, MO: Author.

Lewin, K. (1958). Group decision and social change. In E. Maccoby (Ed.), *Readings in social psychology,* (3rd ed.). New York: Holt, Rinehart and Winston.

Reinkemeyer, A. 1970. Nursing's need: Commitment to an ideology & change. *Nursing Forum, 9*(4), 340–355.

SUGGESTED READINGS

Archer, S.E. (1984). *Implementing change in community: A collaborative process.* St. Louis: C.V. Mosby.

Bertera, R.L. (1990). Planning and implementing health promotion in the workplace: A case study of the DuPont Company experience. *Health Education Quarterly, 17*(3), 307–327.

deVries, H., Weijts, W., Dijkstra, M., & Kok, G. (1992). The utilization of qualitative and quantitative data for health education program planning, implementation, and evaluation: A spiral approach. *Health Education Quarterly, 19*(1), 101–115.

Ervin, N.E., & Kuehnert, P.L. (1993). Application of a model for public health nursing program planning. *Public Health Nursing, 10*(1), 25–30.

Lippitt, G. (1973). *Visualizing change: Model building and the change process.* La Jolla, CA: University Associates.

Lippitt, R., Watson, J., Westley, B. (1951). *The dynamics of planned change.* New York: Harcourt, Brace and World.

10

Implementing a Community Health Program

Objectives

Implementation is the action phase of the nursing process: carrying out the community-focused plan. Implementation is necessary to achieve goals and objectives, but more importantly, the implementation of nursing interventions acts to promote, maintain, or restore health; to prevent illness; and to effect rehabilitation.

This chapter discusses the process of implementing a community-focused health program. Intervention strategies are presented, as well as resources that are helpful in program implementation.

After studying this chapter, you should be able to

- Suggest strategies to the community for implementation of health programs

In partnership with the community, you should be able to

- Implement planned programs
- Review and revise interventions based on community responses
- Use interventions to formulate and influence health and social policies that have an impact on the health of the community

Introduction

Once goals and objectives have been agreed on and recorded during the planning stage, all that remains for implementation is to actually carry out those objectives. This probably seems straightforward and simple. Indeed, at this point you will have spent considerable time assessing, analyzing, and planning a program. You will be ready and eager to begin. But this very eagerness (and the associated impatience of the intervention stage) is a danger. You must take time to consider how you can promote community ownership, a unified program, and a clear health focus.

TAKE NOTE

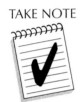

This chapter focuses on the process *of intervention and provides you with some general resources that may prove helpful in your community work. Many excellent examples of interventions in which the community health nurses work together as a partner with the community are included in Part III.*

Community Ownership

Essential to achieving the desired outcomes of the interventions is the active participation of the community. The meaning of partnership and collaboration was discussed in the preceding chapter, but the present concern is *ownership.* The people of the community need to feel a sense of ownership of the program or event, which can only come with their full participation in the decisions regarding planning as well as their assuming some responsibility for implementation. Herein lies a potential conflict. The profession of nursing is one of nurturing, sustaining, and caring for others. It is part of our profession to do for others what they would do for themselves if they were able. Indeed, most nurses interact professionally with people during an altered health state that requires nurses to do for others; but this is not true in community health nursing. Stepping into the community requires an attitude of doing *with* the people, not doing things to them or for them. When things are done to us or for us, our emotional commitment remains limited.

How might you ensure community ownership for a proposed program and planned interventions? How can you facilitate involvement? In Rosemont, the Rosemont Health Promotion Council functioned to coordinate interagency planning for a community-focused health-promotion program. When the planning had been completed, the council directed its attention to the coordination of activities for the program's implementation. The important point in this example is that a coordination group was already in place. Usually the planning committee can coordinate implementation.

TAKE NOTE

When the Rosemont Health Promotion Council and designated staff in charge of program implementation reviewed the program objectives and needed resources, it was evident that before the program could proceed, resources had to be selected. (Resources means audiovisual aids, pamphlets, and other material for presentation of the program.) Council and staff members began to ask where such materials could be obtained. What was available in Rosemont? What could you have suggested at this point?

Examining the initial assessment of Rosemont, it was noted that the United Way listed 42 private and publicly supported social service agencies located in Hampton or Jefferson County. The United Way listing included identifying information for each agency as well as services and fees. Reviewing the list with the council and participating staff, the community health nurse suggested that selected agency representatives be invited to discuss programs and resources that they could make available, such as films and speakers. It was found that several could provide relevant material. The March of Dimes was sponsoring a campaign in Hampton to increase public awareness of the importance of a healthy pregnancy for the birth of a healthy child. The Mental Health Association had developed teaching modules on effective parenting, and the police department and the Woman's Center were offering programs on crime prevention. All of these programs had recently received a brief description, including the names of their contact persons, in the *Hampton Herald*. At this point, it was decided to complete program and learning objectives for each of the health-promotion goals established by the Rosemont Council. Therefore, as various agency personnel discussed their program with the council, decisions could be made on the appropriateness of the material for the Rosemont Community.

TAKE NOTE

Do not panic at this point and feel that you must be knowledgeable about all 42 agencies and their programs in the community that you have assessed. At the implementation stage, do refer back to your initial assessment and consider logically which service agencies may have resources helpful to the planned program(s). Then contact selected agencies, request information on their purpose and present programs, share with the agency your community-focused program plans, and solicit recommendations with regard to materials and resources. In the displayed material, a list is presented of voluntary organizations that have professional staff at the national and local levels and an affiliated or community linkage structure. These voluntary organizations have

Voluntary Organizations

Name of Organization

American Association of
  Retired Persons
American Cancer Society
American Heart Association
American Lung Association
American Red Cross
Association of Junior Leagues, Inc.
Boy Scouts of America
Boy's Clubs of America
Cooperative Extension Service
Girl Scouts of America
Girls' Clubs of America, Inc.

March of Dimes
National Board of the YMCA of the U.S.A.
National Coalition of Hispanic Mental
  Health and Human Services
  Organizations (COSSHMO)
National Council of Alcoholism
National Health Council
National Kidney Foundation
National Safety Council
National Recreation and Parks Association
National Urban League
United Way of America

ongoing programs for a wide variety of health issues, and most acknowledge health promotion as a vital part of their mission. The list is not inclusive and is meant to serve only as a guide.

In addition, the Office of Disease Prevention and Health Promotion (ODPHP), located within the Public Health Service (PHS) (which, in turn, is located within the U.S. Department of Health and Human Services [DHHS]), publishes a tremendous amount of information that is designed to promote health and prevent disease among Americans. Special attention is given to facilitating the prevention activities of the five public health service agencies: the Alcohol, Drug Abuse, and Mental Health Administration; the Centers for Disease Control (CDC); the Food and Drug Administration (FDA); the Health Resources and Services Administration (HRSA); and the National Institutes of Health (NIH). Several special programs, termed *initiatives,* are sponsored by the Office of Disease Prevention and Health Promotion. A partial listing of the initiative programs, services, and information available, as well as addresses and phone contacts, are listed in Table 10-1.

TAKE NOTE

Several libraries are designated as government depositories and therefore have many government publications. The government also has bookstores located throughout the United States. Make yourself familiar with the nearest govern-

TABLE 10-1 *Office of Disease Prevention and Health Promotion: Special Initiatives*	
Initiative	**Description**
Community/Media Health Promotion Initiative	The National Health Promotion Program has used media-based efforts to mobilize community resources for health promotion. Activities for the general public include the HealthStyle campaign as well as the Healthy Mothers Healthy Babies program. Now attention is being directed to older Americans with the initiative Health Promotion for the Elderly. This initiative is designed to use the media and community organizations to enhance the health practices of older people with respect to diet, exercise, smoking, alcohol use, and appropriate use of medications and preventive services.*
National Health Information Clearinghouse (NHIC)	The NHIC responds directly to requests for health information from both the general public and health professions. The clearinghouse is a central source of information and referral for health questions. It answers questions in two ways: by retrieving information from the NHIC's onsite library and database or by forwarding requests to other organizations for direct response. The NHIC staff only provide health information; they cannot give medical advise, diagnose, or recommend treatment. Materials available from the NHIC include health-risk appraisals and a list of physical fitness organizations and centers concerned with health topics.*
School Health Initiative	Focus is to enhance the health of schoolchildren by undertaking comprehensive health-oriented efforts such as the assessment of the fitness level of schoolchildren, development of a special review on the use of computers for health education, and an evaluation of curricula developed for school health education. Summary reports on school health are available as well as information material for a school health program. A listing of reports and published material are available from the Office of Disease Prevention and Health Promotion.*
Put Prevention Into Practice (PPIP)	This is a prevention implementation program that works in cooperation with major health-related voluntary groups and provider organizations (for example, ANA). Its purpose is to help achieve the HP/DP objectives for the nation in *Healthy People 2000*. Clinicians are provided a kit of materials to assist them in the performance of a broad range of clinical preventive services.
Worksite Health Promotion Initiative	Focus is to enhance the health of employees and their families by offering materials to assist in the development of worksite programs, case studies of the health promotion activities of businesses, a national survey of worksite health promotion activities, and projects to explore the future of work and health. Summary reports on worksite health are available as well as information material for a worksite health program. A listing of reports and published material are available from the ODPHP.*

Additional information about these activities and other ODPHP publications may be obtained from the Office of Disease Prevention and Health Promotion, P.O. Box 1133, Washington, DC 20013-1133; Telephone (202) 245-7611.

ment depository library and bookstore. The Suggested Readings list for this chapter contains several government publications that are focused on disease prevention and health promotion.

Having discussed the importance of community participation and ownership of the program, the remaining issues to consider are a unified presentation of the program and an emphasis on health, not the program.

Unified Program

Because of limited resources, staff constraints, and other situations beyond the control of the planners, many good programs are implemented in a piecemeal fashion that minimizes their impact. A *unified program* requires collaboration and coordination between the agency personnel who will implement the program and the program's recipients (the target population). Allowing plenty of time for publicizing the program (and how you perform the mechanics of publicity—the *how, where,* and *to whom*)—can make a crucial difference in whether people attend and what the subsequent impact will be.

After a time and place have been selected (based on initial input from the survey questionnaires), how might you publicize a program? Public service announcements, notification in the newspapers, bulletin inserts for civic and religious associations, flyers sent home with school-age children, and posters and notices in community service buildings and local shopping centers are some of the methods to consider. The Rosemont Health Promotion Council decided to publicize the first program on child health by sending home a flyer with each child at Temple Elementary. The flyer thanked the parents for their participation during the survey and invited them to programs at the Third Street Clinic and the YMCA Indo-Chinese Refugee Center. Public service announcements were made on the radio, and feature articles about the Rosemont Health Promotion Council and upcoming programs appeared in the Vietnamese and Spanish newspapers as well as in the *Hampton Herald* and Rosemont Civic Association's newsletter. Posters were placed in local grocery stores, churches, and gathering places. Because the parents on the Rosemont Health Promotion Council had expressed a concern that parents with young children might not be able to attend programs, arrangements were made for infant and toddler childcare, and a separate health program for preschool and school-age children was planned during the adult programs. The program publicity was focused on health promotion for the *whole family* and not just on programs for selected family members.

The idea of a health program based on unified goals and objectives is central to the document *Healthy People—The Surgeon General's Report on Health Promotion and Disease Prevention* (1979), the first overall health policy statement from the U.S. government. This same concern underpins the sequel documents by the U.S. Department of Health and Human Services, *Promoting Health/Preventing Disease: Objectives for the Nation* (1980) and *Healthy People 2000—National Health Promotion and Disease Prevention Objectives* (1990). These comprehensive plans are not federal plans, to be administered from Washington, but rather plans to be implemented by the citizens of every community. Attainment of the goals and objectives of the latest plan by the year 2000 depends on the participation of state and local health agencies and organizations (both public and private), such as the one you will be working with in your practice as well as the Rosemont Health Promotion Council. Because the national goals and objectives offer guidance for local health program implementation, the following text discusses the specifics of some of them.

Healthy People

In *Healthy People 2000,* three major goals were identified:

- Increase the span of healthy life for Americans
- Reduce health disparities among Americans
- Achieve access to preventive services for all Americans

In addition, age-related objectives were formulated. The following are the age-related objectives relevant to the Rosemont community:

- For *infants,* the goal is to reduce the infant mortality rate to no more than 7 per 1,000 live births. (NOTE: "Infant mortality rates provide a summary measure of the effects of major health threats to the developing fetus and newborn baby. But for every 10 babies who die, 990 live. Some of those who live have been harmed, often permanantly, by unhealthy beginnings. The quality, not just the quantity, of their lives is a function of health during both the prenatal and infant periods" [U.S. Department of Health and Human Services, 1990, p. 9]).

Other important goals for infants are

—To reduce low-birth-weight incidence (the greatest single hazard to infant health is low birth weight)

—To reduce congenital anomalies (the leading cause of infant mortality)

- For *children aged 1 to 14,* the goal is a 15% lower death rate (this would be fewer than 28 deaths per 100,000 population by 2000, compared with 33 in 1987). The leading cause of death in childhood is unintentional injury.

- For *adolescents and young adults, aged 15 to 24,* the goal is a 15% lower death rate (this would mean decreasing the death rate from 99.4 per 100,000 population in 1987 to fewer than 85 in 1990). (NOTE: "The dominant preventable health problems of adolescents and young adults fall into two major categories: injuries and violence that kill and disable many before they reach age 25 and emerging lifestyles that affect their health many years later" [Ibid., p. 17].)

- Subgoals for adolescents and young adults are related to reducing death and disability from motor vehicle accidents and from the misuse of alcohol and drugs.

- For *adults aged 25 to 64,* the goal is a 20% lower death rate (decreasing from 423 per 100,000 population in 1987 to fewer than 340 in 1990).

- Subgoals focus on the reduction of the number one killers: cancer, heart disease, and stroke.

- For *adults aged 65 and over,* the goal is to reduce to no more than 90 per 1,000 people the proportion who have difficulty in performing two or more personal care activities (a reduction of about 19%), thereby preserving independence.

- Related subgoals focus on the improvement of functional independence and quality as well as length of life.

The same report identified improvements in 21 priority areas that are necessary in order to reach the goals. The target areas fit into three categories: health promotion, health protection, and their preventive services. A listing of the three categories and their priority areas is included in the accompanying displayed material.

Priority Areas Identified in Healthy People 2000

Health Promotion

1. Physical activity and fitness
2. Nutrition
3. Tobacco
4. Alcohol and other drugs
5. Family planning
6. Mental health and mental disorders
7. Violent and abusive behavior
8. Educational and community-based programs

Health Protection

9. Unintentional injuries
10. Occupational safety and health
11. Environmental health
12. Food and drug safety
13. Oral health

Preventive Services

14. Maternal and infant health
15. Heart disease and stroke
16. Cancer
17. Diabetes and chronic disabling conditions
18. HIV infection
19. Sexually transmitted diseases
20. Immunization and infectious diseases
21. Clinical preventive services

(From U.S. Department of Health and Human Services (1990), p. 7)

Health promotion denotes programs to educate the public about the risks that are involved in health abuses and to increase public commitment to sensible lifestyles that can add years to life expectancy (and quality to life). *Health protection* includes the efforts made by government, industry, and other organizations to reduce health hazards in the environment. *Preventive services* are usually offered by health care providers and mostly to individuals.

Objectives for each area were developed by a process of including as many people as possible. Hearings were held across the nation, and experts were invited to provide documentation and testimony as well as to give opinions on realistic and relevant targets for the goals. Extensive public review was incorporated into the many drafts of the goals and objectives.

The objectives are keyed to the priority areas in the three groups mentioned previously (personal preventive services, health protection, and health promotion). Each includes a percentage or proportion of people targeted, a measurable outcome, and, when available, baseline figures. The time frame for each objective is understood to be the year 2000, because that is the overriding end point. An example is the following: *Reduce pregnancies among girls aged 17 and younger to no more than 50 per 1000 adolescents.* (Baseline: 71.1 pregnancies per 1000 girls aged 15 through 17 in 1985). NOTE: The objectives are population-based (that is, all persons in the targeted population are included). If we look at a segment (or special set) of the population, for instance, black teenage girls, then the baseline figure is quite different (actually 186 in 1985, not 71.1), and the objective would need to be modified accordingly (120, not 50). If we use the objectives as guides as we work in our own community, we need to be sure we are dealing with comparable groups.

The target areas that particularly need local involvement and programs are those in health promotion. Health promotion is the most difficult area in which to achieve change and to measure progress, because it requires that millions of citizens change their daily habits and modify their lifestyles. The relationship between smoking and health is obvious and proven, yet millions of Americans continue to puff away their lives. Misuse of alcohol and drugs, control of stress, and violent behavior are additional examples of major target areas that must be addressed to promote health.

Cities, counties, regions, and states have used this list of objectives for the nation in many interesting ways. Health agencies are using them to assess existing programs, to determine where additional programs are needed, and to restructure existing programs. A complementary document is *Healthy Communities 2000: Model Standards,* published by the American Public Health Association, which "puts the objectives into practice and encourages communities to establish achievable community health targets" (American Public Health Association, 1991, p. ix). This publication offers formats for setting specific community objectives. For example, the following format appears:

By _____ (year to be filled in) the incidence of motor vehicle-related disabling injuries for children under 15 years will be reduced to _____ (level to be filled in). (American Public Health Association, 1991, p.15)

This type of format allows each community flexibility in setting both its time frame and level of accomplishment. (References to all three documents plus additional federal documents dealing with national health objectives have been included in the Suggested Readings list at the end of this chapter.) Use the national goals and objectives as well as the model standards to guide your own participation in developing community intervention programs that are unified and relevant.

TAKE NOTE

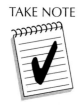

We are reminded in the Healthy Communities document that there may be a tendency to use the national objective targets as targets for community standards. Each community, its authors point out, needs to determine an appropriate and useful target for the future, and one way to do this is to look at past trends. Have you been able to compare trends in your own assessment?

Are the goals and objectives for your community realistic in terms of the past and in relation to trends over time? Do the goals and objectives for your community-focused program further the national goals and objectives? When the Rosemont Health Promotion Council reviewed its goals and objectives, each was found to be congruent with the national plan as well as with Rosemont's state health department objectives for improved health.

Health Focus

There is one remaining question to ask before initiating the program: Does it focus on health? This may seem to be a strange question. You might wonder, don't all community health programs focus on maintaining, restoring, or promoting health? Frequently, the answer is *no*.

In Rosemont, the council and designated staff had become very involved in planning specific activities and information modules associated with the community health program. Several programs had been enlarged to include screening and health fairs; additional activities were suggested at each council meeting. The initial goal of promoting the health of Rosemont residents had seemingly changed to providing Rosemont residents with lots of activities and information *about* health.

What had happened? Remember, we discussed the impatience and eagerness that is often associated with new programs. This situation is normal. Committees tend to overemphasize activities and knowledge and forget the initial reason for the program—to improve health. But it should be remembered that it is the sustained day-to-day use of knowledge and lifestyle practices that improve health. Frequently, a program begins with enthusiastic momentum; media publicity attracts people to screening and information sessions—and then the program is over. Objectives are evaluated as having been achieved successfully, and another program is planned and implemented. But was there any real improvement in health? Did the participants *change lifestyle practices?* Will the changes be maintained and continued for a week? a month? a year? Most importantly, are the changed lifestyle or health practices supported by the surrounding *environment and culture?*

Environmental and Cultural Support

Many parents in Rosemont responded affirmatively to the survey questions about discipline. These parents had felt that they or another person had hurt a child when the child was punished; the parents wanted to learn ways to keep from hurting children when adults were angry. The Rosemont Health Promotion Council responded with a series of programs on effective parenting that included information on various non-physical strategies for disciplining youngsters as well as role-playing and open-discussion periods. However, as part of the community assessment, the community health nurse had recorded that the Hampton Independent School District used physical punishment as a primary discipline method. Youngsters at Temple Elementary were hit on the buttocks with a wide board that frequently left large bruises. The conflict between the effective parenting programs and punishment methods at Temple Elementary was obvious. What could be done? What would you suggest?

In Rosemont, part of the planned effective-parenting classes included discussion sessions on the difference between discipline and punishment and the importance of inquiring as to disciplinary and punitive procedures when parents left their children for supervision, for example, at childcare facilities and schools or with babysitters. Parents were asked to voice their feelings about the school district's policy on physical punishment. Although some parents were unaware of the school district's policy, most were aware of the punishment but felt the procedure could not be changed. After a discussion of parental rights and responsibilities, a group of parents made an appointment with the principal of Temple Elementary to discuss the situation. (Following additional meetings with school board members, an open public hearing on public school discipline, and letters to state school board officials, the Hampton Independent School District changed the discipline policy to exclude physical punishment. The process took two years.)

Countless such incongruencies exist between healthy lifestyles and existing environmental and cultural practices and policies. Here is one additional example: Recall that one community nursing diagnosis for youngsters at Temple Elementary was a high prevalence of dental caries. During the effective-parenting discussions, several parents commented that their children were given hard candy, usually suckers, as a reward for good behavior. When the nurse at Temple Elementary was contacted, it was verified that children exhibiting good behavior were given hard candy. This practice was done daily.

TAKE NOTE

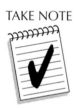

Identify the environmental and cultural practices and policies that are in conflict with the proposed community-focused health program that resulted from your community assessment. What can be done to increase community awareness of these conflicts, and how can change begin? To focus on health and the maintenance of healthy lifestyles, all of the community must be involved.

The best way to maintain a focus on health and not on the activities of the program is to use your nursing practice model as a guide. The nursing practice model built and described in Chapter 6 (see Figure 6-2) defines intervention as primary, secondary, and tertiary levels of prevention. Do the programs proposed for Rosemont address these three levels of prevention?

Levels of Prevention

Recall that *primary prevention* improves the health and well-being of the community, making it less vulnerable to stressors. Health-promotion programs are primary prevention, as are programs that focus on protection from specific diseases. Usually health promotion is nonspecific and directed toward raising the general health of the total community (for example, teaching youngsters about nutritious foods or conducting adult exercise/fitness and stress-reduction sessions). Primary prevention can also be very specific, such as providing immunization against certain diseases. Additional primary prevention measures include the wearing of seatbelts and the purification of public water supplies.

Secondary prevention begins after a disease or condition is present (although there may be no symptoms). Emphasis is on screening, early diagnosis, and treatment of possible stressors that may adversely affect the community's health. The tine test for tuberculosis, the Denver Developmental Screening test for developmental delays, blood pressure assessments, and breast self-examinations are secondary prevention interventions.

Tertiary prevention focuses on restoration and rehabilitation. Tertiary prevention programs act to return the community to an optimum level of functioning. Adequate shelters for battered women and counseling and therapy programs for sexually abused youngsters are examples of tertiary prevention.

The distinction between prevention levels is not always clear. Is a program on the assessment of fever in children (and the prevention of febrile convulsions and dehydration through use of tepid baths and extra fluids) secondary or tertiary prevention? How would you classify an effective-parenting program? support groups for single parents? a crime prevention program? sessions on stress reduction and physical fitness? Can some programs be primary, secondary, and tertiary depending on the needs of the persons who attend? Certainly effective-parenting classes for the parent with a child who has a behavior problem will have a different purpose than classes designed for expectant parents of a first child. Likewise, the corporate executive who has been diagnosed with cardiovascular disease and placed on a low-cholesterol diet has very different nutritional learning needs from those of the senior citizen on a fixed income. Few programs are purely on one level of prevention.

The important point is to evaluate your programs (the implementation phase of the nursing process) and ask if the nursing interventions are consistent with the nursing practice model. If the focus is prevention, then are the programs directed towards prevention?

Summary

Having considered the importance of *community ownership* of the program, the need to offer a *unified program,* and maintaining a *focus on health,* there remains one step in the process—*evaluation.* Before a program is implemented, the manner in which it is to be evaluated must be established. The following chapter explains why this final stage of the nursing process is essential *before* implementation.

REFERENCES

American Public Health Association. (1991). *Healthy Communities 2000: Model Standards* (3rd ed.). Washington, DC: Author.
  Puts the national objectives into practice; an excellent guide for local and regional planning.
U.S. Department of Health and Human Services. Public Health Service. (1990). *Healthy People 2000: National Health Promotion and Disease Prevention Objectives.* Washington, DC: U.S. Government Printing Office.
  The latest goals and objectives for the nation's health. (Full report—GPO Stock No. 017-001-0047-0; Summary report—GPO Stock No. 017-001-00473-1); Superintendent of Documents, GPO, Washington, DC 20402-9325.)
Background for *Healthy People 2000:* U.S. Office of the Assistant Secretary for Health and Surgeon General. (1979). *Healthy People: The Surgeon General's Report on Health Promotion and Disease Prevention.* GPO Stock No. 017-001-00416-1. Washington, D.C. Government Printing Office.
  Sets forth priorities for the nation's health by identifying specific goals in 5 stages of human development and 15 priority areas.
U.S. Office of the Assistant Secretary for Health and Surgeon General. Publ. info: (1979). *Healthy People: The Surgeon General's Report on Health Promotion and Disease Prevention—Background Papers.* GPO Stock No. 017-011-00417-1. Washington, D.C. Government Printing Office.
  A series of articles that examine the past successes, future challenges, and unanswered questions relating to key topics in prevention. Also discussed are psychological factors influencing health and the economic dimensions of prevention.
U.S. Office of the Assistant Secretary for Health and Surgeon General. (1985). *Proceedings of Prospects for a Healthier America: Achieving the Nation's Health Promotion Objectives.* Washington, D.C. Government Printing Office.
  Provides background papers and recommendations from meetings of groups from health care settings, business, voluntary associations, and schools. Helps to identify approaches to developing materials, initiating programs, and stimulating collaboration to implement the health-promotion objectives set forth in *Promoting Health/Preventing Disease: Objectives for the Nation.* (Copies free from the National health Information Clearinghouse.)
U.S. Office of the Assistant Secretary for Health and Surgeon General. (1980). *Promoting Health/Preventing Disease: Objectives for the Nation.* Stock No. 017-001-00435-9. Washington, D.C. Government Printing Office.
  Identifies specific and measurable objectives for the 15 areas set forth in *Healthy People.*

SUGGESTED RESOURCES

Anderson, E.T., Gottschalk, J., & Martin, D.A. (1993). Contemporary issues in the community. In D.J. Mason, S.W. Talbott, & J.K. Leavitt. *Policy and politics for nurses: Action and change in the workplace, government, organizations and community.* Philadelphia: W.B. Saunders.

Beddome, G., Clarke, H.F., & Whyte, N.B. (1993). Vision for the future of public health nursing: A case for primary health care. *Public Health Nursing, 10*(1), 13–18.

Chavis, D.M., & Florin, P. (1990). Nurturing grassroots initiatives for health and housing. *Bulletin of The New York Academy of Medicine, 66*(5), 558–572.

Dahl, S., Gustafson, C., & McCullagh, M. (1993). Collaborating to develop a community-based health service for rural homeless persons. *Journal of Nursing Administration, 23*(4), 41–45.

Jenkins, S. (1991). Community wellness: A group empowerment model for rural America. *Journal of Health Care for the Poor and Underserved, 1*(4), 388–404.

Kinne, A., Thompson, B., Chrisman, N.J., & Hanley, J.R. (1989). Community organization to enhance the delivery of preventive health services. *American Journal of Preventive Medicine, 5*(4), 225–229.

Labonte, R. (1993). Community development and partnerships. *Canadian Journal of Public Health, 84*(4), 237–240.

Rutherford, G.S., & Campbell, D. (1993). Helping people help themselves. *Canadian Nurse, 89*(10), 25–28.

Scott, S. (1990). *Promoting Healthy Traditions Workbook: A Guide to the Healthy People Campaign.* St. Paul: American Indian Health Care Association.
Indian-specific objectives as well as culturally sensitive approaches to community wellness promotion.

In addition to the exemplars presented in Part III of the text, the following program descriptions illustrate community intervention programs:

Durpa, K.C., Quick, M.M., Andrews, A., Engelke, M.K., & Vinvent, P. (1992). A collaborative health promotion effort: Nursing students and Wendy's team up. *Nurse Educator, 17*(6), 35–37.

Farley, S. (1993). The community as partner in primary health care. *Nursing & Health Care, 14*(5), 244–249.

Perino, S.S. (1992). Nike-footed health workers deal with the problems of adolescent pregnancy. *Public Health Reports, 107*(2), 208–212.

Primomo, J. (1990). Diapering decisions: A community education project. In *Notes from the field.* H. Tilson (Ed.), *American Journal of Public Health, 80*(6), 743–744.

Wardrop, K. (1993). A framework for health promotion. *Canadian Journal of Public Health, 84* Suppl. l:S9–13.

Woodard, G.R. & Edouard, L. (1992). Reaching out: A community initiative for disadvantaged pregnant women. *Canadian Journal of Public Health, 83*(3), 188–190.

11

Evaluating a
Community Health Program

Objectives

Evaluation is measurement. During evaluation, information is collected and analyzed to determine its significance and worth. Changes are appraised, and progress is documented. This chapter discusses evaluation and the nursing practices that are necessary to plan and implement it. After studying this chapter, you should be able to act in partnership with the community to

- Establish evaluation criteria that are timely and comprehensive
- Use baseline and current data to measure progress toward goals and objectives
- Validate observations, insights, and new data with colleagues and the community
- Revise priorities, goals, and interventions based on evaluation data
- Document and record evaluation results and revisions of the plan
- Participate in evaluation research with appropriate consultation

Introduction

The nurse evaluates the responses of the community to a health program in order to measure progress that is being made toward the program's goals and objectives. Evaluation data are also crucial for revision of the database and the community nursing diagnoses that were developed from analysis of the community assessment data.

Do you feel as if we are talking in circles? Evaluation is the final step of the nursing process, but it is linked to assessment, which is the first step. Nursing practice is cyclic as well as dynamic, and for community-focused interventions to be timely and relevant, the community database, nursing diagnoses, and health program plans must be evaluated routinely. The effectiveness of community nursing interventions depends on continuous reassessment of the community's health and on appropriate revisions of planned interventions.

Evaluation is important to nursing practice, but of equal importance is its crucial role in the functioning of health agencies. Staffing and funding are frequently based on evaluation findings, and existing programs are subject to termination unless evaluation evidence can be produced that answers this question: What has been the program's impact on the health status of the community? Recent years have witnessed a growing focus on program evaluation; training programs on evaluation have become commonplace, and evaluation has become big business. Unfortunately, evaluation is sometimes practiced separately from program planning. It may even be tacked onto the end of a program just to satisfy funding sources or agency administration. The problems of such an approach are evident. Effective community health nursing requires an integrative approach to evaluation; it is a unique aspect of the field.

The Evaluation Process

When evaluation is discussed, the terms *formative evaluation* and *summative evaluation* are used. Formative evaluation focuses on measuring the daily functions and activities of a program. Its emphasis is on immediate data gathering and analysis to improve the program and its management. For example, when the first effective-parenting training program was offered in Rosemont from 8 to 9 P.M., only five parents attended. They stated that the time was too late for them to return home and complete bedtime activities for their school-age children. As a result of this formative evaluation, the time was changed to 7 to 8 P.M., and attendance increased to 20 parents. Summative evaluation, in contrast, refers to activities that are associated with long-term effects of a program (for example, did the program change the participants' health practices, attitudes, or knowledge?). In the case of effective-parenting classes, summative evaluation criteria might include parental self-reports of changes in their attitudes toward physical punishment and disciplinary practices before and following the program, any alteration in discipline policies at Temple Elementary, and change in the number of reported incidences of child abuse. Both types of evaluation are important, and strategies exist to obtain each.

Before considering specific evaluation strategies, it is important to consider the "evaluability" of the program. To do this, review the program plan and ask yourself the following questions:

- Are program activities stated in precise words whose concepts can be measured?
- Has a time frame for attaining the change been included?
- Are the direction and magnitude of the change included?
- Has a method of measuring the change been included?
- Are the data that will be needed to measure the objectives available at a reasonable cost?
- Are the program activities that are designed to meet the objectives plausible?

If you find in your practice that any of these questions cannot be measured in one of your plans, review Chapter 9 and amend the plan to make it as concise and complete as possible.

TAKE NOTE

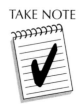

A positive response to each of the above questions would be an ideal state that few programs attain. Therefore, do not despair if your program is less than perfect but rather strive to increase your sensitivity to the issues that need to be considered in program planning in order to achieve optimum program evaluation.

Components of Evaluation

Why collect evaluation data? To whom will the evaluation data be given, and for what purpose will it be used? What programs or activities will result from or be discontinued as a result of evaluation data? Before a strategy or method of evaluation can be selected, the reasons for and uses of the evaluation data must be established. An evaluation strategy appropriate for answering one type of evaluative question would not be useful for another. For example, if the Rosemont Health Promotion Council wanted to know the *relevancy* to community needs of a program on crime prevention, then questions would be asked of the participants concerning the usefulness and adequacy of the information that was given. Possible questions would cover a range of topics: Did the information make a difference as to how residents protect themselves from crime? What protection behaviors do the residents practice now that were not practiced before the program? Did the program answer the residents' questions? Did the program meet *perceived needs?* However, if the council wanted to know the *impact* of the crime prevention program (such as if the program decreased the incidence of crime experienced by the participants), then self-reports and community crime statistics would be monitored. Usually questions of evaluation focus on the areas of *relevancy, progress, cost-efficiency, effectiveness,* and *impact.*

Relevancy

Is there a need for the program? *Relevancy* determines the reasons for having a program or set of activities. Questions of relevancy may be more important for existing programs than for new programs. Frequently a program is planned, such as a blood pressure screening, to meet an expressed community need. Then it is continued for years without an evaluation of relevancy. The question should be asked routinely—is the program still needed? Clearly, evaluation is not necessary just for new programs but for all programs. A common constraint to beginning a new program is inadequate staff or budget. A remedy to that constraint can be a relevancy evaluation of existing programs. Staff and budgets from a program that is no longer needed can be redirected to the new program.

Progress

Are program activities following the intended plan? Are appropriate staff and materials available in the right quantity and at the right time to implement the program activities? Are expected numbers of clients participating in the scheduled program activities? Do the inputs and outputs meet some predetermined plan? Answers to these questions measure the progress of the program.

Cost-Efficiency

What are the costs of a program? What are its benefits? Are program benefits sufficient for the costs incurred? Cost-efficiency evaluation measures the relationship between the results (benefits) of a program and the costs of presenting the program (such as staff salary and materials). Cost-efficiency evaluates whether or not the results of a program could have been obtained less expensively through another approach.

Effectiveness

Were program objectives met? Were the clients satisfied with the program? Were program providers satisfied with the activities and client involvement? Effectiveness focuses on formative evaluation and the immediate, short-term results.

Impact

What are the long-term implications of the program? As a result of the program, what changes in behavior can be expected in six weeks, six months, or six years? Effectiveness measures the immediate results, whereas impact evaluation measures whether or not the program activities changed the initial reason for the program. The fundamental question is this: Has health improved?

Evaluation Strategies

Several methods exist to evaluate programs. No one method is best, and neither does any one strategy address all the issues of relevancy, progress, cost-efficiency, effectiveness, and impact. For example, the case-study method is designed to focus on program relevance but has limited use in evaluating cost-efficiency. Similarly, cost-benefit analysis evaluates cost-efficiency but does not adequately address any of the other issues. Even evaluative research, which is frequently revered as the pinnacle of evaluation techniques, is of little use for answering questions of progress or cost-efficiency. Program evaluation requires a knowledge of the various evaluation methods and careful decision making as to which method can meet evaluation goals.

Case Study

A *case study* looks inside a program to determine its adequacy to meet stated needs. The case-study method provides insight into an entire program and unlike many forms of evaluation can be started at any time during the program. The type of data that is collected during a case study includes observation of program activity, reports prepared by the program, unstructured conversations with program personnel, statistical summaries of program activities, structured or unstructured interview data, and information collected through questionnaires. *Subjective data* and *objective data* can both be collected. Subjective data include information collected primarily through observations of participants or program staff. Objective data are collected from organization or program documents or structured questionnaires and interviews. The distinction between subjective and objective is not readily perceptible. All questionnaires, regardless of how carefully written, have a subjective component, and likewise, "objective" records or documents are all written by people and therefore introduce a subjective factor. It is optimum to have a mix of both objective and subjective data.

Observation

Observation is one method of collecting data for a case study. Observation can be *participatory* or *nonparticipatory*. The participant observer assumes a working role in the agency or organization and collects data about the program while working within the group. The nonparticipant observer remains an "outsider," does not assume a working role within the agency, and reviews and examines the program for designated periods.

The types of observations that are made are determined by the questions that have been asked about the program. For example, if the question is one of relevancy, the observer would concentrate on the *who, what, why,* and *when* of the program. *Who* is using the services? Record the demographics of age, ethnicity, geographic location, educational level, and employment status. *What* services are the participants receiving? (For example, what services are offered in the well child clinic? Immunizations? Physicals? Health teaching? Screening? How often are the services offered and what are the ages of the children who use the services?) *Why* is the population using the offered services? (Availability? Affordability? No other options?). Lastly, *when* are the services accessed? (Do people come at appointed times or only when they are ill? Or do people tend to cluster at opening and closing times?)

Some data can be collected from agency records, other information can be collected by informal conversations with the participants—both the professional health care providers and the clients. When interviewing, always have a checklist of topics you want to consider, arranged in a logical sequence, along with the who, what, why, and when questions. Informal conversations, sometimes referred to as "unstructured interviews," afford the opportunity to *explore* with the participants their perceptions of the program. The results of unstructured interviews provide specific areas from which a "structured" interview can be developed. Recall from Chapter 9 that an interview is administered by an interviewer as opposed to a questionnaire, which is self-administered. (If a questionnaire is written, review the process in Chapter 9.) Observations and interviews share the problem of selective perception.

Selective Perception.   *Selective perception* is the natural tendency of everyone to consciously classify into categories the behaviors or statements of others. These categories have been established by our cultural values, learning, and life experiences. To a certain extent, this process is desirable because it limits the number of observations that need conscious consideration and permits the rapid and effective handling of information. For example, if it was observed that a client waited one hour for a scheduled appointment, most people, based on the common orientation to time, would classify that observation as a negative aspect of the clinic's functioning.

Herein lies the major problem of selective perception. Statements and behaviors are classified according to the selective perception of the observer, which may be completely different from the selective perception of the client or the health care providers. The most dangerous effect of selective perception in program evaluation is when the observer has a preconception that a program will be successful or unsuccessful. This can produce a self-fulfilling prophecy because the biased observer may unconsciously record only data that support the preconceived belief. Both selective perception and self-fulfilling prophecy are sources of subjective data that were discussed earlier. Perhaps the most important point is that you should be aware of the problem of selective perception and share your observation and interview data with a mixed group of clients and health care providers. Ask the group for categorization and summation implications.

Interactiveness.   *Interactiveness* is an additional event to be aware of during all observations. When an observer, whether participant or nonparticipant, observes and records program activities, the person's presence affects and shapes the activities observed. Productivity may increase because staff members are aware of being observed or because they are concerned about client satisfaction or dissatisfaction. All evaluation strategies can have an interactive component, but perhaps the interactive consideration is strongest in case studies because of the presence of an observer.

Two additional techniques of the case study method are *nominal group* and *Delphi technique*. (References to both techniques and examples of their application are presented at the conclusion of this chapter in the Suggested Readings list.) Both techniques are based on the belief that the individuals in a program are the most knowledgeable sources on its relevancy.

Nominal Group

The nominal group technique uses a structured group meeting, during which all individuals are given a judgmental task such as to list the functions of the program, problems of the program, or needed changes in the program. Each member is asked to write a response on paper and to not discuss it with other people. At the end of 5 to 10 minutes, all members present their ideas, and each idea is recorded (without discussion) so that everyone can see all the suggestions. Once all ideas have been presented, a discussion is begun, during which ideas are clarified and evaluated. After the discussion, a vote is held to determine the order in which the group wants to address different areas. The nominal group technique allows all individuals to present their ideas before the entire group. Involving the entire group both decreases selective perception and promotes individual cooperation with the group's decisions because people feel themselves to have been involved in the decision-making process.

Delphi Technique

The Delphi technique tends to be used in large survey studies but is also useful as a case-study method. It involves a series of questionnaires and feedback reports to a designated panel of respondents. An initial questionnaire is distributed by mail to a preselected group (this could be all nursing staff members, a group of clients, or program administrators). Independently, respondents express their thoughts through the questionnaire and return it. Based on the responses of the group, a feedback report and a revised version of the questionnaire is sent to the respondents. Using the feedback information, the respondents evaluate their first answers and complete the questionnaire again. The process continues for a predetermined number of feedback rounds.

Usefulness to Evaluation

The case-study method of program evaluation can help answer questions of *relevance*. Questioning clients and health care providers helps explore perceptions of how well the program is meeting its defined goals as well as ascertaining problem areas and possible solutions. The case-study method would not point to any one solution but rather would offer several possible choices.

Questions of *progress* can also be addressed through the case-study method. The extent to which a program is meeting predetermined standards of service indicates progress. Because the case study provides an examination of the program, much can be learned if program activities are already in place.

Cost-efficiency of the program is difficult to evaluate using a case-study method. First, to evaluate if the program could have been offered more economically, a comparable program must exist; and second, the case-study method is designed to look at only one program. The method is not formatted to look at two programs and compare them. However, judgments can be made as to the operating efficiency of the program. These must be based on the experience and knowledge of the evaluator and cannot be based on comparisons with other operating programs.

Effectiveness determines if the program has produced what it intended to produce immediately following the program, as opposed to *impact*, which measures long-term consequences. Although the case-study method may determine aspects of effectiveness such as whether or not the aims of the program have been met in the short run, it is very difficult to measure long-term consequences unless the case-study method is conducted over a long period that allows a retrospective at the program.

Surveys

A *survey* is a method of collecting information and can be used to collect evaluation information. Surveys are usually completed by self-administered questionnaires (the process used in Rosemont to determine community perception of health information needs) or by personal interviews. Surveys are formulated to describe (*descriptive surveys*) or to analyze relationships (*analytic surveys*). (Actually, most surveys can be used to both describe and analyze.)

Surveys can be used to describe the need for a program, the actual operations of a program, or a program's effects. Along with the descriptive information, questions of analysis can be answered through a survey. For example, a survey could be used to *describe* the composition of the groups that attend crime prevention or weight reduction classes as well as to *analyze* the relationship between descriptive data of sex and weight reduction success.

Surveys are usually performed for summative evaluation. Did the program accomplish what it was proposed to do? Was the program perceived as successful by clients? by personnel? If the program was considered successful, what parts were most helpful? least helpful? What should be changed? left unchanged? The questions asked by the survey are determined by the initial list of questions about program evaluation.

Like the case-study method, the answers on surveys come from the perceptions, values, and belief systems of the respondents. The response given to questions of program usefulness by the nurse who planned and implemented the program may be very different from the answers of the participants. Awareness of perception bias can direct evaluation efforts to consider the perceptions of all persons (providers, clients, and management) involved in program implementation.

Surveys that are used to measure program evaluation must be concerned with the *reliability* and *validity* of the information collected. Reliability deals with the repeatability, or reproducibility, of the data (that is, if the same questions were asked of the same people one week later, would the same responses be recorded?). Validity is the correctness of the information. If questions are written to evaluate knowledge, and the answers of the respondents reflect behaviors, then the questions are not valid because they do not measure what they claim to measure. (Refer to Chapter 2 for further explanation of issues of reliability and validity and for methods that can be used to evaluate the reliability and validity of your questionnaire or interview schedule.)

Usefulness to Evaluation

Surveys can be very valuable to answer questions of *relevance,* or the need for proposed or existing programs, especially if the perceptions of clients, providers, and management are solicited. In like fashion, *progress* can be measured. People critiquing surveys as an evaluation strategy may be concerned with the subjectivity of the survey—indeed, individual perception affects every response to every question. However, most decisions are based on subjective judgments, not objective reality. The important concern is to understand whose subjective impression is being used as a basis for judgment; it is imperative for community health nurses to ensure that clients' perceptions are represented alongside those of health providers and management.

Cost-efficiency, effectiveness, and *impact* are difficult to measure by using a survey. Although a survey can measure the perceived efficiency of the program or ideas on alternative ways of operating to make the program more cost-efficient, these perceptions are formed only in the context of the existing program—there is no other comparison program against which recorded perceptions can be measured. A survey can provide information on the characteristics of program activities that are perceived by the respondents to have caused changes in their health status, *but* these impressions are reported in the absence of any comparison group. A comparison group is especially important with regard to effectiveness and impact because it is impossible to tell if an alternative program (or no program at all) might have been more or less effective in accomplishing the same objectives.

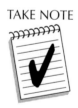

TAKE NOTE   *You may be wondering—if a comparison group is so important and if perceptions cloud the evaluation with subjective impressions, then why use surveys at all? Two pluses exist in surveys: A great deal of information for program evaluation can be obtained, especially about the activities of the program from the perception of several groups, and important evaluation data can be inferred if the instrument (questionnaire or interview schedule) is reliable and valid. Once again, you are referred to Chapter 2 for a review of the importance of reliability and validity as well as information on how to establish the reliability and validity of any questionnaire, interview, or test.*

Experimental Design

Completed correctly, an experimental study can provide an answer to the crucial questions: Did the program make a difference? Are health behaviors, knowledge, and attitudes changed as a result of the program activities? Is the community healthier because of the programs offered by the Rosemont Health Promotion Council? However, the problem with experimental studies in program evaluation is that they require *selective implementation,* meaning that people who participate are selected through a process such as random assignment to a control group and an experimental group. For many ethical, political, and community health reasons, selective implementation is difficult to complete and is sometimes impossible. Despite these problems, the experiment remains the best method to evaluate summative effects of a program and the only way to produce quantified information on whether the program made a difference.

TAKE NOTE   ***Refer to Chapter 2 and review the steps of the research process.***

Indeed, each issue—such as a theoretical framework, sampling, reliability, and validity—must be addressed if an experimental design is proposed for evaluation.

The following designs are the most feasible and appropriate to health care settings. Apply the research process to each design.

Pretest-Posttest One-Group Design

The pretest-posttest design applied to one group is illustrated in Table 11-1. Two observations are made, the first at Time 1 and the second at Time 2. The observation can be the prevalence of a health state (for example, the percentage of adults in Rosemont who exercise regularly, the teenage pregnancy rate, cases of child abuse, and so on), knowledge scores, or other important health facts in the community. Between Time 1 and Time 2, an experiment is introduced. The experiment may be a planned program aimed at a target group, such as teen sexuality classes, or with a community-wide focus, like a crime-prevention program. The evaluation of the program is measured by considering the difference between the health state at Time 1 and the health state following the program at Time 2.

TABLE 11-1   *Pretest-Posttest One-Group Design*

	Time 1		Time 2
Experimental group	Observation 1	Experiment	Observation 2

If the experiment in Table 11-1 was teen sexuality classes for 10th-grade girls at Hampton High School, Time 1 was a teen pregnancy rate of 5 per 100, and Time 2 (one year later) was a teen pregnancy rate of 3 per 100 among the girls taking the classes, then would you agree that the teen sexuality program was responsible for the decrease in teenage pregnancies? What other information do you need to know in order to decide? (Are there other factors that could account for the decrease in the teen pregnancy rate? Perhaps family-planning programs have been focused on teenagers, or maybe local churches and social service agencies have sponsored teen sexuality programs. Teen access and use of contraceptive methods may have increased, or laws regarding teen access to contraceptive methods may have changed.) Each of these factors cannot be eliminated as unassociated with the decrease in the teen pregnancy rate. To eliminate other possible explanations for program effectiveness, a control group must be added.

Pretest-Posttest Two-Group Design

A pretest-posttest with a control group design is illustrated in Table 11-2. The design has both an experimental group and a control group. At Time 1, an observation is made of both the experimental and control groups. Between Time 1 and Time 2, an experiment is introduced with the experimental group. At Time 2, second observations are made on both the experimental and control groups. Program evaluation is the difference between Observations 1 and 2 for the experimental group when compared to the comparison group (which has been selected to be as similar as possible to the experimental group). Will the pretest-posttest with a control group design eliminate the effect of outside factors that occurred simultaneously with the experiment and that might account for the change between Observation 1 and Observation 2, the very problem that plagued the pretest-posttest one-group design? The answer is yes, *if* the experimental and control groups are similar.

TABLE 11-2   *Pretest-Posttest Two-Group Design*

	Time 1		Time 2
Experimental group	Observation 1	Experiment	Observation 2
Control group	Observation 1		Observation 2

To explain, let's return to Rosemont and the idea of a teen sexuality class for 10th-grade students at Hampton High School. If a group of 10th-grade students, similar in social, economic, and geographic characteristics, were randomly selected and then randomly assigned to the experimental or control group, then it could be assumed that any other factors that influenced the experimental group would also affect the control group. However, frequently the decision is made that all students must be given the same program, thereby eliminating a comparison group. At the Rosemont Health Promotion Council, when the information was received that *all* 10th graders must be given a teen sexuality program that had been proposed by the school nurse as a response to an increasing number of teen pregnancies, the suggestion was made that perhaps another high school could be used as a control group. How would you respond to that suggestion? Perhaps another high school class of 10th graders could be used, *if* the students were similar in social, economic, and geographic characteristics to the students at Hampton High (an unlikely situation). Another possibility mentioned by the Rosemont Health Promotion Council was to offer the program in one school year to one half of the Hampton High 10th graders (using the other half as a control) and then in the following year to offer the program to the remaining students. This method would ensure that all students would be given the program but would also allow for an experimental pretest-posttest design for evaluation. A third method that was suggested to ensure an experimental design was to give the control group sexuality education and give the experimental group sexuality education *plus* assertiveness training. The assertiveness training would differentiate the groups and allow an experimental design. All the suggestions were discussed with school officials, and it was decided to offer a traditional sex education class to half the 10th grade students (the control group); the remaining students (the experimental group) would get the traditional sex education material but would also receive classes on assertiveness training and values clarification. This design will not allow for evaluation of traditional sex education classes versus no information, but it will provide all students with the health information (an ethical compromise) and allow for evaluation of a traditional program on sexuality versus that traditional program plus assertiveness and values clarification information (an approach to reduce teenage pregnancies that is supported in the literature).

TAKE NOTE

Notice that the decision to offer information on assertiveness and values clarification as part of teen sexuality classes was based on documentation from the literature. Rosemont is not the first community to offer health-promotion programs. Many communities have assessed the health status and perceived health needs of the residents and have followed up with planned and implemented programs that have been evaluated, with the results reported in the literature. One contribution that the community health nurse can make is to review and synthesize the results of similar programs and present this information to the community for use in decision making. After the program topics have been decided, you should begin a literature review to study the ways in which other communities have addressed and evaluated similar programs.

Usefulness to Evaluation

When completed correctly, the experimental design is the best evaluation technique for assessing the effectiveness and impact of a given program. No other evaluation approach can assess the true value efficiency, effectiveness, and impact. An experimental design can yield data on whether or not a program has produced the desired outcomes when compared to the absence of such a program or, alternatively, whether one program strategy has produced better results with regard to the desired outcomes than some other strategy. However, the experimental design is not useful for evaluation of program progress or program cost-efficiency.

Monitoring

Monitoring measures the difference between the program plan and what has actually happened. Monitoring focuses on the sequence of activities of the program, specifically, *how* the program is to be implemented (the activities), by *whom* (the personnel and other resources), and *when* (the timing of activities). Monitoring is usually done with a chart, and although there are several different styles of charts, all arrange activities in a sequence and specify the time allotted to complete each task. Figure 11-1 shows an example of a monitoring chart.

Monitoring Charts

To construct a monitoring chart for your program plan, information is needed on the *inputs* (resources necessary to carry out the program such

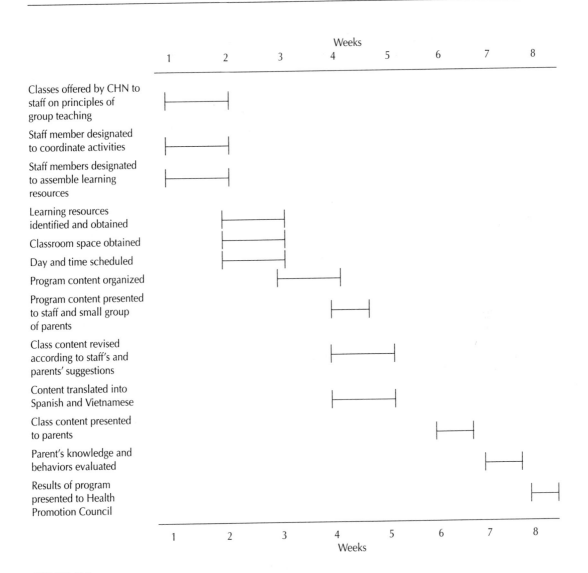

FIGURE 11-1
Sequence of events for program: Common health problems of children.

as personnel, equipment, and finances), the *process* (the program activities, their sequencing, and timing) and *outputs* (the expected results of the program, including immediate and long-term health effects). It is helpful to make a list of inputs, processes, and outputs.

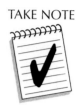

TAKE NOTE   *You have already recorded this information as part of your program plan. Refer back to Chapter 9 and note that* resources, program activities, *and* learning objectives *were listed for the proposed class on common health problems of children.* Resources *are the same as* inputs; program activities *correspond to* processes; *and* learning objectives *designate expected* outputs. *So all that remains is to place the data into a chart for monitoring.*

Figure 11-1 lists the inputs, processes, and outputs for the proposed program in Rosemont, along with a time sequence for beginning and completing each event.

It is difficult to decide on the amount of time that will be needed to complete any task. After assessing the organizational structure and management methods of the agency, you can determine the approximate amounts of time that will be needed to complete the activities of the program. Monitoring charts are easy to formulate and provide useful information for measuring program evaluation *if* the chart is realistic. The publications in the Suggested Readings list include references to several other types of monitoring charts, including the Gantt, Program Evaluation and Review Technique (PERT), and Critical Path Method (CPM). These provide a slightly different variation of the basic time-sequencing, activities-monitoring chart that appears in Figure 11-1.

Usefulness to Evaluation

A monitoring chart measures progress and can be used to evaluate whether or not a program is on schedule and within budget. Perhaps no other evaluation method is as perfectly suited to *progress evaluation* as the monitoring chart. In addition, monitoring can provide information on the *cost-efficiency* of the program by measuring the average cost of the resources required per client served. The effectiveness of the program can be measured by monitoring the chart if the chart records outputs achieved. Monitoring charts cannot determine program relevance or the long-term impact of a program.

Cost-Benefit and Cost-Effectiveness Analyses

Much has been written and discussed about the escalating cost of health care services and on ways that cost can be reduced. The turmoil over health care reform in the United States and the intense debate regarding the pros and cons of various alternative approaches to health care delivery was testimony to the need to contain cost and yet increase access and maintain quality. Every program has a dollar price both in terms of the resources (for example, personnel and equipment) needed to offer the program and the dollar benefits to be gained from improved health (such as increased worker productivity).

Two of the most common methods of analyzing the economic costs and benefits of a program are *cost-benefit analysis* (CBA) and *cost-effectiveness analysis* (CEA). Both CBA and CEA are formal analytic techniques that list all costs (direct and indirect) and consequences (negative and positive) of a particular program. The distinction between CBA and CEA is based on the value that is placed on the consequences of a program. In CBA, consequences or benefits of a program are valued in dollar terms; this makes it possible to compare different projects, because all measurement is made in dollars. Therefore, the worth of a project can be judged by asking if dollar benefits exceed dollar costs and, if so, by how much. In contrast, CEA does not place a dollar value on either the consequences or the costs of a project. Another outcome is used for programs whose benefits or costs are difficult to measure. (For example, how could a dollar value be placed on each suicide prevented by a primary prevention program to decrease teenage suicide?) Therefore, CEA, unlike CBA, does not determine if total benefits exceed total costs.

However, CEA can be used to compare programs with similar goals and objectives. (For example, two different primary prevention approaches to decrease the incidence of teenage suicide share the same benefits, so only costs need be compared—a CEA.) A CEA can also be used if the costs of alternative programs are the same or if only a given amount of money exists and the objective is to select the program with the greatest benefits (not measured in dollar terms). The decision is obvious—select the program that produces the most effectiveness, that is, the most benefits per dollar spent or the least cost for each unit (individual, family, or community) benefited.

The choice between CBA and CEA depends on the type of questions and programs considered. Neither technique is superior to the other. Both techniques can be used in planning for future programs or as an evaluation strategy of present or past programs. The actual procedures for completing a CBA or CEA are beyond the scope of this book; however, several references that include the procedural steps are listed in the Suggested Readings list. Obviously both CBA and CEA are strategies for measuring program cost-efficiency and do not address the issues of relevancy, progress, effectiveness, or impact.

Summary

Several methods of evaluation have been presented and discussed. No one method will evaluate components of *relevancy, progress, cost-efficiency, effectiveness,* and *impact* equally well. It is important to be knowledgeable about different methods of program evaluation and to discuss the benefits and limitations of each with the community as the program is being planned and *before* program implementation occurs. Table 11-3 presents a summary table of appropriate evaluation methods for program components. Once evaluation components. Once evaluation methods are selected, then the methods (case study, experimental design, or monitoring charts) become part of the program plan.

You may be wondering which evaluation methods were used to evaluate the health-promotion programs in Rosemont. A variety were used. To evaluate the relevancy of the health-promotion programs (crime prevention and effective-parenting classes), nominal group meetings were scheduled, and both health care providers and consumers attended. In addition, the use of rates and demographics of the participants using the health-promotion programs were assessed, as were the participants' perceptions of the value of the information. Program progress was evaluated with monitoring charts such as the one presented in Figure 11-1. The effectiveness and impact of individual programs was evaluated with knowledge, attitude, and behavioral intent

TABLE 11-3   *Examination of the Appropriateness of Different Evaluation Methods for Program Components*

	Method			
COMPONENTS	*CASE STUDY*	*SURVEY*	*EXPERIMENTAL*	*MONITORING*
Relevancy	yes	yes	no	no
Progress	yes	yes	no	yes
Cost-efficiency	no	no	yes	yes
Cost-effectiveness	some	no	yes	some
Impact	no	no	yes	no

surveys (that is, questionnaires, interviews, and tests) given to participants before the program, immediately after the program, and at predetermined follow-up times (six weeks and three months following the program). As often as was feasible, an evaluation research design was followed, such as a one-group pretest-posttest. Additional measures of effectiveness and impact were community statistics on crime, child abuse, and teenage pregnancies before as compared to after the program as well as health policy changes that affected the residents of Rosemont (for example, access of minors to contraceptives, disciplinary practices in the public schools, and financial eligibility requirements for health services). Cost-effectiveness analysis was completed on several of the programs.

You are ready *now* for program implementation and the reinitiation of the nursing process, namely, assessment of the program's effects. As you implement the planned program, data will be added to the community assessment profile, which will demand addition, deletion, and revision of the community nursing diagnoses and the associated program plans and interventions. Let's take a final look at the community-as-partner model (see Figure 6-2) and ask: Will the planned programs assist the community to attain, regain, maintain, and promote health? strengthen the community's ability to resist stressors? enhance the community's competence and self-reliance?

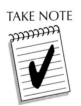

TAKE NOTE *It is fitting that the final chapter of this section on the application of the nursing process in community health nursing end with questions. Community health nursing is the constant questioning, prodding, probing, and pondering of the health status of a population. Although individual and family health are always important, the uniqueness of our field is the application of nursing techniques to the health of a community. Each community is unique and special. There is no other community quite like the one in which you are applying community health nursing. We have enjoyed sharing the uniqueness of Rosemont with you and the application of the nursing process to community health nursing.*

SUGGESTED READINGS

Allen, J. (1993). Impact of the cholesterol education program for nurses: A pilot program evaluation. *Cardiovascular Nursing, 29*(1),1–5.

Birch, S. (1990). The relative cost effectiveness of water fluoridation across communities: Analysis of variations according to underlying caries levels. *Community Dental Health, 7*(1), 3–10.

Finnegan, J.R., Murray, D.M., Kurth, C., & McCarthy, P. (1989). Measuring and tracking education program implementation: The Minnesota Heart Health Program experience. *Health Education Quarterly, 16*(1), 77–90.

Kohler, C.L., Dolce, J.J., Manzella, B.A., Higgins, D., & Brooks, C.M. (1993). Use of focus group methodology to develop an asthma self-management program useful for community-based medical practices. *Health Education Quarterly, 20*(3), 421–429.

O'Brien, K. (1993). Using focus groups to develop health surveys: An example from research on social relationships and AIDS-preventive behavior. *Health Education Quarterly, 20*(3), 361–372.

Thompson, J.C. (1992). Program evaluation within a health promotion framework. *Canadian Journal of Public Health, 83* Suppl. 1:S67–71.

Tonglet, R., Sorogane, M., Lembo, M., WaMukalay, M., Dramaix, M., & Hennart, P. (1993). Evaluation of immunization coverage at local level. *World Health Forum, 14*(3), 275–281.

Wheeler, F.C., Lackland, D.T., Mace, M.L., Reddick, A., Hogelin, G., & Remington, P.L. (1991). Evaluating South Carolina's community cardiovascular disease prevention project. *Public Health Report, 106*(5), 536–543.

Part III

Exemplars of Community as Partner

12

De Madres a Madres: Community Empowerment and Health Through Collaborative Partnerships and Coalitions— Houston, Texas

John Fehir

Community Assessment: The Beginning

In a primarily residential neighborhood near the north side of downtown Houston, Texas, several community health nurses completed a thorough community assessment in 1989 (Mahon, McFarlane, & Golden, 1991). The people in this community are similar to those living in other inner-city areas in that they are socially and financially isolated, stricken with poverty, and underserved in comparison to the general population. The assessment revealed that only 60% of the women received early prenatal care. As a result, low birth weight, infant mortality, and pregnancy complications are more prevalent in Houston, the fourth-largest city in the United States, than in other regions of the country.

The community is located just 2.5 miles from the headquarters of some of the wealthiest energy and financial corporations in the world. Census tract data, socioeconomic data, and clinic use rates provided evidence and were used to validate that the community assessment was entirely correct. Ninety-five percent of the population is Hispanic, and 34% of the women are of childbearing age. Within the group of pregnant women, 27% are either teenagers or older than 34, which puts them at high risk for pregnancy-related health problems. The median income of the neighborhood residents is just over $12,000, and 19% of the families receive public assistance.

By the end of 1989, the nurses had formed a partnership with some of the women in the community to do something about the health care deficiencies revealed in the assessment. Together, they started de Madres a Madres, a volunteer-based primary health care program that disseminates information on how to get prenatal care to pregnant women in the neighborhood. The volunteers are local mothers who are willing to help.

The De Madres a Madres Program was initially funded to do its work for two years by a $111,763 grant from the March of Dimes Foundation. In 1991, the program was fortunate enough to secure funding from the W.K. Kellogg Foundation for three additional years to further the program's development and at the same time evaluate its effectiveness.

By mid-1991, the women of the de Madres a Madres Program needed a space of their own, so they leased a house in the neighborhood to serve as a base of operations. The volunteer mothers began to work from this house, which was named the de Madres a Madres Center.

Mission Statement and Purpose of the de Madres a Madres Program: Implementation of a Collaborative Plan for Success

A collaborative partnership was established between the community health nurses and the women of the community. Freire (1993) discussed this approach at length. Members of the partnership helped determine what problems they wanted to solve and what actions were necessary to do so. After reaching agreement, the volunteer mothers drafted the program's mission statement:

> de Madres a Madres is an organization of volunteers, promoting mother to mother support for at risk pregnant Hispanic women through caring, sharing information, and developing a safety network for a healthier community.

This explains the name they have chosen for themselves—*de madres a madres* means "from mother to mother." Initially, the information sup-

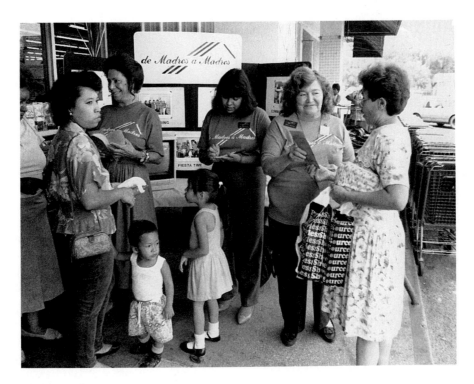

FIGURE 12-1
Volunteer mothers distribute information at an outreach booth.

plied by the volunteer mothers concerned accessing the health care system and getting prenatal care (Rodriguez, McFarlane, Mahon, & Fehir, 1993). Now the scope has expanded to include information about nutrition, food, housing, clothing, jobs, legal aid, shelter for battered women, and social service assistance.

The volunteers of the de Madres a Madres Program contact other women at many public places in the neighborhood, for example, small businesses, schools, and community events. The volunteer mothers also regularly set up and stay at booths at local grocery stores. There they contact other women of the neighborhood who are doing their shopping (Figure 12-1). Members of the program also walk around the neighborhood to contact and talk with other mothers. These volunteers travel in pairs (or sometimes groups of three) for safety's sake and because the work they do is more fun with other people.

Building Community Coalitions

The volunteer mothers took their mission statement and went to the people of the neighborhood to explain the purpose of the de Madres a Madres Program. Agreements were reached as to what the volunteers would do, where they would do it, and when they would do it. For example, as regards the information booths in local supermarkets, the volunteers have agreed to talk to women and offer information about getting prenatal care near the entrance to the store (but out of the way enough so that safety is not compromised) one or two afternoons a week. Perhaps hundreds of women pass a de Madres a Madres booth and are reached by the program's volunteers during each of those afternoons.

Similar coalitions were built by the de Madres a Madres women with

- Neighborhood businesses such as bakeries, banks, grocery stores, and the like. If the business is owned by a local resident, the owner and family are contacted; in other cases, the day-to-day manager was contacted. The women have formed strong alliances with local businesses and have permission to contact and talk to their customers on the sidewalks, in lobbies, and at entrances.
- Elementary, intermediate, and high schools. The teachers and staff as well as the students and their parents are contacted and have access to information about pregnancy, early prenatal care, and additional information about other health matters.
- Local private and public service organizations such as churches, food banks, libraries, the neighborhood police officers at their storefront station, and other community-based agencies.
- Registered nurses and other health-related professionals at neighborhood health care clinics, both private and public.
- Local community events such as health fairs and disease prevention screenings.

Activities and Accomplishments
of the de Madres a Madres Program

The de Madres a Madres Program has been very successful and has received many accolades for its achievements. Some of its more signifi-

Community Coalitions Benefit Pregnant Women:
Reaching Out to the Pregnant Women in the Community

The de Madres a Madres Program has had an extremely successful history. In just one year

221	high-risk pregnant women were visited periodically by volunteer mothers.
376	people, mostly pregnant women, received eligibility for government-funded health care, owing to assistance by the volunteers.
1,938	people, mostly women, stopped by the de Madres a Madres Center to request health-related and other information or assistance with accessing services.
2,263	telephone calls were received by the volunteers from people requesting information regarding parental care, health, sources of food, nutrition, housing, shelter, clothing, legal aid, counseling, education, and employment opportunities.
3,642	people, mostly women, were contacted and given a program brochure.
8,440	= Total number of people helped by the volunteers

cant accomplishments, affecting the lives of not only the targeted population of pregnant women in the community but also everyone living there, are discussed in the accompanying display.

Through the years, other healthy outcomes affecting the originally assessed and community-identified problems have been achieved:

- No low-birth-weight baby has been born to a woman followed by a de Madres a Madres volunteer.
- The rate of infant mortality for the neighborhood fell from 16.5 in 1989 to 11.4 in 1993.

The Community Coalitions Benefit Community Development

Many aspects of the neighborhood have been enhanced and improved because of the tremendous amount of work the de Madres a Madres volunteers have completed in their activities:

- Better communication exists among the community residents.
- Stronger ties have been made between the program participants; community residents; and community businesses, churches, organizations, and institutions.
- Local, state, and national political activity and experience for the community have greatly expanded.
- Each passing year has seen an increasing amount of community pride, for its own sake and for what it offers to residents. They know about and are justifiably proud of the work done by the de Madres a Madres Program volunteers for the community's pregnant women and of the program itself.
- Each year has seen an increasing amount of community unity, probably due in part to the previously mentioned factors acting synergistically to unite the residents in a common cause or identity.

The people in the neighborhood bakeries, grocery stores, restaurants, schools, and churches are outspoken about their pride for the de Madres a Madres Program. Because the program has helped so many thousands of women, reports of it have disseminated widely into the community. Radio stations, newspapers, and television stations have given the program and its volunteers much coverage, so now even more people in the community know and talk about it.

Community Coalitions: Growth and Development of Women

The community's women have benefited from their experiences and participation in the de Madres a Madres Program, both collectively and individually. For example, the women of de Madres a Madres have been called upon to make many decisions about their own, as well as others', health, finances, community partnerships, political stances, and social networks.

Another factor benefiting the women is their involvement in collaborative efforts with local businesses, schools, and other institutions and organizations. The result has been increased levels of health for local pregnant women and their newborns. This has been an empowering experience for the women; they have seen how powerful they are in local as well as regional and national activities and arenas (Kelly, McFarlane, Rodriguez, & Fehir, 1993).

The following are some other significant experiences that the women have had:

- *Local, state, and national political activity.* The women lobbied successfully with health care delivery administrators to change eligibility processing of women for prenatal care.
- *Mortgage and investment activities, insurance negotiating and procurement, arts and craft production and marketing, business negotiation and production, and working toward financial independence and liquidity.* The volunteers run a successful small business in arts and crafts and another in food catering. The profits from all of these activities are used to run the program and increase outreach to pregnant women.
- *Grant and funding resource procurement, improved writing and reading ability, and acquisition of computer literacy.* Several of the women began work on their GEDs (General Equivalency Diplomas) and college degrees. In 1993, they procured grants totaling over $100,000 for the 1994 operating budget for the continuation and expansion of the program's functions.

These experiences have had a synergistic, not summative, effect on the women's lives. Thus, an underlying function of the de Madres a Madres Program is the enhancement of each individual women's self-esteem, self-confidence, and power within her own family as well as the community at large.

Leadership at de Madres a Madres

Since its inception, the de Madres a Madres Program has been fortunate to have a style of leadership that has ensured, maintained, and supported its existence. It has been referred to as *democratic, participatory, shared governance,* or *shared leadership* in the literature. Its distinguishing characteristics are a decentralized decision-making process, mutual commitment and trust among all people involved, a supportive and understanding environment in which people's mistakes are not regarded negatively, and an emphasis on collaboration and communication in team work (Manz, 1991; Peters & Austin, 1985; Peters & Waterman, 1993). True authority and power is then shared among the people involved. This leadership style has been demonstrated not only by the professional community health nurses involved with the program but also from the community's women themselves. The women at the de Madres a Madres Program have excellent managerial abilities; they have adapted to the demands and changes that constantly challenge the program.

The program was indeed lucky to have such leadership as it underwent a planned transition from being dependent on external financial and professional support to becoming totally community based, community led, and community managed. All staff and volunteer members of the program are now community residents. This shift in structure was a learning, growing, and developing experience because of the democratic leadership style.

Continuation of Community-Based Programs

The de Madres a Madres Program has an impressive and unbroken record of successful activities, but as Winston Churchill once observed, "Success is never final." And so the program's work continues, both with regard to supplying information and support to pregnant women and to ensuring its own sustainability over the next few months or years. A number of factors contribute to the likely probability that community-based programs will continue to grow and serve the people of the community:

- As time passes, more people and organizations find out about the program, and this dispersed knowledge helps stabilize it.
- Professional and community leaders have to trust in the community residents to decide for themselves what is best and most needed (Freire, 1993).
- Professional and community leaders must continue to involve individual community residents in every decision.
- Professionals must have respect for and sensitivity to the concerns of the community. They must realize their limits and that they (someday) have to leave (Kelly, McFarlane, Rodriguez, & Fehir, 1993).
- The power base must be dispersed and diversified. Women and minorities in the community must be involved to obtain, share, and maintain power to make decisions and to earn money.
- Community leaders and others need to develop their inherent skills to work with government to increase their own power

base, their own health, the health of their families, and thus the health of their community.

Initiation of Community Partnership Programs Similar to the de Madres a Madres Program

Most people who have heard about the de Madres a Madres Program have responded enthusiastically. In addition to offering compliments, some are genuinely interested in how the program could be replicated elsewhere. Compelling reasons other than outright need exist for similar programs to be set up in other communities. For example, health care reform, which is likely to consume many years of debate and political maneuvering, calls for it.

Some proposed health care reform bills currently being considered by Congress do little or nothing to promote public health and prevent disease from a community perspective (*A look,* 1994; *PHS plans,* 1993); many other bills have proposed specific goals and objectives that the de Madres a Madres Program has already met and achieved. Most of the proposed health care reform bills advocate consumer participation in some capacity (Citizen Action, 1994). The de Madres a Madres Program—and others like it—already has the neighborhood residents' participation in many different ways. Although the Public Health Service plans to expand primary care in underserved areas across the nation (*PHS plans,* 1993), the de Madres a Madres Program is already meeting the health care information needs of pregnant women in its own underserved inner-city area.

What does it take for a program like de Madres a Madres to get started in a community? The following is a list of basic requirements:

- A certain amount of professional community or public health nursing expertise is necessary at the beginning. The leadership style exercised by these people must be democratic and participatory: they must identify and involve the community leaders. The nurses are needed to establish connections, coalitions, and rapport with members of the community and their leaders.
- An assessment of the community (and validation of assessment results) must be done with the community people. The assess-

How a Community-Based Program Can Address Health Care Issues

Health Care Issues	**de Madres a Madres Response**
Health care benefits must be increased in underserved areas.	The program increases early prenatal care in its own underserved neighborhood.
Financial barriers must be eliminated.	The program was successful in relocating financial eligibility for prenatal care into its own neighborhood.
Health promotion must be implemented.	The program's volunteers already do this by offering prenatal, nutrition, nonviolence, antidrug and alcohol, housing, and education information free to all people in its neighborhood.
Service delivery must be nondiscriminatory.	The program's information and help are given to everyone in the neighborhood.
Consumers must get education.	The program's volunteers offer education to parents of school children and to other adults in the neighborhood.
Nonfinancial barriers to service must be eliminated.	The program's volunteers help pregnant women translate the eligibility forms for prenatal care for food and housing assistance. They also help by giving information on how to use public transportation.
Consumers must participate in planning and evaluation.	The program's volunteers already comprise 50% of its advisory board of directors and actively participate in all decisions.

ment should be used only if the community residents themselves verbalize the same problems found in the assessment.

- Everyone involved must work toward empowerment of women and minorities.
- Doing all of the above takes a long time, perhaps three to five years.
- $$$$$. This is a legitimate concern because both private and public budgets are severely constrained. A little bit of financial support will help, but long-term commitments must not be made

to any person(s), institutions, or organizations that grant money or funding. Money is ultimately always linked to power and control. The community residents must always be in complete control of their own program.

An excellent videotape and accompanying monograph have been prepared to outline strategies for initiating and sustaining programs similar to de Madres a Madres. For further information, contact the de Madres a Madres Center, 1108 Paschall, Houston, TX 77009.

REFERENCES

A look at public health provisions of major reform bills. (1994, February). *The Nation's Health,* pp. 1, 5.

APHA rates major planks in White House health plan. (1993, October). *The Nation's Health,* pp. 1, 20.

Citizen Action (1994, January). Comparison of key congressional health care reform bills—1993. *The Nation's Health,* pp. 14–16.

Freire, P. (1993). *Pedagogy of the oppressed* (rev. ed.) (M.B. Ramos, Trans.). New York: Continuum Press. (Original work published 1973).

Kelly, E., McFarlane, J., Rodriguez, R., & Fehir, J. (1993). Community health organizing: Whom are we empowering? *Journal of Health Care for the Poor and Underserved, 4,* 358–362.

Mahon, J, McFarlane, J., & Golden, K. (1991). De Madres a Madres: A community partnership for health. *Public Health Nursing, 8*(1), 15–19.

Manz, C.C. (1991). *Mastering self-leadership: Empowering yourself for personal excellence.* Englewood Cliffs, NJ: Prentice-Hall.

Peters, T.J., & Austin, N.K. (1985). *A passion for excellence: The leadership difference.* New York: Random House.

Peters, T.J., & Waterman, R.H., Jr. (1993). *In search of excellence.* New York: Warner Books.

PHS plans to expand primary care in underserved areas. (1993, December). *The Nation's Health,* p. 5.

Rodriguez, R., McFarlane, J., Mahon, J., & Fehir, J. (1993). De Madres a Madres: A community partnership to increase access to prenatal care. *Bulletin of the Pan American Health Organization, 27,* 403–408. (Published in Spanish in *Boletín de la Oficina Sanitaria Panamerica, 116*(1), 82–87.)

13

Partnership Building in a Rural Community— El Dorado, Arkansas

Mary Wainwright

The Rural Community

The name of the town is El Dorado. The state is Arkansas. The ebb and flow of life here moves to a distinctively rural rhythm mingled with a surprising air of sophistication. It is the smallest town in the United States to have its own symphony and public broadcasting radio station. El Dorado also has an arts center with an artist-in-residence. Each year the picturesque town square is closed off for four days to host a music festival. El Dorado has a significant medical center that boasts the largest number of on-staff physicians in southern Arkansas. As a secondary referral center for smaller communities, the medical center, in turn, refers people needing tertiary care to Little Rock, the state's capital and largest city.

Arkansas is a sparsely populated, primarily rural state of 2.5 million people, 25% of whom live in Little Rock. El Dorado is 110 miles south of Little Rock in an area of the state whose economy is based largely on agriculture, oil, and chemical industry. It has a population of 23,000 people. Typical of southern Arkansas, the racial mix consists of African Americans (30%), Asians (1%–2%), a scattering of migrant hispanic farm

For an old-timer/newcomer, an insider/outsider, a transient passerby or a temporary resident, it is difficult to say goodbye to a community like El Dorado and to all the partnerships rooted there. The author wishes to thank the community for lessons learned and experiences shared.

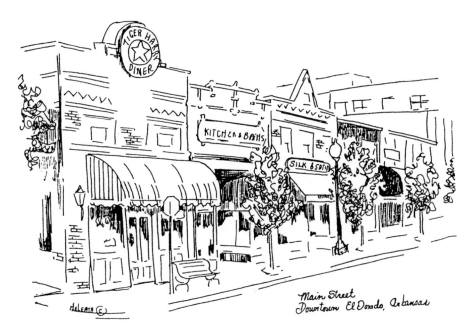

FIGURE 13-1
El Dorado Town Square. (Artist: De Leath Ludwig)

workers, and an Anglo majority. Between a large impoverished segment and a small wealthy philanthropic cluster is a solid core of middle-class residents. El Dorado has a well-defined, Southern culture and an independent, conservative attitude. Isolated 70 to 100 miles from the nearest large town, El Dorado is more rural than urban, despite its cultural achievements. (See Figure 13-1.)

Rural Nursing Theory

This southern Arkansas town demonstrates many of the characteristics that researchers attribute to rural communities. In rural nursing theory development work, Long and Weinert (1989) have identified the following key concepts relating to rural dwellers:

Work beliefs and health
Isolation and distance

Self-reliance
Lack of anonymity
Outsider/insider designation
Old-timer/newcomer mind-set

Work Beliefs and Health

Rural dwellers define health in terms of ability to work. A logger in El Dorado probably considers himself in good health as long as he is able to work. He will try home remedies and neighborly advice before he seeks professional help. Only when the remedies and advice fail will the logger consult a physician. Treatment that will get him back to work is his dominant medical care expectation. Nichols (1989) described rural residents' health care orientation as present-time and crisis oriented. As such, the minimal interest in health maintenance/disease prevention activities among El Dorado residents is consistent with their work/health beliefs. Only small numbers participate in smoking-cessation programs, and tobacco chewing, obesity, and disregard for regular exercise are common.

Isolation and Distance

Residents accept and adapt to isolation and distance, which were major factors in the midcentury, oil-money–facilitated investment in cultural pursuits and health care facilities. Distance is integrated into everyday life. Residents anticipate and even relish shopping trips that require one to three hours one way. With little hesitation, a neighbor may devote a day to driving the distance required for a sick friend's specialty doctor appointment. However, even with significant adaptive strategies, distance is a barrier that increases the likelihood of deferring health care until one is very ill. Furthermore, recovery times and optimal rehabilitation are compromised by inadequate and untimely treatment.

Mrs. R. was diagnosed with breast cancer. She trusted doctors in Little Rock, where she was sent for further evaluation. For more than six months she made the five-hour round trip to receive surgery and chemotherapy. Many times discomfort forced her to lie quietly in the back seat on the way home. When she lost her hair, the closest wig shops to her were in Little Rock, too. Mrs. R. continued to work throughout her illness. She refused to give in to pain and discomfort, and after every therapy trip ordeal she returned to work the next day. Consistently, Mrs. R. never complained about the inconvenient medical care that exacted energy and time from her limited reserves.

Self-Reliance

For survival, isolation and distance require the development of strong self-reliant attitudes. The high value placed on self-reliance is readily observed both in individuals and the community as a whole. For example, the development of a secondary regional medical center—and the necessary financial commitment—is part of the community's autonomous demeanor. Individual self-reliance can be seen in behavior such as Mr. K.'s response to his elderly wife's immobility. Rather than place his wife in a skilled-care setting, Mr. K. fed, bathed, and changed her decubitus dressing as best he could. He maintained the exhausting care until he himself developed pneumonia and had to be admitted to the hospital.

Lack of Anonymity

Rural communities are fishbowls. Everyone knows about everyone. The all-too-real quote "You know you are in rural America when you find out the results of your daughter-in-law's pregnancy test before she does" describes the lack of anonymity in El Dorado. Each person is observed and judged based equally on his or her personal life and professional ability. A health care provider is known throughout the community, and privacy may therefore, be difficult to obtain. In all settings, such as the grocery store, school, or church, the provider is expected to deal with health care issues. Because persons with advanced education or leadership skills are often lured to larger cities, the role of health care provider in a rural community frequently has expectations of leadership attached. This additional visibility magnifies the fact that credibility, trust, and effectiveness as an agent of change are dependent on the community's judgment of the person as a whole.

Insider/Outsider and Old-Timer/Newcomer Designation

Rural community residents tend to be less mobile than their urban counterparts. Several generations live within close proximity, and friends grow up together. People are identified in the context of their relationships: "You know her. She's Mr. Gray's daughter-in-law." If one's great-grandfather was the town drunk, one is always known as the grandchild of the town drunk. This is often expressed in comments such as "Jill has done well in spite of the fact that she's old man Jones's granddaughter." In a similar vein, it's easy to learn who is an insider and who is an outsider by listening to comments like "Make sure you include Mr. W. on your invitation list. He's on every money-raising committee in town," or "Why are you inviting Mrs. E.? She's never been involved in this kind of meeting before."

In fact, newcomers may not join the ranks of old-timers for as long as 15 to 20 years. Mrs. T. came to El Dorado when she was first married and was referred to as "the lady from Missouri" until her grandchildren were born. Lenz and Edwards (1992) stated that these distinctions usually produce more favorable consideration for insiders and old-timers. However, the outsider position is sometimes advantageous when issues of confidentiality arise and emotional distance is preferred. Acceptance of the person and his or her community role is influenced by the insider/outsider, old-timer/newcomer mind-set.

As a typical rural town, El Dorado demonstrates the characteristic rural concepts described by Long and Weinert (1989), but it also has unique qualities that distinguish it from others. This individuality is typical of rural towns; if you've seen one, you haven't seem them all.

The Partnership

South Arkansas Area Health Education Center

Initiated out of concern for underserved populations and workforce supply and distribution, the South Arkansas Area Health Education Center (AHEC) is a community-based health care education institution. Its mission is to provide primary care to a majority of El Dorado's indigent population through its Family Practice Residency program.

In an effort to develop a broader array of services responsive to the community, AHEC created a new position, director of nursing education. The position required a master's degree in nursing. Southern Arkansas had no nurses with that qualification except those employed by a school of nursing in the next town. The position was filled by an outsider who had moved to El Dorado from another state. AHEC administration designed the nursing position to be autonomous and with few boundaries. The primary goal of the director of nursing education was to develop programming that was responsive to the community and create a community/AHEC partnership. Providing health care services responsive to the community as a whole was a new experience for director of nursing education, hereafter referred to as the AHEC nurse. However, as with individual and group clients, assessment of the community's defined needs and priorities was the first step in partnership building.

In the Beginning

A community mentor advised, "Don't *do* anything for six months." This proved to be valuable wisdom, although difficult in practice for any action-oriented nurse. Rural community partnerships can't be rushed. The quiet start was an important time to become acculturated, to assess the community, and to establish relationships. These were all essential foundations for developing a community-oriented program. The nurse's relationship with the community became based on many public and personal aspects. The rural lack of anonymity noted by Long and Weinert (1989) was evinced by the community's awareness of the nurse's civic/church activities, personal reputation, and communication skills. Even her husband's management position and her two children's athletic involvement contributed to her establishing a positive image in the eyes of the rural community.

As an outsider, the AHEC nurse needed a community sponsor who could identify key community resources and leadership. A physician who was highly esteemed by the community for both his established family background and altruistic care provided the important entrée into the community. The doctor enlisted several other key persons to act as catalysts, and together they introduced the AHEC nurse to the community and vice versa. With the outsider/newcomer barriers mitigated somewhat by the sponsor, community residents shared their interests and concerns about health care. The assessment process was informal and often began with "You ought to have lunch with so-and-so." As an example of the characteristic informality of these meetings, the AHEC nurse met with the spouse of a prominent school board member at the local deli.

From this spouse's insider/old-timer position, a deep concern for the high rate of adolescent pregnancy in El Dorado was expressed. The health and future of "children having children" was a recurring theme from the beginning of the assessment process. A civic leader explained the phenomena by stating that "girls have babies just so they can get more welfare money." When introduced to the AHEC nurse, residents would often respond by saying "Oh, nurse educator . . . can you do something about all these pregnant teens? They need education." Clergy offered statements such as "We have got to stop this sexual immorality." Parents repeatedly commented, "I really do not know what to do." Frequently, teenagers discussed the numbers of their classmates who had children or were pregnant with both incredulity and resigned acceptance.

Consistent with its historically high rate, in 1990 Arkansas had the second-highest percentage of births to teenagers in the nation (*MMWR*, 1990), and southern Arkansas, including El Dorado, has a higher rate of births to teens than the state average (Arkansas Vital Statistics, 1990). Adolescent birth rates represent tremendous health risks and costs. Long-term effects take their toll on society through a greater incidence of poverty and reduced productive contributions associated with adolescent childbearing. On the strength of the community-identified theme and quantitative statistical evidence, AHEC explored the possibility of addressing adolescent pregnancy issues. It carefully considered El Dorado's conservative culture, with its emphasis on "family values" and its sensitivity to sexuality. The acute awareness of the potential controversy and negative response that insensitive programming could precipitate caused trepidation in the AHEC. However, convinced that the community had identified the priority need, AHEC made a commitment to developing a comprehensive plan to address the problem of adolescent pregnancy.

The Circuitous Journey to Primary Prevention

Obviously, the least expensive and most efficacious treatment for premature parenting is primary prevention. Nevertheless, the rural community's lack of active health promotion and disease prevention amplified the barriers relating to sexuality issues. Thus, sex education and pregnancy prevention were not the primary objectives in early phases of the plan for intervention. Instead, the plan began with the path of least resistance. Once a girl was pregnant, prenatal care was universally accepted for the health of the girl and her unborn child. Staying within community-defined axioms, much-needed prenatal classes for adolescent mothers became the focus of early activities.

Designing the prenatal class curriculum was the first task. Although the AHEC nurse's clinical background was predominately in adult critical care, she had acquired generalist skills from other rural experiences. Strengthened by the awareness that she surely knew more than the teens knew, she augmented her limited obstetrical experience with AHEC library resources. Research and content literature (Alexander, Peterson, Hulsey, & Gibson, 1987; Lineberger, 1987; Slager-Earnest, Hoffman, & Beckman, 1987; Fuller, Lum, Sprik, & Cooper, 1988; Hardy & Repke, 1987) gave direction to prenatal curriculum development. Objectives for the class included the following:

1. Provide age-adapted educational content regarding childbearing, with emphasis on content that discourages repeat pregnancies
2. Promote rapport development and continuity of contact with a health care provider
3. Establish an environment conducive to peer support and interaction

Implementing the planned classes involved a number of community resources. Lay volunteers were recruited to assist with hospitality and support activities. AHEC identified and recruited speakers such as professionals from the health department and hospital OB unit as well as a local lawyer. Because the nature of the program required willing, motivated faculty, recruitment was always a soft sell. No arm-twisting was used or required. Only those who really wanted to be involved were enlisted.

The director of the hospital's OB unit was particularly supportive and enthused about the classes. She spoke of teens who came to labor and delivery terrified of the unknown. When she conducted tours of the hospital, the director always made an effort to greet the girls personally, provide special refreshments, and encourage the young mothers about their birthing experience. Yet the director noted with frustration that it was rare for a teen mom to participate in traditional prenatal classes.

Involving the Community

Those community persons directly or indirectly involved in the prenatal classes and the teen participants became the program's best marketing agents. They shared with others the purpose and specific arrangements of the classes. Both young mothers and other people became aware of the classes through word of mouth. The classes were also marketed through schools and doctor's offices. The largest numbers of participants came from AHEC Family Practice Clinics. Eventually, several private physicians began to send their patients after the classes were well established. However, the process of marketing the prenatal classes in schools again demonstrated community cultural constraints. The school superintendent arranged for student access to transportation to prenatal classes but would not allow announcements about the classes to be posted at the school or fliers to be distributed to students. School policy forbade teachers to initiate discussion with any student regarding pregnancy. Only if a student requested information could a teacher then make a referral. Even with somewhat guarded marketing, AHEC was able to contact many potential students for the prenatal classes.

Once AHEC developed the curriculum and recruited faculty and clients, weekly classes began on a continuous basis. A girl could begin attending classes at any time during her pregnancy and attend as long as she wished. Many showed up regularly throughout their pregnancy, drawing on the group for support. Some even brought their new babies to a few sessions. No one was discouraged from attending. Sporadic boyfriends, supportive mothers, curious cousins, and sisters were all welcome. One mother of a pregnant teen also brought another of her daughters to classes. The mother seemed aware that the younger sister was at higher risk for adolescent pregnancy, as are all siblings and close friends of pregnant teens. In hopes of influencing behaviors, the class openly discussed this "catching" phenomenon and the greater risks of repeat. Although the effectiveness of such discussions is difficult to document, even the possibility of reduced premature childbearing as a result is worth the effort.

Program Outcomes

Within limits, the teen prenatal classes met planned objectives. Teen mothers often expressed their feelings that the classes were an important source of information and support. On a personal note, some young mothers developed strong attachments to class faculty and kept in touch long after they delivered their babies. One young mother brought the program faculty a senior prom picture of herself and her baby daughter in dazzling, matching red formals. Periodic formative evaluation demonstrated consistent gains in knowledge about reproduction, the birth process, and other curricular subjects. As a component of support activities, program faculty encouraged the teenagers to stay in or go back to school. With great satisfaction, program faculty and advocates attended high school graduation ceremonies of many teen mothers in the program.

The classes impacted clinical outcomes. Physicians and OB nurses reported that there was a significant difference in the labor and delivery management between a teen who had participated in the classes and one who had not. Class attendees had less fear and a more positive experience. Although there was no study to verify the observation, some clinicians noticed that the knowledgeable, more controlled teen moms had lower cesarean section rates.

Experience with the prenatal classes and related activities helped to raise community awareness. Understanding about issues related to adolescent childbearing began to increase. After a year of prenatal programming, AHEC brought together community leaders for the purpose of exploring further strategies. The climate was not yet conducive to emphasizing prevention. However, teens who were already parents had undeniable special needs. Consequently, the second phase of programming focused on strategies relating to teen parents.

The Program Expands to Address Additional Community Needs

The realization of the circular nature of adolescent childbearing (teen mothers are often children of teen mothers) led community leaders to look at the parenting skills of teen parents. Many of the leaders believed that interaction between young parents and their children was less nurturing than average and was sometimes abusive. One leader expressed anger at a scene she had observed. She spoke disgustedly of a young mother who had jerked her child into the air, shook the child violently, and screamed, "I wish you was never born. If you don't stop that cryin', I'll give you to the Boogie Man." Each leader spoke of similar heart-wrenching stories. Research demonstrating a higher incidence of child abuse and poor parenting skills in adolescent parents validated the leaders' observations. Research also showed that parenting skills improve as the teen parent matures. However, that improvement does not compensate for the potential loss of important nurturing for very young children. Directed by personal observations and supporting facts, representatives of 26 community agencies agreed to establish an informal collaboration to advocate parenting-skills development in teen parents. They encouraged the AHEC nurse to develop a Teen Parents Program and pledged their support.

Partnerships With Businesses

Building on the base established by the prenatal classes, wider community resources were invested in the development and long-term delivery of the Teen Parents Program. Resources came from many different directions. At an associates team rally, Wal-Mart employees agreed to donate $746 from their employee fund, which is generated from car washes, bake sales, and so forth. One of the associates spoke in support of the project by observing that "good parenting skills would make those teen parents better potential employees for Wal-Mart." Several others stated that many Wal-Mart employees had been teen parents and that they wanted to help. To encourage attendance by young parents, other businesses either donated or gave discount prices to AHEC on incentives such as movie passes, donated by the theater, and cosmetics, discounted by the drug store. A big hit with the young parents was pizza frequently donated by Pizza Hut. Arkansas Power and Light was another business partner. It donated funds toward purchasing educational material from their Stay-in-School Challenge Grant Program.

Partnerships for Essential Resources

Other diverse sources contributed support. The South Arkansas Developmental Center, which serves developmentally challenged children, donated classroom space and use of video equipment. A church donated food for refreshments from its large community garden pantry. The South Arkansas Health Education Foundation provided continuing support for personnel and operations expenditures. Grant funds from the regional March of Dimes purchased Bavolek's Nurturing Program (Bavolek & Bavolek, 1987), a skills-development program targeted specifically toward teen parents.

In a short period of time, there were enough resources to begin the program. First, AHEC needed a teacher. Newspaper advertisements attracted an expressive African-American educator to fill the position. Mrs. S. had put herself through college and graduate school while supporting her family of four children and her disabled husband. She held three jobs: two part-time, at Eckerds and Wal-Mart, and one full-time, as an elementary school counselor. She later became the first African-American female school principal in southern Arkansas. Many residents spoke of Mrs. S. as an inspiration. A graduate nursing student said that she was encouraged by Mrs. S. to continue her advanced education. The student further related how young African-American women in the community looked to Mrs. S. as a role model. She explained how Mrs. S. symbolized what hard work and high goals can accomplish even against tough odds and how everyone wanted to be like Mrs. S. Mrs. S. brought dignity, respect, and a deep commitment to helping young people to the Teen Parents Program.

Partnerships for Financial Funding

After six months of successful parenting classes, the United Way was asked to contribute to funding for the project. United Way board members reviewed the project proposal and interviewed the AHEC nurse. The informal meeting revealed high interest and concern from the United Way board regarding adolescent pregnancy. Funds were usually committed to traditional programs such as Girl Scouts. But the board felt that the parenting classes proposal had merit and decided to contribute funds to the nontraditional program as requested. The next year, a United Way community assessment revealed adolescent pregnancy as a community-wide priority of concern. The Teen Parents Program was the only service supported by United Way that dealt directly with adolescent childbearing. Consequently, United Way increased its contributions to the Teen Parents Program. The following year, the Teen Parents Program received support from a competitive research grant and did not require United Way funds. Reluctant to withdraw support, United Way officials actively followed the progress of the project and pledged further funds when needed.

Partnerships With the Media

This movement of the community to address adolescent childbearing problems continued to grow slowly. Little by little, during the development of the adolescent prenatal and parenting classes, AHEC and others made efforts to address public awareness and opinion. Utilizing health care providers, a local radio station produced public service announcements that encouraged prenatal care. Television also played a role in building public awareness. The AHEC nurse developed a positive relationship with the regional TV news reporter assigned to El Dorado. When the reporter needed background information for health-related stories, the AHECs nurse's assistance strengthened their relationship. The reporter had a genuine interest in issues of adolescent childbearing. She related observations from her own high school experience; with obvious disapproval, the reporter told of her school's most popular cheerleader's several abortions that "no one seemed to care about." Subsequently, the reporter contributed several broadcast news stories that focused on adolescent childbearing. One particularly effective series featured a touching interview with an adolescent mother who had participated in the Teen Parents Program. The usually timid young mother convincingly articulated the knowledge and parenting confidence she had gained from parenting classes. One parenting concept she specifically spoke of was nonabusive discipline: "My little girl and I have learned to use 'time-out' when she's bad. 'Time-out' was hard for her at first, but it works better than a spankin' most of the time."

Partnerships With Education

In another awareness-raising activity, the school system participated in an AHEC-designed descriptive study involving all eighth-grade students. Although the study had a career-selection focus, a small section of the survey tool elicited student perceptions of the consequences of adolescent childbearing. Consistently over 2.5 years, 21% of the students surveyed did not think that having a child before completing high school would interfere with their career plans. AHEC reported the results of the study to school administration, teachers, and board members. They recognized that a poor grasp of cause-and-effect relationships in a pubescent population has serious health-risk implications. Realizing that the study was of their own students and not some "out-of-state, big-city kids" multiplied the stunning effect.

One group's concern took a different direction. Touched by the plight of pregnant adolescents and committed to providing alternatives to abortion, the group established a home for unwed mothers. Ironically, the expensive residence, developed primarily to serve others in the state, did little to assist those in the immediate community. However, these activities contributed to the overall community perceptions, motivations, and awareness that the problems of adolescent pregnancy are serious and worthy of attention.

Changing Community Attitudes

Further evidence of the community's changing attitudes came through requests for information from youth service organizations, which began as a trickle and progressed with regularity. These calls asked for presentations from health care providers relating to adolescent sexuality and childbearing. Teachers requested information and supportive literature to incorporate into their health lesson plans. A high-profile long-term community resident, also a registered nurse, became a significant factor in increased activity. Mrs. C. had not worked as a nurse for 20 years, but she had a long list of credits for community civic contributions. The community acclaimed her 25 years of teaching creative Sunday School classes to high school students. Her work with the Salvation Army youth program was also widely known and admired. People enthused, "If Mrs. C. is involved with a project, then it must be good." Mrs. C. wanted to be involved in the comprehensive programming for premature, adolescent childbearing. With extensive experience with children, including having raised four girls, Mrs. C. developed presentations that captured the attention of both children and parents. She was able to communicate the most sensitive information with accuracy and acceptance. With that ability and effectiveness, she became the point position for primary prevention programming. Her stature in the community and energetic passion for making things happen added momentum to the community's changed attitudes.

In the most difficult arena of change, local school board public meetings discussed the possibility of a sex education curriculum. Although the majority of the school board's members were ultraconservative, the board was accused of promoting sexual immorality and causing the deterioration of traditional families by discussing these issues. Although the meetings generated loud protests from an extremely conservative and vocal community sector, the school board quietly formed a study task force. The school board asked the task force to evaluate the current curriculum and recommend changes that would result in compliance with state-legislated requirements in essential sex education for grades K–12. Over several years, the school system took steps to integrate acceptable sex education elements in the curriculum. Teachers usually delivered information regarding sexuality within the framework of traditional family values. They emphasized the "just say no" option for preventing pregnancy and gradually other critical prevention education material began to appear with less and less publicity and protest.

Primary Prevention Is Achieved

Thus, over several years, the community partnership implemented the third phase of the programming: primary prevention. Adaptation to cultural constraints and gaining support from community personalities continued as prudent strategies in the development of primary prevention education. There were no ostentatious blitzes or fanfare, just the thread-by-thread weaving of a fabric, as it were, that could be used by the community for protection and growth.

Building comprehensive programming for this community's adolescent childbearing problems included secondary, tertiary, and finally, primary prevention. Visible, AHEC-generated activities were a stimulus for the community to initiate its own actions in each focal area. Certainly, what the partnership accomplished was only a beginning; much more work remains to be done. Results of the initial programming cannot be truly evaluated for another 10 to 15 years. There are notable individual triumphs such as Tricia, a third-generation premature mother, who managed to go to college. Tricia has great hopes that her daughter, Alicia, will break the pattern of adolescent parenting and poverty. But success stories such as this can be countered with disappointments such as the little sister who got pregnant within a year after attending prenatal classes with her mother and pregnant sister.

Community Empowerment

Perhaps the most immediate and significant outcome from the community/AHEC partnership was community empowerment. The process of empowerment began with the community identifying its own needs and priorities. Purely objective assessment based on statistics and comparisons to other national standards could have elicited other health care priorities. But gathering subjective data from community residents demonstrated outsiders' confidence in the community's self-determination ability. An additive benefit of early community involvement was the reduction of resistance to change. Community involvement in each step of the planning process helped to establish an appropriate model for strategic and long-term problem solving. A planning model further empowered the community by reducing potential squandering of resources from reactionary jumping from one issue to another.

Both in and of itself and as a component of the planning process, action is an empowering force. High rates of adolescent pregnancy have existed in El Dorado for several generations. Poverty, also indigenous to southern Arkansas, is very highly correlated to adolescent pregnancy rates. Although no one likes the situation, it has been that way for as long as most people can remember. A long-standing complex problem can be overwhelming, like a room that is so dirty that one closes the door and pretends it's not there. But each specific positive action fosters a sense of control, a dynamic power that enables the next step. Whether it be the initiation of prenatal classes or a small contribution toward a teen graduating from high school, momentum alone gives encouragement for chipping away at mountainous challenges. With each layer of action, El Dorado took greater control over the daunting problems of adolescent pregnancy.

Summary

Layers of action and change are achieved by individuals. One person does make a difference. To create community change, start by finding a committed, action-oriented individual. El Dorado had many such individuals. Enlisting the synergistic forces of people like Mrs. S. and Mrs. C. facilitated community empowerment. Linking individuals in collaboration is the essence of partnership building.

Building a community partnership that can generate empowerment requires adaptation to the culture, sensitivity to community values, and allowance of adequate time. The initial activities ascribed to the El Dorado, Arkansas, partnership required five years to accomplish. In many places, but particularly in rural settings, it is often best not to begin something if one cannot see it through. False starts increase resistance to future change movements and perpetuate acceptance of unhealthy situations. A realistic assessment of the resources and time that one is willing and able to commit should be taken at the beginning of a community partnership. Although it requires significant time to begin the community change process, once inertia is overcome, the winds of change may have cascading effects. For example, in El Dorado the same community/AHEC partnership that began adolescent childbearing programming also facilitated the development of advanced nursing education, fulfilling a 25-year-old community goal. Even with adequate time allowances, successful community partnership building can only be achieved within the boundaries of that community's values. Strategies that do not accommodate the community's prevalent values and philosophy have limited outcomes. They are not likely to either engage or empower the community. Furthermore, rural community partnerships are molded within the framework of rural concepts such as those outlined by Long and Weinert (1989). To ignore rural concepts is to risk being dismissed as a "meddlin' outsider." However, when incorporated into the building design, rural concepts strengthen the partnership.

Building partnerships can be a life-changing adventure and possibly a habit. Although it is both worthwhile and humbling, it is not for those who require immediate gratification or lack perseverance. The builder will need the tools of patience and faith in empowerment and patience for the process. Equipped with these tools, those who are willing to try and willing to learn can experience the rich reward of rural community partnership building.

REFERENCES

Alexander, G., Petersen, D., Hulsey, T., & Gibson, J. (1987). Adolescent sexual activity and pregnancy in South Carolina: Trends, risks, and practice implications. *Adolescent Pregnancy, 80*(5), 581–587.

Arkansas Department of Health. (1990). *Arkansas vital statistics 1990.* Little Rock: Center for Health Statistics and Division of Vital Records.

Bavolek, S., & Bavolek, J. (1987). *Nurturing program for teen parents and young children.* Eau Claire, WI: Family Development Resources, Inc.

Fuller, S., Lum, B., Sprik, M., & Cooper, E. (1988). A small group can go a long way. *Maternal Child Health, 13,* 414–418.

Hardy, J., & Repke, J. (1987). The Johns Hopkins Adolescent pregnancy program: An evaluation. *Obstetrics & Gynecology, 69*(3), 414–418.

Lenz, C., & Edwards, J., (1992). Nurse-managed primary care: tapping the rural community power base. *Journal of Nursing Administration, 22*(9), 57–61.

Lineberger, M. (1987). Pregnant adolescents attending prenatal parent education classes: Self-concept, anxiety, and depression levels. *Adolescence, 22*(85), 179–193.

Long, K., & Weinert, C. (1989). Rural nursing: Developing the theory base. *Scholarly Inquiry for Nursing Practice: An International Journal, 3*(2), 113–127.

Morbidity and Mortality Weekly Report (*MMWR*) (1990). Teenage pregnancy and birth rates—United States, 1990. *MMWR, 42*(38),734–735.

Nichols, E. (1989). Response to rural nursing: Developing the theory base. *Scholarly Inquiry for Nursing Practice: An International Journal, 3*(2), 129–132.

Slager-Earnest, S., Hoffman, S., & Beckmann, C. (1987, November/December). Effects of a specialized prenatal adolescent program on maternal and infant outcomes. *Journal of Obstetric Gynecologic and Neonatal Nursing*, Nov/Dec, *17*(6), 422–429.

14

Refugee Health and Community Nursing—Dallas, Texas

Charles Kemp

Since 1975, at least 1 million refugees have come to the United States (Office of Refugee Resettlement, 1992). The first and largest wave of refugees came from Vietnam, Cambodia, and Laos as a result of the war in Southeast Asia; later groups of refugees coming to the United States included persons from Ethiopia, Cuba, Eastern Europe, and Iraq (the Kurds). There are also unknown numbers of people from Central America, Haiti, China, and other countries who, although not legally classified as such, have many or all of the characteristics of refugees.

Characteristics of Refugees

Although there are individual variations, people who are members of refugee communities share certain characteristics regardless of ethnicity or social class (Kemp, 1993). Descriptions of some of these characteristics are presented in the following sections.

Displacement

Refugees leave their homeland and culture without hope of return. Culture shock is thus overwhelming and unrelenting. A lifetime of memories, familiarity, and accomplishment is abandoned, and a completely new and often incomprehensible and hostile world is entered. The language, customs, and values of the new world not only are different from those of the refugee but also are perceived by many refugees as superior. Adjustment to the new culture is often more difficult for refugees than for immigrants (Lipson & Meleis, 1985).

War/Trauma Experience

War is the most brutal experience in the world; it is simply unimaginable to those who have not experienced it. Caught in the middle and burdened by family and possessions, refugees often experience far greater brutality than do the actual combatants. Common experiences include the following:

- The home and all possessions are destroyed. Any valuables retained are usually stolen by soldiers, bandits, or refugee camp guards or traded for food or medicine.
- Family members are killed or wounded. During fighting, separation of family members may occur, and for various reasons some may be abandoned.
- Rape and other assaults are far more common than is generally reported (Granjon & Deloche, 1993), and torture is also common (Jacobsen & Vesti, 1989). The norms of war are dominance and humiliation.
- Hunger is widespread. Food (or its lack) is a classic and effective weapon of war, and civilians, of course, are the last priority for receiving food and the first to have it taken away.
- Health is compromised. Risk factors include nutritional deficiencies, shortages of medicine, shortages of health personnel, and lack of facilities. Health problems are discussed in a later section.
- Life in a refugee camp is usually difficult. Conditions in most camps are primitive and dangerous, with many camps similar to third-world prisons.

Post-traumatic stress disorder (PTSD) or combat stress reaction (CSR) are common responses to war trauma (Mollica, Caspi-Yavin, Bollini, Truong, & Lavelle, 1992; Solomon, 1993). Refugees are *always* on the side that loses and suffers the most in a war. The accompanying display explains the process of becoming a refugee.

Becoming a Refugee

The process of becoming a refugee begins when an individual, family, or community is displaced from the homeland by war and/or repression. To avoid death, torture, or imprisonment, it becomes necessary to seek refuge, usually temporary, in another country, which is called the "country of first asylum." Food, shelter, and health care are provided most often by the United Nations High Commissioner For Refugees (UNHCR), private or nongovernmental voluntary agencies (VOLAGs or NGOs), and the country of first asylum. Stays in these countries are usually temporary and characterized by hardship.

While in the country of first asylum, refugees are screened by the immigration and naturalization services of potential host countries. Those who pass the screening (and many do not) are then eligible to go to a permanent home in the host country or "country of second asylum." Transportation is funded by the host government or a VOLAG, and the refugee is responsible for paying back the price of transportation.

Refugee resettlement in the United States takes place under the auspices of VOLAG resettlement agencies (the sponsors) such as Catholic Charities, International Rescue Committee, or Church World Service. With grants of $200 to $300 per refugee, these agencies provide living expenses and casework services for two to three months and then, in most cases, discontinue services. Refugees who are resettled through churches or similar groups tend to receive services for longer periods of time. Volunteer, mutual aid groups, and health and social service providers play essential roles in providing support to refugees after resettlement agency services are discontinued.

Note should be made of persons classified by immigration services as "nonrefugees" or "economic refugees." These are people judged to not be in danger of repression if returned to their country of origin or who seek to leave their home country for economic reasons only. People from El Salvador and Haiti are examples of those who have been unable to achieve legal refugee status but for all practical purposes can be considered refugees.

Grief

Through war and displacement, refugees lose their home, possessions, and often loved ones. Any one of these losses might result in severe grief. Other losses that may be less obvious include the following:

- The unconditional loss of a war, that is, complete dominance by a hostile force, may be a shattering blow to individual and community esteem.
- Decisions made during war or flight from war may come to haunt refugees as they shift from circumstances of war to those of peace. What seemed right and necessary at one time may later be perceived as wrong and perhaps unnecessary.
- Old ways of life are seldom valued in the new life. The respected family or village elder becomes irrelevant, impotent, or even an object of ridicule. Relations within families or groups undergo irrevocable change. Rituals, ceremonies, and perhaps religions are out of synch with the mainstream culture and may thus lose at least some of their power. Adjustment to the new culture, highly valued by many, means losing the old while never quite gaining the new. These losses may be complicated by difficulty in articulating them to others.
- Loss of future is a subtle and little-understood phenomenon. For many refugees the future seems at best uncertain. Once safety is reached, there is a sense of great relief, but relief is often followed by persistent and well-founded uncertainty and anxiety about the future.

Health Problems

Refugees frequently exhibit a poor health status typified by serious physical and mental health problems (International Council of Nurses, 1991). In countries of first asylum, the leading causes of morbidity and mortality among refugees are measles, diarrheal diseases, respiratory infections, and in some locales, malaria (Centers for Disease Control, 1992). The severity of these illnesses is markedly increased by malnutrition.

Common communicable diseases of refugees in countries of second asylum include tuberculosis, other upper-respiratory infections, gastrointestinal infections, and familiar childhood infections. Chronic illnesses commonly include hypertension, arthritis, and stress-related disorders such as gastrointestinal distress and headache. The long-term sequelae of tuberculosis, hepatitis B, and malnutrition are an emerging problem (Frye, 1990a). Especially during the early stages of resettlement prenatal care, family planning services, and child health services are underutilized. Mental health is compromised, with anxiety disorders such as

PTSD and CSR and affective disorders such as depression or dysthymia predominating. Family violence and substance abuse are not uncommon. These health problems may all be complicated by long-term nutritional deficits.

Access to care frequently becomes a problem after the initial two to three months of service delivery by resettlement agencies and before independence is achieved. Problems of access include finding and getting to a source of care, communicating accurately with the provider, following instructions, and obtaining follow-up or specialty care.

The Refugee Health Project

Beginning in 1981, large numbers of Cambodian refugees were resettled in "cluster projects" in several locations in the United States. These projects consisted of 500 to 1,500 refugees placed in apartment complexes in low-income areas of such cities as Los Angeles, Houston, Dallas, New York, and Boston. By 1985, approximately 150,000 Cambodians were resettled in the United States (Frye, 1990b). With only a few exceptions, the pattern of resettlement services was the same: After providing minimal services to families for a few months, refugee agencies turned to newer arrivals and left previous arrivals to fend for themselves. Cut off from American society and services by language, cultural, knowledge, and transportation barriers, the Cambodians found themselves in difficult and sometimes desperate circumstances. Problems were compounded by refugee agencies having failed to communicate with health and social service providers about the presence or any characteristics or problems of Cambodian refugees.

Volunteer and community groups worked to meet the needs of Cambodians, the most deeply traumatized population since the survivors of the Nazi holocaust. In Dallas, where 3,000 to 4,000 Cambodians were resettled, the effort was initiated and sustained through nurses and nursing students in partnership with refugees and community groups, most notably the Association for the Salvation of Cambodian Refugees (a refugee self-help or mutual assistance agency [MAA]) and the Dallas chapter of the National Council of Jewish Women.

The Beginning: Services and Assessment

The Refugee Health Project began as an effort of student nurses and faculty going to apartments where we knew large numbers of refugees were living. The initial undertaking was twofold:

- To find refugees or other people who needed health care and provide or find the care
- To assess the community

Operating in two-person teams, students went door to door, inquiring about the problems and needs of families and individuals. By the end of the first day, two students had helped deliver a baby, and all students had found at least one family needing assistance with health care. Every day of the experience, we found people with health needs that we could meet, primarily through helping overcome problems of access, teaching, and case management–related activities. Few women were receiving any prenatal care, and about 20% of Cambodian women were having home births for the sole reason that they did not know how to get to a hospital (Sargent & Marcucci, 1984). Almost every home had at least one person with upper-respiratory or gastrointestinal infections. Food, clothing, and blankets were frequently lacking, and hunger was not uncommon. It was not long before we had people waiting for us every day we came to the community. All referrals to students were from the refugee community itself.

For the first month the project operated out of the back of one faculty member's pickup truck, which was parked in a refugee apartment lot. As the weather cooled, we moved into a Cambodian family's apartment. By the end of the semester, we had found a refugee agency at a church that was willing to let us use its office and phones.

Because of language and cultural barriers, communication was an ongoing problem. The accompanying display cites some of these barriers to addressing the needs of refugees or similarly underserved populations. Through the first and following semesters, we moved gradually from utilizing neighbors and family members for translation to identifying key individuals who were able to translate with accuracy. Eventually, through grants and agreements with mutual assistance and refugee agencies, we were able to pay for translating services for students.

It soon became clear to faculty and students that (1) the primary individual, family, and community problem was access to services and (2) if we did not provide or find the services, nobody would. We also realized that needs were so apparent and great that conducting a community assessment first (or alone) seemed unethical. However, it was also clear that a community assessment was essential to obtaining services beyond those we were able to provide.

Frequently Cited Barriers to Addressing the Needs of Refugees or Similarly Underserved Populations

In discussing this learning experience with community health nurses, especially those serving as faculty, we repeatedly heard concerns about perceived barriers that kept them from seriously considering an experience such as this. Those concerns were so widespread and so disturbing that they deserve to be addressed in specific terms. Perceived barriers to working to meet the needs of this or similarly underserved populations and responses to those barriers include the following:

- There is a language barrier. Our experience with Cambodian, Kurdish, and other non-English-speaking people however, is that there is always a way around this barrier. Neighbors may speak some English, and sometimes refugee agencies or other organizations will help. Because of language differences, health histories may not be 100% accurate, but something is better than nothing. A blood test and a pelvic examination during one or two visits are infinitely better than no prenatal care at all. Through the process of providing care, translators are identified, and other means of communication are developed.

- There is no agency providing care. The lack of a health provider for a population does not mean that nurses should not get involved! Too often, nurses let others decide who receives services and how they will be delivered. The mission of community health nursing is to apply the nursing process to populations, not to provide services according to the existence of health care agencies. Populations with the greatest health needs often are the least connected to providers. It is sometimes necessary to create health resources.

Students in that first semester completed a community assessment. Although the assessment met course objectives, the faculty felt that it would not adequately serve the purposes we had set for it of (1) informing the broad community of Dallas health and social service providers about the realities of life in the Cambodian community and (2) being a fund-raising tool. Moreover, the Cambodian community did not lend itself to quick assessment. There were no health statistics and almost nothing in the literature on Cambodian health care beliefs and practices. The larger resettlement agencies were uncooperative with both students and Cambodian mutual assistance groups.

The assessment done in the first semester was therefore revised and expanded by the second-semester students, who used the knowledge generated by the first-semester students to develop a deeper beginning understanding of the community. Second-semester students were thus better able to *immerse themselves in the community and culture.* This deeper understanding and immersion worked synergistically and led to improved relations between students and refugees and thus to a community assessment with "soul"—a living document that spoke to health providers, educators, social service providers, church-sponsored agencies, and others and that was clearly based on first-hand experience. This is in contradistinction to what the assessment could have been, a report that provided primarily biostatistical and secondary data. We obtained a small grant to print several hundred copies of the community assessment and distributed these to appropriate individuals and agencies.

We eventually concluded that providing services, especially case management, should be an essential component of most serious community assessments, that is, assessments intended to lead to implementation of a plan to address the health needs of a community. Community-based case management as part of assessment allows the assessor to understand the health care and social service systems from the community's perspective.

Analysis

Although access to services was the primary community problem and the overriding focus of efforts throughout the life of the project, there were, of course, compelling family and individual problems as well. Students and faculty found themselves face to face with people who had been starved and tortured and who had seen loved ones starved, tortured, and killed. There was a constant refrain of death: "Soldiers Pol Pot kill all. Kill all! Family all die. Now me one person." ("Soldiers Pol Pot" refers to soldiers of the communist Khmer Rouge, led by a man named Pol Pot.) In many cases abandoned by their sponsors and living in a tough urban environment, families struggled to survive with dignity.

With a very few exceptions, students effectively identified and analyzed family and individual problems. Diagnosing community problems occurred in clinical group meetings and was an ongoing and difficult process. Besides group agreement on the diagnosis, at least some degree of community agreement was also required. Thus, a diagnosis agreed upon by students was presented to people in the community so that they could verify its accuracy. Among the community diagnoses (Kemp, 1994) were the following:

- A risk of health deterioration, related to barriers to access to health care services
- Negatively altered nutrition, related to lack of knowledge
- Ineffective coping on the part of the community, related to lack of knowledge and post-traumatic stress
- Negatively altered parenting, related to difficulties in adapting to the new culture

Several of these diagnoses were not widely regarded as significant problems among the Cambodians—for example, poor nutrition, which was not perceived by some Cambodians as being of concern except as it applied to families who did not know how to obtain adequate food. Students and faculty, on the other hand, saw a problem in the rapid shift among some children from indigenous foods to sweetened cereal, soft drinks, and the like and in the widespread, rapid shift from breast- to bottle-feeding. A lack of response among the Cambodians to efforts aimed at changing nutritional patterns indicated that community agreement about problems was important.

Planning

Plans to meet health and other needs of families and individuals usually focused on instruction and helping with access to services. Three basic directions evolved in plans to meet community health needs:

- Resource development
- Providing knowledge to the Cambodian community about health-related matters, especially what services were available and how to access them
- Providing knowledge about Cambodians and other refugees to health and social service providers

Plans evolved from semester to semester; the resource development plan was developed and enacted over the course of eight semesters. Each of the basic directions is discussed below.

Resource Development

Acting as advocates, nursing students were able to obtain care for Cambodians, but the Cambodians had tremendous difficulty in obtaining care for themselves. Only naive students would consider starting a clinic as a means of ensuring community access to services, and only a nurse committed to community health would ask, "Why not?" It seemed clear, however, that developing community resources would be the best means of addressing problems of access to health care services, and community support for resource development was unanimous among Cambodians. And once viewed outside the artificial constraints of semesters and changes in student clinical groups, setting up a clinic seemed possible.

Planning began with revising and expanding the community assessment so that it could serve as a fund-raising tool. The assessment also helped identify potential resources that might help with fund-raising or other aspects of resource development. Ultimately, the resources section of the assessment served as a blueprint for individuals and organizations that would participate in the coalition that developed the clinic.

Rather than make detailed plans for services, we planned primarily to build a coalition of individuals and organizations with whom we could work to create services. A broad-based coalition was needed. Along with the Cambodian community itself, we needed people or organizations with the ability to interact effectively with foundations and politicians. Because of their history and experience with their own holocaust, we identified the Jewish community as a natural constituent of the effort to address the health and well-being of Cambodians who themselves had survived a holocaust. (We were careful to not draw too many parallels between the holocausts except to say that both groups had suffered immensely.) The participation of the Dallas chapter of the National Council of Jewish Women (NCJW) and a large synagogue was the crux of the development process. The coalition of Cambodians and Jews was a powerful and effective symbol to which many individuals and organizations responded.

We found, as have others (for example Muecke, 1983), that Cambodians were usually reluctant to openly advocate or speak out for anything that might generate conflict. On the other hand, there was significant participation among Cambodians and respect for that participation behind the scenes and within the Cambodian community.

The partnership of Cambodians, Jews, nursing students and faculty, and other individuals and organizations had a name: We were the East Dallas Health Coalition. With assistance from volunteer attorneys and others, we applied for and received all the necessary state and federal

Assistance in starting a nonprofit organization can be found through local chapters of the National Council of Jewish Women, the Junior League, and other service groups. Some cities have organizations whose only purpose is to assist others in starting and maintaining nonprofit organizations. The following steps may vary somewhat from locale to locale.

- Determine the purpose of the organization and initiate a limited series of planning/organizing meetings. Writing a mission statement is important. The fewer the meetings, the better; too many meetings may result in a loss of focus and interest. Find an attorney. Keep minutes of all meetings.
- Tasks that must be accomplished early in the process include writing bylaws, filing for incorporation, developing a preliminary program plan and budget, and planning fund-raising. Several of these tasks require an attorney, and all usually require a committee with an involved and organized chair.
- Establish an initial board of directors. Many organizations start with a small board, later expand it, and still later reduce its size. This has to do with board politics and is far beyond the scope of this chapter.
- File for articles of incorporation.
- Draft bylaws. It is helpful to use an IRS 1023 form to be sure that legal requirements are met.
- Write goals and objectives, services plan, and management plan.
- Develop a budget.
- Develop a comprehensive fund-raising plan.
- Hold a formal organizational meeting to elect officers, accept articles of incorporation, adopt bylaws, authorize tax-exemption application, authorize necessary financial transactions if necessary, and continue planning. Meetings such as this must be carefully planned and orchestrated to avoid confusion and political battles.
- Establish a bookkeeping/accounting system. Keep in mind that a complete financial audit will be required by most funding sources within the first two years of operations.
- Find a reputable insurer and apply for board and organization liability insurance.
- File an IRS 1023 application for designation as a nonprofit 501(c)(3) organization.
- If necessary, file Charitable Trust Registration with the state.
- File for federal and state Employer Registration.
- If appropriate, apply for state sales tax exemption.
- Implement management, fund-raising, and initial service plans.
- Register with state unemployment insurance program after paid staff are present.

legal and nonprofit designations. The accompanying display outlines the steps taken to initiate a nonprofit organization.

Throughout the planning and other phases, students were providing services to Cambodians and reporting (1) needs and problems and (2) successes in addressing those needs and problems.

TAKE NOTE

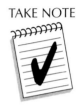

There are many communities with problems, and the presence of a community with problems is not the primary issue in community development. The primary issues are (1) that human problems exist and (2) that something can be done to help with those problems.

Fund-raising, development of volunteer services, and similar activities were conducted primarily by NCJW volunteers. Planning health services was a joint effort of all parties. Student activities in the Cambodian community were an enormous influence on the planning process. By this time, students had been working in the Cambodian community for about two years. They had a strong sense of mission in knowing that they were an essential part of a process leading to something much bigger than their own individual work. At the same time, they were keenly aware that their individual work was making an enormous difference in people's lives.

Providing Knowledge in the Cambodian Community

Most Cambodians came to the United States with little knowledge of U.S. life, customs, or languages. They also brought with them community handicaps that included universal refugee and concentration camp experience and having had their secular and religious leadership (teachers, military, priests, physicians, businessmen, and so on) systematically murdered by the communist Khmer Rouge regime. The eradication of the leadership meant, among other things, that many Cambodians were illiterate in their own language as well as English. The use of familiar teaching tools, including common life experiences/culture, a common language, written materials, and electronic media, was thus denied to the students.

After several semesters, students developed a teaching technique that included these characteristics:

- Classes or teaching "parties" were held in Cambodian apartments.

- Learners and teachers were of the same gender, and groups were small, ranging in size from 5 to 15 people. The teachers also became learners in these groups.
- Topics discussed had been identified by refugees themselves as concerns (sometimes other topics were included). Nearly all topics were directed toward increasing independence.
- Because many Cambodians, especially women, could not read, printed materials were kept to a minimum. Demonstrations and practice were the primary means of communication.
- "Favors" such as thermometers and perfume were always given.
- Follow-up to determine what was learned was included.

Many refugees learned how to prepare homemade oral rehydration solution, how to read a thermometer, how to take oral contraceptives, and other essentials of life in the United States. Central to all educational activities was encouraging the learners to teach others in the community. Increasing independence and empowerment was always a goal.

Providing Knowledge to Health and Social Service Providers

Primarily through faculty but sometimes through Cambodians and students as well, we provided in-service and other educational services to health and social service providers and community leaders. We found that small (less than 20 participants) one-day seminars in the refugee community were an effective way to educate Americans about the Cambodian community.

Implementation

From the beginning of this project, students delivered a variety of services to families and individuals. Community work was focused primarily on (1) education to improve health and increase independence and (2) development of community resources, in particular, opening a community-based clinic.

Despite great effort on the part of students and Cambodian and American volunteers, many health needs remained unmet for the first several years of the project, and everyone concerned felt a sense of urgency about opening the clinic. As the search for funding and other resources went forward, we found space that a neighborhood school was willing to donate for two evening clinics a week. Thus, in the sixth semester (year three) of the project, a community clinic opened for Cambodian refugees, which was staffed by a paid registered nurse and volunteer physician. The administrative "office" was located on an internal balcony overlooking the lobby of the YWCA a half mile from the clinic. Patient records were kept in cardboard boxes carried back and forth from the office to the clinic in the trunk of the nurse's car.

After working out of the school for about eight months, we were able to move the clinic to a renovated storefront. This was the dream: a "real clinic" in the heart of the refugee community staffed by a full-time pediatric nurse practitioner, part-time physicians, and a full-time (Cambodian) community health worker. The Cambodian mutual assistance association continued to furnish volunteers, as did the NCJW. The sign out in front of the clinic read, "East Dallas Health Coalition." The refugees gave the clinic a name a little less grand—the "two-dollar clinic"—and they came.

The clinic provided primary care five days and two nights a week. Computer links were established with the county hospital so that referrals and appointments could be made without difficulty. Direct referrals to the local women's clinic were also possible for family planning and prenatal care. The nursing students continued to work in the community, providing outreach, follow-up, and health education services. Follow-up was especially important because compliance remained a challenge even when instructions for medications or treatments were given through a translator.

Growth sometimes takes on a life of its own, and the East Dallas Health Coalition was no exception. Tension developed within the board about whether to expand the scope of the clinic and move to a larger facility further away from the refugee community or to stay small and in the heart of the community. There was logic to both positions. The clinic moved to the larger, more distant location.

Today, the East Dallas Health Coalition is incorporated into the Dallas County Hospital District Community-Oriented Primary Care (COPC) System. As part of the agreement to merge, the original governing board devolved into an advisory board, which has significant input into the policies of what is now called the East Dallas COPC Health Center. The board also raises money for equipment, services, and for the salary of a staff refugee outreach worker. Refugees continue to utilize the center's services.

Evaluation

We accomplished most of what we set out to do. Through the hard and sustained work of a coalition of diverse community groups, an essential and permanent resource was created. The health status of Cambodian refugees was markedly improved. Although we did not conduct formal research, home visits 10 years after Cambodians began coming to the United States showed the following results in Dallas:

- More than 90% of children under five years of age in surveyed families were properly immunized. Readers should note that these children were all in a very low-income neighborhood, in which 90% immunization is a high rate.
- Home births are almost unheard of.
- All families surveyed knew how to access services at the East Dallas Health Center.

Follow-up in 1994 showed that significant problems still exist. In particular, children and youth are at risk for the many problems typical of inner-city, low-income neighborhoods. The diagnosis that will determine the direction of much of the future work is the potential for developmental delay related to a lack of knowledge on the part of families and the community regarding positive child development in urban America.

Lessons Learned in Working in Refugee Health Care

Providing Care Across Cultures

Cultural characteristics and health-related beliefs exist in a matrix of individual, social, economic, gender-based, experiential, and other influences. Thus, although it is important to learn the common characteristics of the cultures in which one is working, it is essential to remember that individual and even community variations always exist. The great challenge in working across cultures is dealing with attitudes or perspectives that are unconscious or otherwise outside of awareness on both sides, in other words, attitudes or perspectives of both the patient or community *and* of the nurse or health care system. What seems obvious and just plain common sense to one may be mysterious and illogical to another.

A number of tools exist to help assess cultural, community, familial, individual, and other health values and beliefs. The tool developed by Tripp-Reimer, Brink, and Saunders (1984) is functional and relatively brief. The following questions are a slight modification of that tool and give insight into patient and family perceptions of health problems:

- What do you think caused your problem?
- Do you have an explanation for why it started when it did?
- What does your sickness do to you; how does it work?
- How severe is your sickness? How long do you expect it to last?
- What problems has your sickness caused you?
- What do you fear about your sickness?
- What kind of treatment do you think you should receive?
- What are the most important results you hope to receive from this treatment?

Tripp-Reimer, Brink, and Saunders (1984) suggested other questions, but given the realities of time constraints in providing care, especially when language barriers exist, the ones listed here serve well.

The key to providing competent care across cultures or belief systems is respect. Respect or its lack nearly always shows through and overshadows whatever knowledge one does or does not possess.

Traditional medical practices are highly regarded by many Cambodians (as well as by other populations), but there is often a concurrent regard for Western or scientific practices. In this pluralistic approach to health and illness, treatment may include traditional and Western modalities without any conflict—at least to the patient (Frye, 1990b). In the United States, the pluralistic approach is increasingly common among people with AIDS as scientific and alternative approaches to treatment are simultaneously utilized.

The Community as Partner

Sometimes it seems like we know better than patients or communities what they need. And indeed, sometimes we do. The abusive spouse, for example, who feels that violence is right and normal needs help to find a better way of interacting. However, the issue in community or other health endeavors is not who knows best but how best to achieve a higher state of health.

Developing a community coalition is challenging. Different individuals and organizations often have significantly different goals or agendas. In refugee and other communities, especially those with little power, the accrual of power is almost always an underlying issue in any endeavor. Thus, the community development process should empower the community as part of the effort to provide services or resources and improve health. To achieve success, it is necessary to involve the community as full partners who participate in

- The hard work that must be done
- The decisions that must be made
- The compromises that are always necessary

Anything other than this sort of full partnership is unlikely to result in the empowerment that is the essence of a healthy community.

The Role of the Nurse in Community Development

The role of the nurse in community development *and anything else not specifically proscribed by law is whatever we choose and are willing to work for.* We are limited primarily by our own imaginations and view of ourselves as professionals. We have tended to let others take the lead in developing community and other health resources. We serve (not to mention, serve *in leadership positions*) on distressingly few governing boards outside our own professional organizations. The amount of grant monies going to nurse-led or nursing research in comparison to that going to research initiated by other professions is pitiful.

A key characteristic of power, such as that wielded by governing boards, funding sources, agency heads, and so on, is that few people are willing to give it away. We, as nurses, must work to take a fair share of power. There should be nurses on every governing board of every community, local, and national health organization in the United States.

One way to begin taking a fair share of power in community health is to implement the community nursing process without regard to what agencies are not providing services. The process to follow is to look to communities in need and then do the following:

- Establish that needs exist and identify the needs.
- Analyze the needs.

- Develop comprehensive and effective plans to meet the needs.
- Implement the plans.
- Evaluate the effectiveness of the plans and, without apology, tell the community about the success.

Baccalaureate Nursing Students and Community Health Services

Nursing students are surely one of the most undervalued and underutilized health resources in the United States. Our experience is that nursing students can play central roles in community assessment, community development, primary care, and other aspects of community health not always considered as student roles. Our experience also is that nursing students have a strong positive response to being valued and making a real and lasting difference in the lives of people and communities.

The Good Fortune of Living in the United States

For all the problems that exist in the United States, we who live here are very fortunate. We worry about violence in the United States, yet compared with the violence of war, violence-related morbidity and mortality here are almost insignificant (statistically, anyway). We worry about homelessness in America while 17 million persons worldwide are homeless refugees without even a country and 16 to 20 million persons are homeless war-related refugees within their own countries (Centers for Disease Control, 1992). We worry about the nutritional status of Americans, yet we have never seen anything even remotely related to the monstrous starvation we keep seeing in places like Biafra, India, Bangladesh, Cambodia, Somalia, and so many others.

We are fortunate that we live in relative safety and prosperity. Most of the world aches to come to the United States. We are fortunate, too, that we can offer refuge to some of the dispossessed of the world and that as nurses we can participate in a concrete manner.

REFERENCES

Centers for Disease Control. (1992). Famine-affected, refugee, and displaced populations: Recommendations for public health issues. *Morbidity and Mortality Weekly Report, 41*/No. RR-13.

Frye, B. (1990a). The Cambodian refugee patient: Providing culturally sensitive rehabilitation nursing care. *Rehabilitation Nursing, 15*(3), 157–159.

———— (1990b). The process of health care decision making among Cambodian immigrant women. *International Quarterly of Community Health Education, 10*(2), 113–124.

Granjon, P., & Deloche, P. (1993). Rape as a weapon of war. *Refugees, 93*, 42–44.

International Council of Nurses: Council of National Representatives. (1991). *Health services for migrants, refugees, and displaced persons.* Geneva: Author.

Jacobsen, L., and Vesti, P. (1989). Treatment of torture survivors and their families: The nurse's function. *International Nursing Review, 36*(3), 75–80.

Kemp, C.E. (1993). Health services for refugees in countries of second asylum. *International Nursing Review, 40*(1), 21–24.

———— (1994). Community health clinical experiences: The primary health care setting. *Public Health Nursing, 11*(1), 2–6.

Lipson, J.G., and Meleis, A.I. (1985). Culturally appropriate care: The case of immigrants. *Topics in Clinical Nursing, 7*(3), 48–56.

Mollica, R.F., Caspi-Yavin, Y., Bollini, P., Truong, T., & Lavelle, J. (1992). Validating a cross-cultural instrument for measuring torture, trauma, and post-traumatic stress disorder in Indochinese refugees. *Journal of Nervous and Mental Disease, 180*(2), 111–116.

Muecke, M. (1983). Caring for Southeast Asian refugees in the U.S.A. *American Journal of Public Health, 73*(4), 431–438.

Office of Refugee Resettlement. (1992). *Refugee Reports, 12*(3), 10–13.

Sargent, C.F., and Marcucci, J. (1984). Aspects of Khmer medicine among refugees in urban America. *Medical Anthropology Quarterly, 16*(1), 7–9.

Solomon, Z. (1993). *Combat stress reaction: The enduring toll of war.* New York: Plenum Press.

Tripp-Reimer, T., Brink, P.J., & Saunders, J.M. (1984). Cultural assessment: Content and process. *Nursing Outlook, 32*(2), 78–82.

15

Promoting Healthy Partnerships With Migrant Farmworkers—Colorado

Rachel Rodriguez

After a long, hard, and hot day in the field,
under the implacable rays of the Father of Life,
my muscles ache and my bones hurt and crack
as though they were crystals breaking.
I'm dirty, thirsty, and hungry.
My body is so tired and sore
that I fear it might crumble
like an old building being torn down

Eugenia Ortiz
Voices From the Fields
(Atkin, 1993)

Introduction

Migrant farmworkers travel thousands of miles each year searching for work in some of the most hazardous occupations in the United States. Dangerous working conditions, exposure to pesticides, and the potential for infectious disease are only a few of the risks associated with migrant farmwork (Wilk, 1986). Low wages and harsh living conditions contribute to the potential for poor health that is virtually inevitable for the migrant farmworker (Slesinger, 1992).

A *migrant farmworker* is described by the federal government as "an individual whose principal employment within the last 24 months

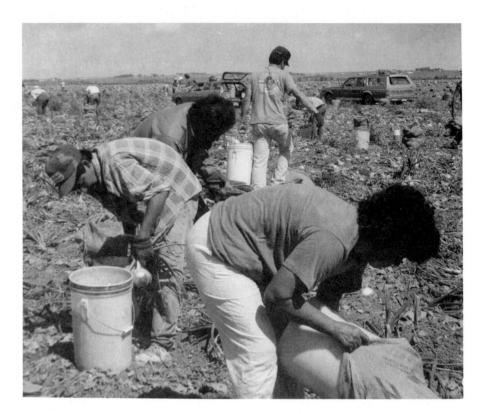

FIGURE 15-1
Long hours in the field, low wages, and temporary employment define the lifestyle of migrant farmworkers.

[has been] in agriculture on a seasonal basis . . . and [has established] a temporary abode for employment purposes" (Migrant Health Program, 1992, p. 1) (see Figure 15-1). Farmworkers travel through three main streams or routes. The western stream encompasses southern California and Arizona to northern California, Oregon, and Washington. The midwestern stream includes southern Texas and progresses to Illinois, Michigan, Wisconsin, Colorado, and most of the midwestern states. The eastern stream begins in Florida, moves through the Carolinas, and ends in upstate New York (Martaus, 1986).

Migrant farmworkers routinely leave their permanent home (home base) and live in temporary housing (labor camps) for approximately six months out of the year while working in northern states. Some families move continuously throughout the year, following the crops. Men sometimes leave their families at the home base and travel alone to work. Often families, particularly extended families, travel together.

Migrant farmworkers are a multiethnic group. Hispanics make up the largest segment (60%). Most are Mexican or Mexican American. Puerto Ricans, Central Americans, Haitians, and African Americans are also among those doing farmwork throughout the country (Zuroweste, 1991; Office of Migrant Health, 1992).

It is estimated that 70% of migrant women work in the fields (National Advisory Council on Migrant Health, 1992). Life in the camps is particularly difficult for women. After working 10 to 12 hours in the field, their work day continues with housework and child care (Rodriguez, 1993b).

Children also work in the fields alongside their parents. Approximately 20% of migrant agricultural workers are under the age of 18 (Atkin, 1993). Children working in the fields often sacrifice their education in order to help support the family (see Figure 15-2).

Health of Migrant Farmworkers

Documentation regarding the health status of migrant farmworkers is lacking. Although there is regional and anecdotal information suggesting that farmworkers are at risk for poor health, there is a paucity of reliable research data. Acccording to Meister (1991), available data documenting the health needs of migrant farmworkers are sparse, incomplete, or inconclusive.

Rust (1990) also illustrated the lack of reliable data through a review of the literature covering a period from 1966 to 1989. Of 485 articles identified over this 23-year period, only 152 were found to relate specifically to migrant families. Rust identified a long list of unanswered questions relating to the health of migrant farmworkers, including questions about population characteristics, mortality and survival data, perinatal outcome data, chronic diseases, health-related behaviors (including domestic violence), and accessibility to health care.

Literature focusing specifically on migrant health reveals the following. A recent review by Dever (1991) of 6,969 patient charts from migrant health centers across the country revealed a listing of the most common

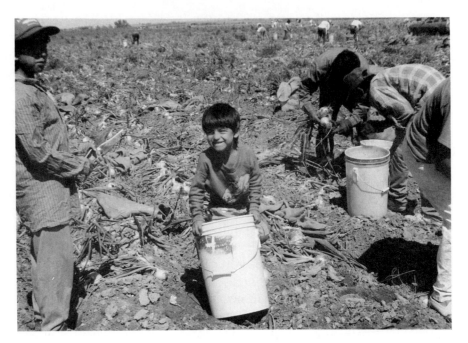

FIGURE 15-2
Even young children are not exempt from working in the fields.

health problems encountered by migrant workers using migrant clinics. He found that migrant farmworkers suffered from a number of complex health problems such as infectious diseases, diabetes, hypertension, and contact dermatitis. He also found that 40% of migrant farmworkers who visited health clinics suffered from multiple health problems.

The health of migrant farmworker children is also discussed by Dever (1991). According to his survey, children aged 1–4 visit migrant clinics for infectious and nutritional health problems. For children aged 10–14, dental disease is the primary health problem.

Another chart review (*n* = 936) by Arbab and Weidner (1986) focused on clinic utilization rates and the prevalence of infectious diseases in migrant farmworkers without access to water and sanitation facilities. An audit of 936 clinic charts found that such farmworkers had a clinic utilization rate for diarrhea that was 20 times higher than that of the urban poor (control group). Fevers of unknown origin were 120 times more common than in the control group.

Chapter 15   **Promoting Healthy Partnerships—Colorado**   383

Medical utilization patterns were also examined by Chi (1985). He found that female migrants were more likely than males to visit a physician. As would be expected, the availability of Medicaid increased the number of physician visits, although only 12% of the sample were covered by Medicaid.

Martaus (1986) conducted a descriptive study of the health-seeking process of migrant farmworkers. The study included a sample of 20 Mexican or Mexican Americans working in northwest Ohio. She offered an illness-focused model beginning with symptom definition and ending with adherence to treatment. Martaus found that migrant farmworkers' explanations for illness could be summarized in three ways. Hot/cold imbalance, germ theory, and emotional origin seemed to explain illnesses in her study population. Sudden onset of symptoms was considered highly credible and a measure of real illness. There were two factors that influenced a person's choice of treatment. First, the most important outcome of the treatment should be quick and effective relief of symptoms. Second, trust in the source of advice for the treatment was the most influential factor in one's use of a remedy.

The health of migrant farmworker women is an area about which little is known. There have been no comprehensive studies focusing specifically on the health of migrant women. Data on pregnancy outcomes and infant mortality rates are scarce. A study in California (Slesinger, Christensen, & Cautley, 1986) found an infant mortality rate of 29 per 1000 among migrant farmworkers, compared to 14 per 1000 in the general U.S. population. This same 1986 study reported a mortality rate of 46 per 1000 migrant children under the age of five. de la Torre & Rush (1989) found that 24% of women in their sample ($n = 148$) experienced one or more miscarriages and/or stillbirths. A survey of migrant farmworkers in Colorado (Littlefield & Stout, 1987) documented that 32.5% of their sample ($n = 120$) experienced at least one miscarriage or abortion. Infant mortality for this sample was reported as 12.5%.

There are no studies currently found in the literature that focus on the prevalence of domestic violence among migrant farmworkers or the consequences of this violence on the health of migrant women. Although published studies do not yet exist, anecdotal information from both migrant health clinicians and migrant farmworker women indicates that domestic violence is a major concern of this population. Along these same lines, the Office of Migrant Health of the U.S. Public Health Service has identified the reduction of violent and abusive behavior, including domestic violence, in its *Migrant and Seasonal Farmworker Health Objectives for the Year 2000* (Office of Migrant Health, 1990).

Access to Health Care

Access to health care is nothing short of a luxury for migrant farmworkers. Across the United States, there are over 100 federally funded migrant health clinics serving approximately 500,000 farmworkers in 40 states and Puerto Rico. This number represents only 12% of the estimated 3 to 5 million migrant farmworkers in the United States today. Current expenditures by the federal government for migrant health are approximately $100 per person per year (National Advisory Council on Migrant Health, 1993).

In addition to the barriers that exist for other disenfranchised populations, for example, cost, transportation, and language/culture differences, there are barriers to access that are unique to the transient nature of migrant life. Examples of these were evident in a recent ethnographic study (Rodriguez, 1993a) with hispanic migrant farmworker women. Examples of these barriers included *lack of time, lack of trust, and women's relationships with men.*

To illustrate the issue of time, women described their typical daily schedule. They arose at 4 or 5 A.M. to prepare the meals and get the family ready for the day. They worked in the fields until approximately 5 or 6 P.M. and then continued their work day with housework and child care. They usually retired around midnight. In the words of one farmworker woman:

> I think that was what was needed, counseling for this (cancer, diabetes) and for the women to check themselves regularly because they don't have time, if they have something else to do, they don't give themselves time. . . . because she wants to get her work done and get some rest, it's more important to wash the dishes or the clothes to finish quickly and get some rest.

Trust is also a barrier to access to health care. Farmworker women described the problem of gossip, which is pervasive in migrant camps:

> A lot of people don't know each other so they don't even share their problems with other people because they don't really know them. . . . I would

look for somebody that doesn't gossip, it's hard though because in the camp a lot of people like to gossip and they go from house to house.

Migrant women's relationships with men exacerbate the isolation that evolves from these barriers of time and trust:

Well, the first thing that comes to my mind is there was a couple last year and we would invite her to come to the group sessions but the husband didn't let her, I mean "your place is right here inside the house" [respondent uses husband's words], and if she wanted to go and hang up some clothes on the clothes line he would go with her, so I think most of that is the husband . . . because there was more people in the camp, like men, you know, looking through the windows or whatever and maybe they think they're looking at the wife.

Men's control over women's activities can also lead to forced avoidance of health care services. Migrant women have reported that men do not allow them to seek health care:

There's times when they're really sick [the women] and they need to go to the doctor, but their husbands just really don't want them to . . . and the husband won't let them because he doesn't want them to and he doesn't have time and won't give them permission and if she doesn't have permission, she can't go.

(Rodriguez, 1993a).

Implications for Nursing and Health Care

Nurses have traditionally been educated within a biomedical framework or model that is based on Western European cultural values. In *The Health of Women*, Brems and Griffiths (1993) described biomedicine as dividing the human being into the "somatic body and intangible mind" (p. 260). They also described how the biomedical model separates the mind from the body and further dissects the body into systems and organs, emphasizing areas of specialization for health care practioners. Brems and Griffiths further stated that "biomedicine has a . . . tendency to divide health from the setting that produces it" (p. 260).

The migrant women interviewed in the ethnographic study (Rodriguez, 1993a) neither separated the mind from the body nor defined health from a biomedical, illness-based perspective. The data indicate that the respondents' definitions of health could not be separated from their lifestyle or their environment, in other words, from the setting that produced them. The culture of their transient lifestyle clearly had an impact on the way these women described and ordered their world and, consequently, could not be separated from how they described and defined health.

The way in which hispanic migrant farmworker women described and defined health is illustrative of the ethnomedical perspective of health and health care. The ethnomedical perspective gives meaning and context to perceptions of health and illness that are not necessarily based on Western medical standards but rather on the culture and values of the people with whom the health care professionals are working (Brems & Griffiths, 1993).

Brems and Griffiths (1993) recommended that listening and talking with women become a fundamental organizing prinicple in the development of women's health programs. They further state that health professionals cannot isolate health as a distinct entity apart from the everyday lives of women.

Partnerships for Health

Partnerships for health evolve at a number of levels. To explain further, I will share some of my experiences as a community health nurse for the Colorado Migrant Health Program (CMHP) during the summer of 1990. The Colorado Migrant Health Program employs nurses and other health professionals for short-term assignments (approximately six weeks to three or four months) during the peak migrant season. Nurses and other health care professionals are assigned to work in rural areas with high concentrations of migrant farmworkers throughout the state.

For this assignment, I worked as a member of a team of health care workers including a community health nurse, school nurse, dentist, and the health service coordinator. Because my role was primarily that of an outreach nurse, I worked in partnership with the CMHP health service coordinator, who was a resident of the area and a trusted ally of the farmworkers. This partnership facilitated my entry into the farmworker community. Traveling with the health service coordinator, I was accepted into the migrant farmworkers' homes and lives.

Another significant partnership developed among the health care workers. The entire health team, including the health service coordinator, nurses, and dentists, would work together to conduct screening clinics. One evening each week we would pack our cars with supplies and conduct screening clinics in areas where migrant families were living and working. This partnership enabled us to provide on-site screening, information, and referral for a number of health concerns.

As I moved through the different levels of partnerships, I was led to the most important one of all, the partnership with the migrant farmworker families, primarily with migrant farmworker women. By spending time with them where they lived and worked, I was able to gain the trust of the women and learn from them the best approach for meeting their health needs. For instance, a diabetic woman was concerned about her blood sugar levels because her work in the fields interfered with her ability to eat at regular hours. Instead of asking her to come by my office, we agreed to meet in the field at 4 P.M. one day to test her blood sugar. This kept her from missing a day's work and driving 50 miles to my office.

Another way of working to promote women's health was to work with the men. For the "solo males," men who came north to work without their families, I kept a hefty supply of condoms in the trunk of my car. Because of the cultural taboo in hispanic culture preventing women from talking openly with men (especially strangers) about sex, I would wait until we had completed our screening (taking blood pressures, filling out forms) and then carefully approach one man in the group and ask if I could speak with him in private. Once at my car, I would open the trunk and ask if he would take a supply of condoms and pass them along to the others. He would enthusiastically accept the offer, discreetly filling all of his pockets, and promise to pass them on to his coworkers.

The most compelling example of the development of the partnership with migrant farmworker women was in the area of domestic violence. Along with my assignment as a community health nurse generalist, I had also agreed to begin examining the problem of domestic violence and learn from the women the best approach for assessment and intervention. Although I heard many stories from the women describing the problem of domestic violence, I was not being successful in assessing individual women for domestic violence.

I had come to Colorado with experience working with urban hispanic battered women and felt I could use the same strategies and skills with this population. Wrong!! I quickly learned that it was difficult for migrant farmworker women to openly discuss such an intimate problem, even though I was becoming a familiar face to the women over time. I had tried every way of asking directly about abuse (asking, for example, if they had ever been hit, slapped, kicked by their partner or if they were afraid when they fought with their husband), and the response was always, "No, everything is fine."

Finally, toward the end of my stay, I decided to take a new approach. I asked one woman, "If a woman came to me as the nurse and told me she was being hit, what would you tell me to tell her?" To this the woman responded, "Well, when it happens to me, I do this. . . ." This was the same woman who had told me earlier in the summer that she had no problems with domestic violence. I continued to use this approach successfully with other migrant farmworker women. The partnership had been established through our unspoken acknowledgment of the women's ways of discussing such a personal and difficult issue.

Development of community partnerships takes time and patience. As the examples cited here have shown, the partnerships evolve through different levels. In your practice you will identify the people who will lead you to your community. As you develop these entry level partnerships with coworkers and community leaders, you are moving toward the most important and rewarding journey of professional practice—working in true partnership with the people of your community.

The Camp Health Aide Program

The Midwest Migrant Health Information Office (MMHIO) is a nonprofit organization working in partnership with migrant farmworkers in the development of community-based health education programs and advocacy. Its mission statement is reflective of its nature and philosophy: "By providing services that are farmworker defined, culturally responsive, and peer-based, MMHIO works to increase contacts, relationships, and power of migrant farmworkers within the health care system" (MMHIO, 1992).

This mission is personified in the Camp Health Aide Program (CHAP). Initiated in 1985 by MMHIO, CHAP was developed to help bridge the gap between the health care system and migrant farmworkers. The active involvement of migrant farmworkers ensures that information and services are offered in a culturally acceptable and appropriate manner. The philosophy of the program is based in the self identification of needs and the self-determination of people to meet those needs. Health care becomes a natural part of everyday life as these women incorporate their work into their daily routines.

Camp health aides (CHAs) make home visits with community health nurses. They also provide health education in the labor camps, provide first aid, and work directly with clinic staff in making appointments, translating, and advocating for migrant health issues. Each woman receives a stipend. The idea behind the program is that because these women are respected as informal leaders in their camps, they can serve as effective liaisons between the formal health care system and migrant farmworkers. One CHA described her work in this way:

> Now I know how people are supposed to be treated. . . . When I call the clinic and talk to the receptionist I expect her to listen to me, to pay attention to me. . . . Then when they can't listen now I have this strength to complain, to say "she's not doing her job." She's not paying attention to the people. I think I have the courage because I was a Camp Health Aide. If I wasn't in this program I would have just let it go, like I've done before. But when you know that something is right and something is wrong you need to tell them.
>
> *(Stewart, 1990.)*

During the time when migrant farmworkers are at their home base, camp health aides work in local clinics and other health facilities. These jobs often lead to the CHAs becoming interested in pursuing health careers. One woman in Texas who received a scholarship from MMHIO in 1990 is currently working toward her degree in medicine.

Camp health aides also advocate for changes in the living conditions in migrant labor camps. For example, one CHA in the Midwest has been successful in improving housing and obtaining day care on site in her camp and recently obtained support for a small library for the camp. Most importantly, this CHA has been key in negotiating with the grower regarding the exposure of farmworkers to the spraying of pesticides.

Summary

Migrant farmworkers face formidable challenges in their struggle to achieve and sustain health. Although they are responsible for bringing most of the fresh fruits and vegetables to our tables, they are often forgotten. They have been called by some the "invisible population."

Evidence of this lack of visibility is the scarcity of current research data regarding the health of migrant farmworkers. Rust (1990) and Meister (1991) highlight the need for research specifically aimed at the many unanswered questions about migrant health. Research with migrant farmworker women must move beyond a focus on maternal-child health indicators and include a wide range of issues important to their health.

Migrant farmworkers, unlike health care professionals, do not consider health to be an entity distinct from their everyday lives. As you develop partnerships with migrant farmworker communities, you will come to understand the interconnectedness of health to the many issues of concern in migrant farmworkers' lives. You will find health to be a common thread in such issues as inadequate housing, exposure to pesticides, and the risks of driving across the country in search of work. You will understand how migrant farmworker women create peace in their lives in order to stay healthy. By living and working with migrant farmworker communities, you will come to know the strengths of this population and the valuable contributions they make to our world.

REFERENCES

Arbab, D., & Weidner, L. (1986). Infectious diseases and field water supply and sanitation among migrant farmworkers. *American Journal of Public Health, 76*(6), 694–695.

Atkin, S. (1993). *Voices from the fields.* Boston: Little, Brown & Company.

Brems, S., & Griffiths, M. (1993). Health women's way: Learning to listen. In M. Koblinsky, J. Timyan, & J. Gay (Eds.)., *The health of women* (pp. 255–271). Boulder, CO: Westview Press.

Chi, P. (1985). Medical utilization patterns of migrant farmworkers in Wayne County, New York. *Public Health Reports, 100*(5), 480–490.

de la Torre, A., & Rush, L. (1989, January–February). The effects of healthcare access on maternal and migrant seasonal farmworker women infant health of California. *Migrant Health Newsline Clinical Supplement.* Austin, TX: National Migrant Resource Program.

Dever, A. (1991). Profile of a population with complex health problems. *Migrant Clinicians Network, Monograph Series,* 1–16.

Littlefield, C., & Stout, C. (1987). *Access to healthcare: A survey of Colorado's migrant farmworkers.* Denver, CO: Colorado Migrant Health Program.

Martaus, T. (1986). The health-seeking process of Mexican-American migrant farmworkers. *Home Healthcare Nurse, 4*(5), 32–38.

Meister, J. (1991). The health of migrant farmworkers. *Occupational Health: State of the Art Reviews, 6*(3), 503–518.

Midwest Migrant Health Information Office (MMHIO). (1992). Information brochure. Monroe, MI: Author.

Migrant Health Program. (1992). Program information sheet. Washington, DC: Public Health Service.

National Advisory Council on Migrant Health. (1992). *Farmworker health for the year 2000.* Austin, TX: National Migrant Resource Program.

———. (1993). *1993 recommendations.* Rockville, MD: Bureau of Primary Health Care.

Office of Migrant Health. (1990). *Migrant and seasonal farmworker health objectives for the year 2000.* Austin, TX: National Migrant Resource Program.

———. (1992). A strategy for reaching migrant and seasonal farmworkers. Washington, DC: Migrant Health Program.

Rodriguez, R. (1993a). *Female migrant farmworkers: The meaning of health within the culture of transience.* Unpublished doctoral dissertation, Texas Woman's University, Houston.

———. (1993b). Violence in transience. *AWHONN's Clinical Issues in Perinatal and Women's Health Nursing, 4*(3), 437–440.

Rust, G. (1990). Health status of migrant farmworkers: A literature review and commentary. *American Journal of Public Health, 80*(10), 1213–1217.

Slesinger, D. (1992, Summer). Health status and needs of migrant farmworkers in the United States: A literature review. *Texas Journal of Rural Health,* 227–233.

Slesinger, D., Christensen, B., & Cautley, E. (1986). Health and mortality of migrant farm children. *Social Science Medicine, 23*(1), 65–74.

Stewart, G. (1990). *Personal and collective empowerment among migrant farmworker camp health aides.* Unpublished evaluation report.

Wilk, V. (1986). Farmworker occupational health and field sanitation. *Migrant Health Newsline—Compendium of Clinical Supplements 1985–87.* Austin, TX: National Migrant Resource Program.

Zuroweste, E. (1991). Migrant Clinicians Network testimony before Hispanic caucus. *Migrant Clinical Supplement.* Austin, TX: Migrant Clinician's Network.

16

Back Lakes Community Health Pilot Project—Alberta, Canada

Karen Titanich

John McDonough

Sandra Woodhead-Lyons

Sharon Snell

Introduction

Providing access to appropriate health services in rural and remote communities has been, and will continue to be, a challenge for many Canadian provinces and territories. Alberta, with large tracts of sparsely populated land, is no exception. In order to better meet the health needs of rural and remote communities, Alberta Health established working groups to develop alternate health services delivery pilot projects in conjunction/cooperation with different and distinct rural and remote communities in the province.

Alternate health services delivery pilot projects can assist in the development of coordinated, integrated, community-based health services delivery systems for the participating communities. These projects examine the broad issues related to the determinants of health and the root causes of disease and injury and seek to enhance and improve access to needed health programs and services. The focus is on the development of community-based programs and services, which are linked into and coordinated with other services provided in the community by visiting service providers and other programs and services available at the district, regional, and provincial levels. Community-based programs and services include entry-level programs and services for health promotion; health protection; disease and injury prevention; support, treatment, and rehabilitation provided through a range of service providers; and access to emergency services, including stabilization, referral, and transport to other levels of health care when needed.

Concepts and Principles

These pilot projects developed through an evolutionary process based on principles of primary health care and the inherent concepts of health promotion and community mobilization and development. The concepts and principles that guide project activities are as follows:

1. Health.
Health is is defined as "the extent to which an individual or group is able, on the one hand, to realize aspirations and satisfy needs, and on the other hand, to change or cope with the environment. Health is therefore seen as a resource for everyday life, instead of as the objective of living" (World Health Organization, 1984).

2. Focus on population health needs.
The focus will be on the health needs and priorities of the community.

3. Focus on health outcomes.
Health programs and services that result will be evaluated for their contribution to the improved health of the population served.

4. Sensitivity to aboriginal health and cultural needs.

5. Primary health care.

Primary health care is essential health [services] based on practical, scientifically sound and socially acceptable methods and technology made universally accessible to individuals and families in the community at a price they can afford to maintain at every stage of their development in the spirit of self-reliance and self-determination. It forms an integral part both of the country's health system, of which it is the central junction and main focus,

Overview of the Process

Phase of the Process	Focus of Attention	Major Tasks During This Phase
● ENTRY PHASE	—The existing situation	Learn about the environment within which the process will happen. Introduce yourself into that environment.
● NEEDS ASSESSMENT PHASE	—Health needs	Gather facts and opinions about community health needs.
	—Public acceptance	Learn what skills and resources already exist. Have key individuals and the public accept that health needs are significant. Gain commitment to action.
● PLANNING PHASE	—How to respond to health needs	Explore and choose methods of responding to the health needs. Acquire necessary resources.
● DOING PHASE	—Community action	Implement plans.
● RENEWAL PHASE	—Evaluation/rejuvenation	Evaluate what worked, what didn't. Determine what has been learned. Foster self-renewal of those involved. Reexamine the existing situation.

FIGURE 16-1
Healthy communities: The process.

and of the overall social and economic development of the community. It is the first level of contact of individuals, the family and community with the national health system bringing health [services] as close as possible to where people live and work, and constitutes the first element of a continuing health process.

(World Health Organization, The Alma Ata Declaration, 1978).

The six principles of primary health care arising from this definition are as follows:

—Provision of essential health services

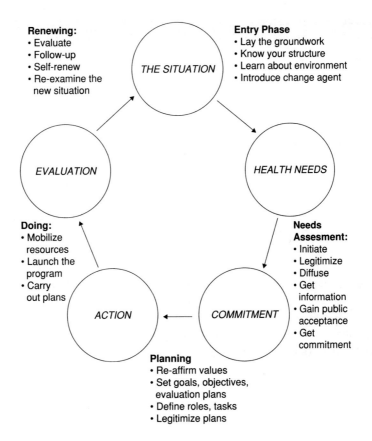

Renewing:
• Evaluate
• Follow-up
• Self-renew
• Re-examine the
 new situation

THE SITUATION

Entry Phase
• Lay the groundwork
• Know your structure
• Learn about environment
• Introduce change agent

EVALUATION

HEALTH NEEDS

Doing:
• Mobilize
 resources
• Launch the
 program
• Carry
 out plans

ACTION

COMMITMENT

**Needs
Assesment:**
• Initiate
• Legitimize
• Diffuse
• Get
 information
• Gain public
 acceptance
• Get
 commitment

Planning
• Re-affirm values
• Set goals, objectives,
 evaluation plans
• Define roles, tasks
• Legitimize plans

*FIGURE 16-1
(continued)*

—Provision of a contact point for consumers with the health
system
—Full participation of individuals and the community
—Accessible health services
—Intersectoral collaboration
—Socially acceptable and affordable methods and technologies

Healthy Communities: The Process (British Columbia Ministry of
Health, 1989) describes a planning process to use when working with
communities that guided the steps in these projects. An overview of the
process is shown in Figure 16-1.

Summary Points About the Community Process

- The process is not all visible. The "doing" phase may be the only activity that is obvious to the public. But just because nothing is visible doesn't mean nothing is happening.
- The "invisible" parts of the process are crucial. Establishing rapport with the community, learning about the needs, and gaining acceptance are the groundwork that generate successful community programs.
- The process is not guaranteed to complete itself. It could end at any step.
- The process is not smooth. Sometimes it's three steps forward and two steps back.

So why are we advocating such a messy process?
- Because it's consistent with the values of health promotion. The community process empowers individuals and communities to identify their own health issues and decide what to do about them. The process gives communities control over their own destiny.
- Because it builds on the strengths of individuals and communities. The process can be carried out using the innate talents and resources of the community. It is not dependent on government or other external help.
- Because it works.

When to use the Community Process:
The process could be applied to
- A total comprehensive community approach to promoting health
- The way a health organization develops and carries out its activities and programs
- A specific community project addressing one health issue
- Some aspect of a professional, board or volunteer role

FIGURE 16-1
(continued)

The Communities

The Back Lakes include the aboriginal communities of Peerless Lake, Trout Lake, and Loon Lake, and the nonaboriginal community of Red Earth Creek in northwestern Alberta.

Red Earth Creek developed during the oil boom of the 1970s and early 1980s. It is an oil field service center with a population of 300 permanent residents plus several hundred seasonal workers, many of whom live in neighboring work camps. Red Earth Creek is situated on Highway 67, 109 miles (176 kilometers) north of Slave Lake, which in turn is 156 miles (251 kilometers) north of Edmonton, the provincial capital.

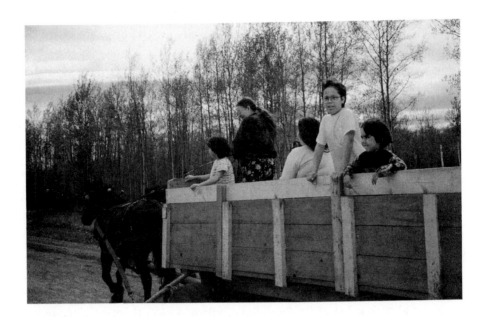

FIGURE 16-2
Riding the Loon Lake school bus together signifies the sense of community the residents have established. (Photo by Anne Givens)

Loon Lake (population 270) is 5 miles (8 kilometers) west of Red Earth Creek. Peerless Lake (population 325) is 48 miles (78 kilometers) east of Red Earth Creek; Trout Lake (population 316) is an additional 16 miles (25 kilometers) away. These communities are connected to Red Earth Creek by a washboard, gravel road.

The inhabitants of the aboriginal communities are Woodland Cree. Less than 40 years ago, these people lived in scattered family groups across the region. They hunted, trapped, fished, and moved with the seasons. The aboriginal people have come together in communities located on provincial crown land (see Figure 16-2).

Health Services

Both federal and provincial governments have responsibilities for health services to the aboriginal people in the region. Each aboriginal community is involved in a land claims negotiation with the federal government that will lead to reserve status. When reserve status is achieved, the responsibility for community health services will shift to the federal government.

Health Canada (Medical Services Branch) provides a noninsured health benefits program to all registered Indians whether they live on or off reserve. These benefits cover a wide variety of health goods and services including prescription drugs, medical supplies/equipment, medical transportation, optometric services, dental services, and Alberta's health care insurance premiums. Nonregistered Indians living in the Back Lakes communities do not receive these services.

A key service is transportation to medical services. Medical Services Branch will cover the cost for registered Indians to travel to other centers for physician-approved referrals. Emergency air and ground ambulance services are provided by Alberta Health for all residents. This does not include the return trips to the communities. A "medical" taxi from Peerless Lake or Trout Lake to Slave Lake costs $500 Canadian. A ground or air ambulance costs double that amount. Even though there is some provision for financial aid for people on social assistance, the cost can be prohibitive for many families.

At present, the Back Lakes communities have limited access to health and social services and no access to 24-hour emergency on-call services. Peerless Lake and Trout Lake have small health centers attached to their local schools (see Figure 16-3). The Athabasca Health Unit provides community health nursing services and some home care services on a monthly basis. Dental hygiene and other school health services are provided at the school. Other specialty services such as speech therapy and early intervention are provided as needed. The Athabasca Health Unit employs community health representatives to provide a range of health promotion services through the community health centers. One physician from Slave Lake flies into Trout Lake weekly to visit the health center. Another flies in biweekly to visit Peerless Lake.

A new health trailer has recently been provided to Loon Lake. Red Earth Creek has no health facility. The Peace River Health Unit provides visiting community health nursing and home care services on a weekly basis to Loon Lake. A physician from Slave Lake flies into Red Earth Creek on a biweekly basis and provides medical services at the health trailer in Loon Lake.

Mental health services are provided by Alberta Health, Northwestern Mental Health Services Region. Some community development

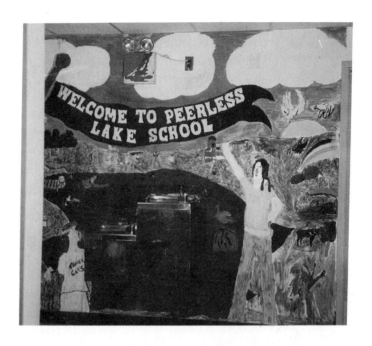

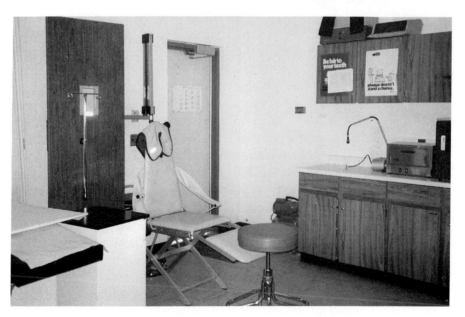

FIGURE 16-3
Health clinic located in the Peerless Lake school. (Photo by Anne Givens)

services are being provided to Peerless Lake to help the community address recent suicides and attempted suicides. Social services are provided by Alberta Family and Social Services, Northwestern Region.

In 1986, the High Prairie District Hospital submitted a request to the Albertan government to construct an ambulatory care facility at Red Earth Creek. Consultations were held with Red Earth Creek and the aboriginal communities. The facility would act as a regional ambulatory care center for all the communities across the Back Lakes. This project was approved in 1989; however, later that year, the project was deferred just before construction began.

Organization of the Project

In the spring of 1992, two unexpected changes occurred in health services to the Back Lakes: The federal government withdrew funding for physician flights into the Back Lakes communities, and a supply of prescription drugs was removed from the health center in Peerless Lake by the Athabasca Health Unit. These changes highlighted the need for a mechanism to address the health needs of these communities in a comprehensive way. In October 1992, Alberta Health reactivated the Red Earth Creek capital project by refocusing it as a health center with outreach services for the neighboring aboriginal communities.

Alberta Health invited the four communities, the five health service providers, and other community services representatives to participate in the creation of an implementation team to assist in planning health services for the communities in a holistic, integrated manner.

Initial reaction was positive. The communities worked with Alberta Health to validate and expand community profiles that had been compiled from available sources. However, two of the aboriginal communities raised concerns about the project. They believed that a Red Earth Creek facility might centralize health services for the area and consequently restrict the potential growth of future health services in their communities.

Alberta Health offered to work with each community to carry out a community needs assessment. The communities indicated they would prefer to conduct the assessments themselves. Alberta Health then provided information and suggestions to the communities, including the following questions to aid in eliciting input, on how to conduct a community needs assessment:

Community Profile

A. Introduction
   —Name, including reason for name
   —Location
   —Population, including age distribution
   —Key elements, including main industries/employers
   —Political representation at local level
B. Land Use
C. Recreation and Tourism
D. Education
E. Community Services
F. Police and Fire Protection
G. Government Services
H. Financial Services
 I. Communications/Media
 J. Transportation
   —Roads
   —Freight services
   —Passenger services
   —Air services
K. Utilities
   —Water
   —Sewer
   —Garbage collection
   —Power
L. Health Facilities
M. Health Services
N. Utilization of Physician and Hospital Services by Community

1. How would you describe your community in order to help people from outside to understand it better?
2. What are the major health concerns facing your community?
3. Of these concerns, which are the most important?
4. What strengths or qualities does your community possess that can be used to improve the quality of health of the people?
5. What advice or suggestions can you provide to make more effective use of existing provincial health resources in this community?

6. What new resources could be used to improve the health of your community?

These questions were designed to work in a community meeting or to guide interviews with key informants. The resulting information, when combined with the community profiles, would create a picture of each community and its particular needs (see the accompanying display).

The assessments were completed by each community. Approaches used included holding community meetings, interviewing key informants, and examining the views of the community leaders involved in the project. The results of the assessments varied widely. Several of them identified services that the communities wanted as well as some of the health and social needs of the communities. Services identified included 24-hour access to nursing services, a community health worker, a transportation clerk, regular physician visits, ambulance services, and availability of prescription drugs. Community needs identified included improvements to water and sewer systems, roads and landing strips, and housing. Further work would be needed on these needs assessments, which was not surprising given these communities' underserviced state. In March 1992, the Red Earth Creek capital project was removed from the deferred list, and approval was given to the High Prairie Hospital Board to design and construct the facility.

The divergent views of the community representatives and the health planners came to a head at an implementation team meeting in April 1993. Alberta Health unveiled its model for a community health center for Red Earth Creek with basic health services provided on an outreach basis to the aboriginal communities by a registered nurse with advanced knowledge and skills in primary health care. These programs and services would be augmented by other visiting service providers based on need. Alberta Health officials were confident that they had the appropriate approvals to build the facility and that their plan would provide substantially improved health services across the area. Members from the aboriginal communities voiced opposition to the plan, which would have them receive their services on an outreach basis. To emphasize their disapproval of the plan, they walked out of the meeting.

The aboriginal reaction shocked most department officials. At the same time, the aboriginal communities were concerned that they might have shut the door to improved health services.

The community of Peerless Lake invited representatives of Alberta Health to visit their community to discuss health issues with their membership. Department officials visited the community, staying overnight in local residences. The officials put aside their previous positions and asked the community to discuss their health needs and to explore ways in which those needs could be met. This new openness and demonstration of respect helped to improve relations between the community and the department.

Based on a better understanding of the communities and their needs, department officials drafted a new proposal. As much as possible, health services and programs would be specific to, and located in, each community. Registered nurses with advanced knowledge and skills in

Community Nurse Practitioners

Community nurse practitioners are registered nurses in advanced nursing practice who have expertise in community health as well as entry-level treatment services, including emergency stabilization and referral. Community nurse practitioners play a key role as members of the primary health care team, providing a broad range of programs and services based on community needs.

The use of registered nurses in rural and remote communities is not new. However, the introduction of these alternate health services delivery pilot projects has helped to formalize the requirements of, and the expectations for, registered nurses in advanced practice in rural and remote areas of Alberta.

The development of guidelines has provided the opportunity for doctors, registered nurses, pharmacists, consumers, and policymakers to identify and begin to resolve issues that must be addressed in order to ensure the successful acceptance and integration of community nurse practitioners into the Albertan health system. The guidelines will provide a framework for practitioners and employing organizations to use and will serve as a fundamental reference document in developing a regulation to support the practice of community nurse practitioners in Alberta.

It has become clear that to provide primary health care services in rural and remote communities, registered nurses require an educational and practical background that includes both community health and entry-level acute care. Registered nurses in advanced practice with competency in these areas are qualified to take on the role of community nurse practitioner.

primary health care, called *community nurse practitioners* in recognition of their unique knowledge and skill, and community health representatives would provide programs and services based in each aboriginal community, and they would work out of the existing health centers. The Red Earth Creek team would be based on a community nurse practitioner and a clerical/administrative support person to work out of the proposed new community health center. (See the accompanying display for a more in-depth discussion of the community nurse practitioner.) The concept of centralized health services being provided on an outreach basis in each community was scrapped. Some predicted changes in service delivery are shown in Figure 16-4.

The minister of health and the local member of the provincial legislative assembly met with representatives of the four communities in Peerless Lake on August 12, 1993. The minister made a commitment that the health services project, including the Red Earth Creek facility, would proceed quickly and that jurisdictional issues between governments and among providers should not stand in the way of progress. The leadership for the project shifted from Alberta Health to the local service providers and communities, with the High Prairie Hospital Board having the facilitative role.

On August 26, 1993, the four communities, the five service providers, other representatives, and Alberta Health met to restart the consultation process and begin planning for community-based health services (McDonough, J., & Woodhead-Lyons, S., 1993). Alberta Health presented its revised model of health services to the communities and providers for their consideration and input. Despite the apparent progress, there was still a good deal of mistrust. Two of the aboriginal communities wanted to stop any progress on the Red Earth Creek facility until there was full agreement on all other health service issues. In addition, one of the five providers was very concerned about the proposed approach, especially its cost, and the proposed role of community nurse practitioners. Although the concept is not new, health services in Alberta have been provided through several sectors in recent years: public health, mental health, hospitals, long-term care, and insured medical services. The concept meant bridging current roles, responsibilities, and mandates into an integrated health services delivery system.

By the end of the August 26th meeting, the communities appeared more satisfied with the model. They created a Community Health Services Working Group, with two members from each community plus

FROM	TO
● Fragmented, episodic health services by several service providers	● Coordinated, community-based, primary health care services
● Health services based on availability and perceptions of service providers	● Health services based on community needs assessment and community input
● Changes in health services based on viewpoints of service providers and the weather, i.e., fog prevents air travel	● Changes in health services based on evaluation of results and health needs
● Address symptoms of problems	● Deal with root causes of problems
● Input-oriented	● Outcome-oriented
● Activity-oriented	● Results-oriented
● Individual health	● Population health
● Traveling long distances to reach acute care services between visits by service providers	● Access to a range of primary health care services in the community with referral and transport as needed
● Jurisdiction for health services split among four boards, two regions, and autonomous service providers	● An administering body focused on the Back Lakes communities to oversee services provided and coordinate access to other needed primary health care services and to other levels of services

FIGURE 16-4
Predicted changes in health services delivery to the Back Lakes communities.

two resource people from the service providers. The Community Health Services Working Group would do the detailed planning for health services to meet the health needs of each participating community, to identify opportunities for cost savings, and to draft an appropriate budget.

The communities also agreed to a coordinating committee that would include representatives from Alberta Health and the five health services providers. The coordinating committee will review the health services plans developed for each community by the Community Health Services Working Group.

Current Status

The revised project appears to be back on track. However, numerous hurdles remain. Some representatives from two of the aboriginal communities continue to be concerned about the role of the Red Earth Creek facility. They fear that the existence of the facility will compromise their chances of receiving the augmented health services and facilities that will be provided by the federal government once reserve status is achieved.

Due to budget cuts, the Red Earth Creek capital project was again deferred on October 4, 1993.

The communities, with the providers acting as facilitators/consultants, have developed the community-based health services plans, which are being reviewed by the other service providers not directly involved in the planning. Alberta Health expects to receive these plans soon.

Observations

The preceding narrative demonstrates some of the complexities and challenges faced by Alberta Health in developing alternative health services delivery models with primary health care as a fundamental underpinning:

1. Territorial issues based on Alberta Health's divisional structure act as barriers to the creation of alternative health service delivery models that cross traditional boundaries. Until 1988, the community-based health sectors, that is, public health and mental health, and the institutionally and medically based sectors, that is, acute care, long-term care, and insured services, were in separate departments. Each of these five sectors has been used to operating autonomously. In Alberta, we call them "stovepipes." The concept of primary health care challenges the various mandates, philosophies, procedures, financial mechanisms, and usual operating methods of staff drawn from these different divisions.

2. Similar territorial issues may exist in the field when more than one health service agency or provider is involved. Agencies providing public health, hospital, and long-term care services are decentralized and have their own local boards. Mental health is centralized and has six regions; one mental health region may contain several health unit boards and dozens of hospital and long-term care facility boards. This structure creates artifical boundaries that can complicate the coordination and integration of services to meet community needs.

3. Department planners and community leaders have very different needs and expectations of community-based planning. Traditionally, departments prefer to have an understanding of the pro-

posed costs prior to serious discussions at the community level. This may mean that preliminary decisions about the nature and scope of the proposed health services will precede community consultations. Communities prefer the widest possible latitude to discuss their health needs and the possible solutions.

4. Political, economic, social, and cultural issues complicate the health services planning process. Governance and economic issues are often more important to community leaders than health services plans. When community leaders in aboriginal communities are involved in far-reaching negotiations with the federal government over land claims and the achievement of band or reserve status, health services may be considered relatively unimportant in comparison.

5. Healthy public policy for aboriginal communities, as with all other communities, needs to concentrate on developing participation in and control of their health and social services planning as well as the delivery, management, and evaluation of health services.

Conclusion

The project represents a challenge to all involved because successful implementation of primary health service delivery requires the development of partnerships among service providers and with community residents. Successful partnerships demand open communication, cooperation, coordination, collaboration, and compromise. This project means new ways of doing business and requires the participation of all involved in a spirit of teamwork.

The alternate health services delivery pilot projects have been an invaluable learning experience for those of us participating. Attempting to do business differently by putting the principles of primary health care and community-based planning into action, by working across sectors, and by having community leaders and residents actively participate has begun the process of change. There is growing recognition and appreciation of the need to address the determinants of health (such as transportation) and not simply health services. Working together, we can develop a coordinated, integrated, holistic, and community-based health services delivery system for the participating communities that better meets their needs.

REFERENCES

British Columbia Ministry of Health. (1989). *Healthy Communities: The Process, a guide for volunteers, community leaders, elected officials and health professionals who want to build healthy communities.* Vancouver, B.C.: Author.

McDonough, J., & Woodhead-Lyons, S. (1993). *One approach to alternative health service delivery—Community nurse practitioners in rural/remote communities of Alberta.* Presentation to a conference in Thunder Bay, Ontario, in fall 1993.

World Health Organization. (1978). *The Alma Ata declaration.* Geneva: Author.

——— (1984). *Health.* Geneva: Author.

17

The Primary Health Care Fieldworker and Town Health Committees—Ghana, West Africa

Jean Mouch

Introduction

The countries of Africa cannot be considered as a whole when the topic of community health is explored. Ghana, in West Africa, falls within the sub-Saharan and "developing countries" classifications. During the time period discussed in this chapter, 1980–1991, the rate of annual growth in Ghana's gross national product (GNP) had been a negative percentage since 1965 (Grant, 1993). It is within the context of an economy of scarcity that the following community partnership experience is presented. It is also presented within the setting of the desire to have a primary health care (PHC) approach to meeting basic health needs for the people of Ghana.

Ghana is on the Guinea coast of West Africa (see Figure 17-1). It gained independence from the United Kingdom in 1957, making it the first African country to emerge from the colonial era. In 1991 Ghana had a population of 15.5 million, with a GNP per capita of $390, a life expectancy of 55 years, and an adult literacy rate of 60%.

The WHO initiative in Alma Ata laid the basis for the implementation on a worldwide scale of primary health care strategies. *Primary health care* is defined as "essential health care, made universally accessible to individuals and families in the community, by means acceptable

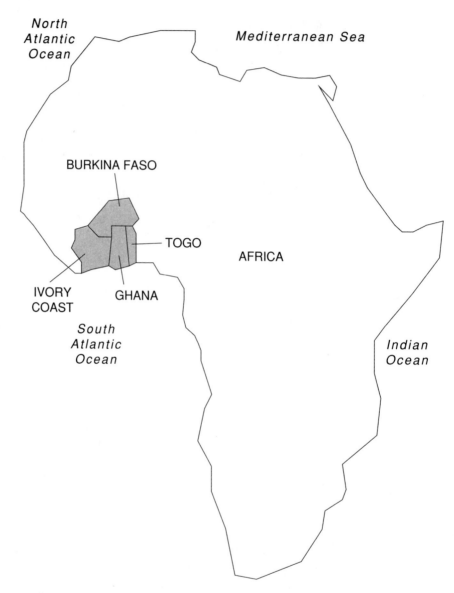

North
Atlantic
Ocean

Mediterranean Sea

BURKINA FASO

TOGO

AFRICA

IVORY
COAST

GHANA

South
Atlantic
Ocean

Indian
Ocean

FIGURE 17-1
Ghana and surrounding countries of West Africa.

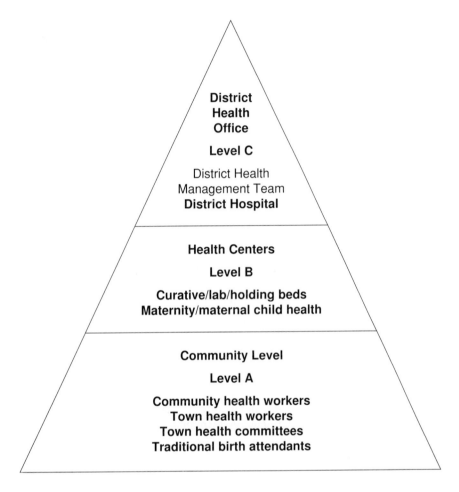

FIGURE 17-2
A three-tiered primary health care system.

to them through their full participation and at a cost that the community and country can afford" (World Health Organization, 1978).

The planning unit for the Ghanian Ministry of Health set overall guidance for health priorities as well as a number of pilot projects and training programs for a PHC strategy, including preparation of traditional birth attendants TBAs and developing a community health worker (CHW) model. Ghana choose to implement a three-tiered PHC system (see Figure 17-2). The three levels were defined as follows:

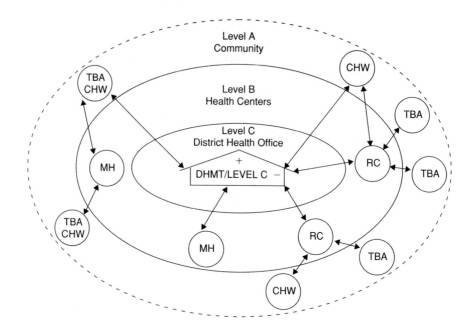

Level A – Community
 CHW = Community health worker
 TBA = Traditional birth attendant

Level B – Health Centers
 MH = Maternity homes/birthing centers
 RC = Rural clinics

Level C – District Health Office
 DHMT = District health management team

FIGURE 17-3
District health levels in a network.

Level A—Small towns or villages with a community clinic staffed by a health provider who is a community health worker or traditional birth attendant

Level B—Larger towns with a health center/maternity unit or a maternity home with trained nurses and midwives

> **Level C**—District centers with a district hospital; full district health
> administration with a district medical officer of health and core
> preventive and promotive health personnel

These district levels were to be administered via a district health
management team. The larger regional level would be coordinating the
district levels and thus provide a regional structure for a country-wide system of health care delivery. Another way to think of this model is in terms
of expanding circles instead of tiers (see Figure 17-3). Level C, the inner-
most circle, is the furthest removed from the people but has the most
advanced technology and the district hospital. Level B houses the maternity and community clinics, and Level A is the domain of the community
health workers. Sometimes a villager in the outermost loop, Level A, will
be referred directly to the district hospital because there is no Level B.

This chapter discusses the experiences of one district in Ghana and
the process of implementing primary health care. The people and geographic setting will be discussed followed by a discussion of the primary
health initiative.

The People

The population of the district, which covers 800 square miles, was
180,000 persons in 1980. Maternal mortality was 10 per 1,000 live births.
Infant mortality was 89 per 1,000 live births, mortality for children aged
5 years or less was 146 per 1,000 population, and life expectancy was 55
years.

The district is centrally placed in the country, and its population
consists of five major ethnic groups that in some areas of the district
speak three languages. The dominant culture is matrilineal, a tradition
that is experiencing strain as traditional ways are changed. For example,
the new inheritance law allows the husband and wife to share in assets
earned and to pass them onto their children. In the matrilineal system,
the inheritance would have stayed within the husband's mother's clan,
and the wife and children would not have been able to access the inheritance.

Traditionally, Ghanaian women can receive a divorce as easily as the
men, and they exercise independence with regard to managing their

farmland. Because families frequently do not have the money to invest in a home, the wife and children live with the maternal grandmother, and the husband rents a room in town. Polygamy is common. These traditional ways clash with Christianity, the largest religion in Ghana, which teaches that the monogamous family unit is divinely ordained.

Education is seen as a way to get the family ahead economically. Early in the westernization of the economy, boys were urged to go to school; however, girls were valued for childbearing and maintaining the farmlands. Consequently, many girls do not finish even six years of education.

Most of the people in the district are involved with farming, which is nonmechanized and completed on small plots. Produce is transported to market by head-load (that is, in a bundle on the head), which can weigh 60 to 80 pounds, often via footpaths. One of the most common images of daily life in Ghana is that of a man with a long knife and a bunch of bananas on his head, carrying a toddler, followed by a woman with a head-load of food, and trailed by two or three children with smaller loads (usually wood to prepare the evening meal) and a grandparent with a water gourd or bottle. On every seventh day, farming is taboo. It is on that day that a town will welcome outreach health services.

The Land

Ghana is about the size of Oregon. It has a varied climate, ranging from the coastal savannah to forest areas, grassland savannah, and sub-Saharan areas in the north. The district described here lies in the transitional terrain of west-central Ghana, between the forest and savannah, on the border with the Ivory Coast. The rainy season comes in two installments: April through July, the major season, and then September and October, the minor season. This district has the highest rate of production of food crops in Ghana, including yam, corn, and banana, with cocoa and coffee raised as cash crops. In recent years, the development of sawmills and export of hardwood has been substantial and has led to deforestation and soil erosion. The condition of the soil and the terms of land tenure directly relate to the health of the people.

Transportation is difficult throughout the country, and it may be impossible during certain times of the year to arrive at the district hospital due to impassable roads. The main north–south road of the district is graded; however, a 50-mile trip from the south to the larger health center with more facilities in the north takes two and a half hours in the dry season and over five hours during the rainy season.

Because of the type of geology, it is difficult to maintain deep borehole wells, which can provide safe drinking water year-round. Many streams and small rivers are dry during the last weeks of the dry season, causing hardship and long walks for water. Most cooking is done with wood or charcoal on open fires, which is often a hazard, especially to young children, who suffer many severe burns. Safe drinking water and adequate food to meet daily caloric demand are primary health care issues.

A Primary Health Care Initiative Begins

In 1980, a two-step goal-setting process for the large nongovernment hospital was initiated to define the development of a PHC strategy for the coming years. The first step was to rename the Public Health Department as the Primary Health Care Department. The second was to appoint an experienced pediatric nurse to be the primary health care fieldworker. Two years later, a doctor with public health training accepted the position of district medical officer of health. The district health care system began to be viewed as a network of health care units including curative care and separate maternal child health outreach efforts.

The Role of the Primary Health Care Fieldworker

The nurse serving as the PHC fieldworker was to develop and expand the services at the community level (Level A) of the health pyramid. This was a new concept. Previously, most resources of management, training, and technology had gone to Level C. The PHC fieldworker was to be a catalyst helping weave together the present health care system and future health care goals.

The PHC fieldworker began by systematically visiting nurses, midwives, rural clinics, health centers, church clinics, private clinics, traditional healers, and spiritualist healers in the district. A diary was kept that included the names of town leaders, active church groups, local birth attendants, teachers interested in health, and traditional healing centers.

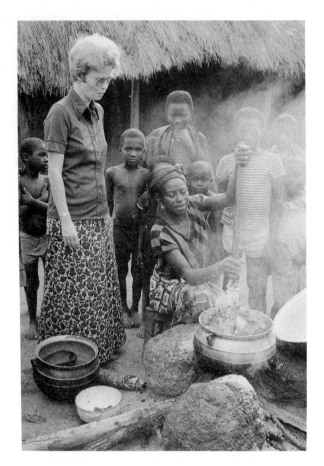

FIGURE 17-4A
The PHC fieldworker visits with women to determine health needs.

This diary style became an excellent source for information over the years and provided personnel from other hospitals or PHC projects with examples of what was involved in PHC.

The PHC fieldworker sponsored meetings of nurses and midwives from small towns, and their needs were surveyed. The fieldworker traveled and stayed with nurses or women's group leaders in isolated places. Town water and sanitation facilities were inspected in every town with a health unit and in each town requesting help from community health workers, traditional birth attendants, and staff at the rural clinics.

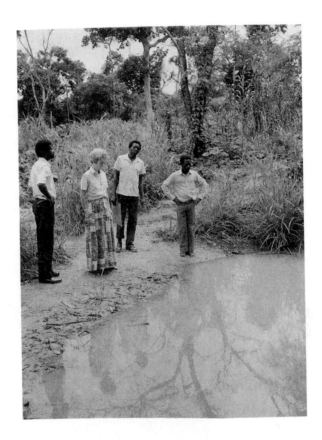

FIGURE 17-4B
The PHC fieldworker evaluates a water source with town leaders and a community health worker.

    Town meetings were held to explain the concept of PHC. Teaching what was different about a primary health care system from the present health care nonsystem was a continuous effort that involved nursing and midwifery students, medical students, church groups, women's associations, political groups, hospital staff, and others. All of the PHC fieldworker's activities were financed by a start-up grant from a Dutch donor organization, except for her salary, which came from the district hospital. Figure 17-4 presents a photographic essay of the PHC fieldworker's daily activities as she worked with villagers and their health issues.

    Strategies to strengthen Level A of the health pyramid included the following:

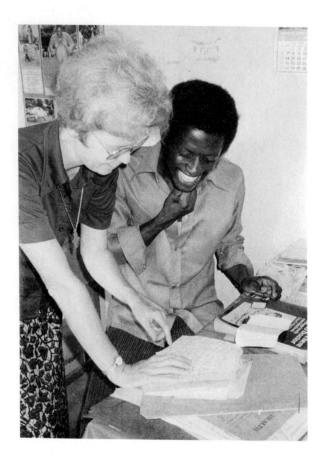

FIGURE 17-4C
The PHC fieldworker helps a community health worker to assess health needs.

- Health education plays and village activities about PHC
- Involvement of mothers in child clinic activities
- District nurse midwives' involvement in village health education
- Development in village women of the skills of traditional birth attendants and traditional healers
- Offering holistic health workshops
- Developing a manual for home care of persons with AIDS

Because the PHC fieldworker came from the church hospital and also was a foreigner, she was not readily accepted by nursing and mid-

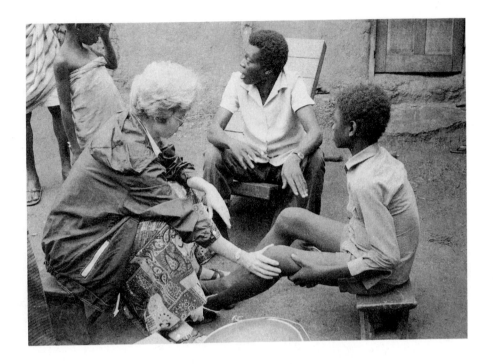

FIGURE 17-4D
The PHC fieldworker evaluates an infection with the community health worker.

wifery units. This underscores the fact that if members of different groups are to work together successfully, trust—as well as a commitment to and belief in community participation—is essential.

Town Health Committees: An Example of Community Participation

The PHC strategy called for the formation of town health committees (THCs). The primary health care worker recommended that at least 3 women be on each committee of 7 to 10 people and that all members focus on working toward a safe drinking water source and adequate latrines for women and men.

Many problems in supporting the development of THCs were encountered. First, a high number of younger persons or couples migrated for six to eight months each year to other parts of the country

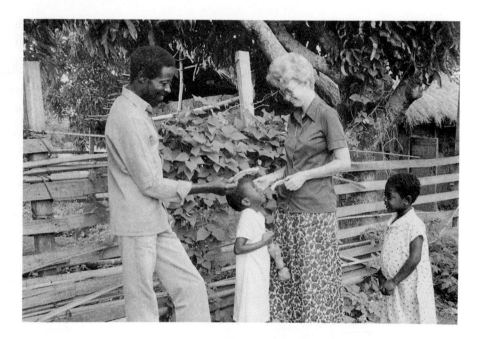

FIGURE 17-4E
The PHC fieldworker visits with a community business leader to discuss health.

to farm or smuggle cocoa. This left older town members and persons
with fewer skills in community mobilization available to participate in
the THCs. Second, PHC stresses increasing the commitment to preventive and promotive health, whereas the previous network of health services had a long history of prioritizing curative care. Third, reorienting
the health staff toward PHC required additional time and personnel if
health staff members were to be part of the daily life and health of local
villages. For example, when the fieldworker reviewed the statistics of
one rural clinic, she noted that over 40 cases of adult diarrhea occurred
in one month's time. When the fieldworker asked the clinic nurse about
the cause of the problem, the nurse replied that he had no medicines to
treat the cases. After much further questioning, the clinic nurse mentioned that a local water source was polluted and that the water pump
was broken. That the clinic nursing role included working with town
members to repair the water pump and teach about making drinking
water safe was a new idea to the clinic nurse.

The town health committees made difficult decisions that affected neighbors and relatives. For example, one clinic was closed because of drug abuse. The elders and leaders were included in the decision-making processs and in the explanation of the verdict. Eventually the clinic was reopened after certain criteria also decided by town health committee representatives had been met. The experience deepened what it means to be involved at the community level for all involved.

Each of the community (Level A) clinics holds its own unique story. There is no easy way to better health if reliance is placed on complete local participation; it is a dynamic process with many ups and downs. At the end of 1991, 11 clinics were functioning, and 4 were having serious problems. At one clinic, problems centered around a key person. In another town, years of effort and joint training sessions failed to make any lasting changes in people's behavior. It would seem that people must be ready to change. We could not find a way to enable people to move themselves through the obstacles of ingrained behavior to a new mind-set. Unenlightened leadership and extreme isolation are additional factors that block change.

Establishing town health committees was intended to accomplish part of the ideal of having local people actively involved in the planning and implementation of the efforts to achieve a better quality of life for their community. However, committees may not work well for a variety of reasons. Sometimes traditional chiefs, with their advisors, could move an issue better. Or church groups, dedicated to having a maternity home in their town, could work more effectively than attempts to elect a THC group when local rival political groups were unable to solve their differences.

With the Strengthening of District Health Services initiative, the problem of local involvement was again identified as a priority. To foster community leadership, a program of education called Town Leaders for PHC was started using Adult Learning techniques and Paulo Freire's (1972) community development and empowerment methods. Both men and women took part in these training sessions, which had the goal of getting more skilled persons involved in THCs. These leadership training techniques come out of the experience of Anne Hope and Sally Timmel (1984) in South Africa and Zimbabwe. The lived realities within the small town or the local women's group became the topics of learning and basis for empowerment. Empowerment means getting people to appre-

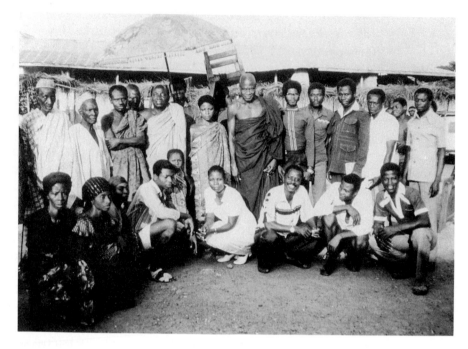

FIGURE 17-5
The town health committee with villagers, health care providers, traditional leaders, and elected members.

ciate the value of their knowledge and to define health or quality of life in their own terms and with their own desires as the starting point. This training for town leaders was begun to achieve quality community participation (see Figure 17-5).

Partnership Strategies to Achieve PHC

Peer Relationships and Empowerment

A *peer relationship* means equality within all professional roles, teams, groups, THCs, clinic staffs, and political organizations. Each person and each committee has something to contribute that is important to discussions of how the practice and mind-set of PHC will be brought into the community. Establishing a peer relationship requires a new attitude, which is best described as being a learner and a listener before bringing suggestions and information; this is particularly true for medical care professionals and public health personnel. One must allow for and actively create a setting in which people can be empowered. This is always a mutual experience between persons and groups, professional people and clients, teachers and students, midwives and mothers, and fieldworkers and town leaders. Public health professionals, particularly, need to study ways of creating such settings and fostering peer relationships in town meetings, classrooms, church discussion groups, women's organizations, and political parties. Empowerment training needs to be part of the reeducation of medical care personnel. Acknowledging people's right to understand and be involved in their own healing process requires a new way of relating.

One example of peer relationships and empowerment was the use of growth charts to monitor the development of children younger than five years. After a number of years of promoting PHC, it was decided that children under the age of five seen in the outpatient department and emergency department would require a growth chart, used by public health and community health nurses at Child Welfare Clinics and available only there, to be seen by the doctor or clinic-trained nurse. In the absence of a life-threatening problem, a mother might be asked to go home for the child health chart. This policy increased the number of registrations in the Child Welfare Clinics by over 30%. It brought the clinical services into the effort of watching for developmental delays, poor nutritional states, and incomplete vaccinations, a problem so widespread that the district health management team had to arrange for daily immunizations for those who needed to catch up. A survey revealed that 91% of children had growth charts. Use of the growth chart as a teaching guide for students and parents continues in combination with a project to have simple scales in the towns so that mothers can do their own growth monitoring. Then during periodic visits, the health team checked these growth measurements.

Integrating Primary Health Care

Primary health care strategies won't be effective if implemented only at the most local level (town, village, or neighborhood). Although local involvement is an essential starting point, as stated and restated by WHO ever since its Alma Ata Declaration of 1978, the local or Level A experience must be linked to a wider system and network composed of all manner of interest groups. The role of basic groups as advocates is crucial, but the role of the middle management level (in this example, Level C), is often overlooked, and little time or money is provided for retraining these health professionals so that they understand the concepts of PHC.

The three-tiered system needs to be supported and developed. An evaluation of the PHC program showed the principal shortcoming of its first five years; Level C, the district health management team, was committed to the training of community health workers, traditional birth attendants, and supervisors for all units and was doing it all on its own. Level B was not involved in training or supervision which limited the number of areas that could be covered. The retraining of Level B staff for training and supervision was a critical need and became a new focus for the future. Training district midwives to themselves train traditional birth attendants was a successful step.

Time

Health providers need time to understand community-based issues in health. I once sat in a meeting with a Nigerian medical doctor who was arguing that the slogan "Health for All by the Year 2000" was impossibly unrealistic. I realized that he understood the slogan to mean *"Medical Care* for All by the Year 2000." Health issues are much larger in scope than mere illness issues. It was helpful when someone articulated the slogan in reverse: "All for Health by the Year 2000."

Preventive-Promotive Equity

One of the most time-consuming issues in PHC is how to set the priorities so that preventive and promotive health concerns are given equal weight in planning, in budgets, and in personnel. Recently, an attempt was made to start a reporting system for basic health services that used a comparison of the number of people seen in a week to the expected population for that preventive service. Health must meet the people's needs—not numbers.

Appropriate Technology

Priorities determine the nature of appropriate technologies. How and for what money is spent is a critical issue, and making the right choice requires a clear understanding of the values involved. When considering appropriate technology, one must remember that quality care does not require sophisticated technologies. Frequently, respected and effective traditional medicines and practices are set aside by developing systems of health care in favor of the science-based medical model. These traditional therapies are often very appropriate, available, and widely accessible. In Ghana, at the ministry level, there is a new office for traditional medicine, and there has been for many years a research unit on herbs. Although the impact of these government agencies on the local health delivery systems is slight, they have begun discussions with people involved in active PHC programs who are including traditional practitioners among primary care providers at Level A.

Summary

Primary health care can be a reality for all if the basis for health care delivery is working with the community as partner. We must build the goals of PHC into the planning, training, and supervisory roles of health care providers.

We must learn from our experiences and make multisectoral problem definition and problem solving a priority in our in-service sessions. We must encourage articulation and inclusion of values stemming from beliefs, culture, and concern for the environment in our planning process.

We must continually ask ourselves this question: Are the issues of local groups connected within the networks of their own neighborhoods, towns, states, countries, and planet? How are we planning to keep the dynamics of these interdependent circles of potential communities open to new possibilities? How are we, as health professionals, considering the degradation of the physical environment (for example, deforestation and soil erosion) as concerns for PHC/community-based health care focus?

Ghana's government has an Agriculture Department and a Forestry Department. Both are heavily involved in developing the country's economic base. Adding an ecological dimension to the PHC perspective would keep its focus one of broad concerns for not only the present population but future generations as well.

Ghana began 20 years ago with a commitment to PHC. The journey has been arduous and wrought with difficulties. Change has occurred, priorities have been reset, and health problems have been viewed from the perspective of those with the problem. The local communities are involved in crafting a PHC system that seeks to share the country's resources to make health for all a reality for all.

REFERENCES

Grant, J.P. (1993). *The state of the world's children 1993.* Oxford: Oxford University Press.

World Health Organization. (1978). *The Alma-Ata declaration.* Geneva: Author.

Freire, P. (1972). *Pedagogy of the oppressed.* New York: Herder and Herder.

Hope, A., Timmel, S., (1984). *Training for transformation: A handbook for community workers,* vols. 1–3. Gweru, Zimbabwe: Mambo Press.

Part IV

The Future:
Nursing Beyond
the Year 2000

WHO Study Group on Nursing Beyond the Year 2000
Geneva, 12–16 July 1993

1. Introduction

A WHO Study Group on Nursing beyond the Year 2000 met in Geneva from 12 to 16 July 1993. Dr Hu Ching-Li, Assistant Director-General, opened the meeting on behalf of the Director-General, and referred to the many changes in health and in the world at large over the previous years. He noted that much of health care, in both developed and developing countries, was provided by nurses, and the profession had gained increasing visibility in both the political and the social arena. Dr Hu hoped the outcome of the Study Group would allow this momentum to be maintained.

The major task of the Study Group was to give direction and advice on how best to meet the challenges of the next century, and to provide a clearer perspective on the role of nursing and midwifery in promoting health and health services beyond the year 2000. The Study Group's work was closely linked to that of a multidisciplinary Global Advisory Group on Nursing and Midwifery which was set up in 1992 to advise the Director-General on:

- developing mechanisms for assessing national nursing and midwifery service needs;
- assisting countries with the development of national action plans for nursing and midwifery services, including research and resource planning;
- monitoring progress in strengthening nursing and midwifery in support of strategies for health for all.

2. Rationale and Objectives of the Study Group

2.1   Rationale

Most planning to date has focused on the goal of health for all by the year 2000. As that year approaches, it has become necessary to summarize past successes and failures and look further ahead. The Study Group was established to provide a global perspective on the role of nursing and midwifery in promoting health and health care services beyond the year 2000.

2.2   Objectives

The objectives of the Study Group were:

- to review the state of nursing and midwifery practice, education and research related to WHO's priorities:
- to recommend, where appropriate, goals for nursing and midwifery practice, education and research beyond the year 2000 in accordance with the recommendations of the first meeting of the Global Advisory Group on Nursing and Midwifery[1];
- to define the goals according to levels of socioeconomic development and cultural diversity across and within regions;
- to identify changes in the organization and delivery of health care services by nursing and midwifery personnel that could lead to greater effectiveness, efficiency and equity;
- to identify strategies required to bring about the needed changes in the organization and delivery of health care.

Study Group members were invited to pay particular attention to three main contextual issues:

- poverty differences within and between countries;
- population displacement, particularly from rural to urban areas, but also due to natural and man-made disasters;
- epidemiological and demographic transitions resulting in the increasing numbers of elderly people, changing and increasing chronic disease patterns, and financial and human resource constraints.

It was stressed that nursing issues could not be addressed in isolation or only within the health sector, but needed to be looked at within a societal perspective to determine how nursing could best contribute to better health.

3. Background

The World Health Assembly resolution WHA45.5 on strengthening nursing and midwifery in support of strategies for health for all[2] sought ways of addressing the following pressing issues:

- the growing demand for, and cost of, health care in countries around the world;
- the continued shortage of nursing and midwifery personnel and the urgent need to recruit, retain, educate and motivate sufficient numbers to meet present and future community health needs;
- the need to increase WHO's nursing and midwifery activities at all levels;
- the need to demonstrate commitment to nursing and midwifery as essential services in all countries, for the development and improvement of health-for-all strategies.

As one of its recommendations, the resolution urges Member States to "identify their nursing and midwifery service needs and, in this context, assess the roles and utilization of nursing and midwifery personnel."

In examining countries' needs for nurses and midwives, current global issues must be taken into account, as must demographic trends, morbidity and mortality patterns, health care needs and available resources as well as the socioeconomic, cultural and political context of health care delivery.

4. Current Global Issues

4.1   Population Growth and Demographic Transitions

A significant slow-down in the growth of the world population which began around 1970 is projected to continue, reaching an annual growth rate of 1.5% by 2000 and 1.0% by 2020.[3] Nevertheless, because three-quarters of people live in developing regions, the burden of population growth in these regions is probably one of the most important obstacles to achieving health for all. One in three people alive today is aged between 10 and 24 years of age. For every young person living in a developed country, there are four in developing areas. Twenty per cent of the world's young people live in China alone. One consequence of the huge increase in the number of young people in the developing world is the prospect of an even greater population expansion in the future. Between 1990 and 2025, the total urban population in developing regions is projected to increase threefold to 4000 million. The trend towards urbanization of populations and the growth of urban centres will have a major impact on the concept and delivery of health care services in the future.

As the rate of population growth has slowed, remarkable gains in life expectancy across the world have resulted in a global aging population profile. The continued decline in mortality has led in developed countries to an increase in the proportion of the population (currently 12.8%) aged 65 and over. By contrast, the proportion of the population aged 65 and over in developing countries is currently only 4.5%. However, the absolute numbers of elderly have risen dramatically in developing countries (to 182 million in 1990) and now exceed the elderly population (145 million) in developed countries.[4] By the year 2000, the overall number of elderly people in the world is projected to reach 423 million, with 250 million living in developing countries. This transition is producing increased global demand for services for the elderly and for the treatment of chronic diseases. Increased affluence may bring not only longer life and the diseases of aging but also the need to provide care for more chronic ill-health throughout a person's life. For example, cardiovascular disease, cancer and diseases related to tobacco, alcohol and drug use are increasing in developing countries, and diabetes is increasing everywhere. Mental health problems and suicide are increasing too, particularly in developed countries.[4]

4.2   Infectious and Parasitic Diseases

Epidemics of infectious and parasitic diseases continue to have devastating effects, especially among the poor. Poliomyelitis, measles, whooping cough and neonatal tetanus represent success stories in terms of immunization programmes, but special efforts are still required to make erad-ication a reality. In 1990, poliomyelitis disabled 200 000 children and the other three diseases accounted for about 2.6 million deaths.[5]

Pneumonia kills approximately 4 million young children each year, often as a consequence of measles or whooping cough or as a result of early cessation of breast-feeding and the inappropriate nutrition of the young child.[5] Cholera, leprosy and tuberculosis continue to result in avoidable deaths or major disabilities. Since 1985 the incidence of tuber-culosis has started to increase in both developed and developing coun-tries as a result of the association of tuberculosis and human immunod-eficiency virus (HIV) infection. In countries most affected by HIV, the tuberculosis problem is assuming dramatic dimensions. In certain areas the number of diagnosed cases of tuberculosis has doubled over the past five years.[4]

The malaria situation is deteriorating in many places compared with 10 years ago. More than 2000 million people, almost half the world's population, are exposed to varying degrees of malaria risk in 100 coun-tries and areas.[4] The most common waterborne parasites cause condi-tions such as schistosomiasis which, although easily treated with inex-pensive modern drugs, lead annually to high levels of pain and severe morbidity for millions of people in Africa and the Indian subcontinent. Lack of safe water supply and sanitation contributes to the diarrhoeal diseases and intestinal worm infections which together make up 10% of the total burden of disease in developing countries.[6]

The acquired immunodeficiency syndrome (AIDS) continues to spread with particular rapidity in developing countries, with major con-sequences for individuals as well as for communities and their economies. WHO projects cumulative totals of over 40 million people with HIV infection, including 10 million children, by the year 2000.[4] Projections show little difference between adult infection rates of men and women by the mid-1990s. In addition, there is a rapidly growing problem of orphaned sick children in communities that are affected by AIDS and that have minimal health care and economic resources.

4.3   Health Needs and the Concept of Vulnerability

A complex array of cultural, political and socioeconomic factors influ-ence the health status of populations. The concept of health-related vul-nerability is reflected in patterns of morbidity, mortality and reproduction and is the product of simultaneous social and economic deprivation of various forms.[7] All the major global health concerns involve groups that are vulnerable in some way in relation to others. This vulnerability can sometimes be the unintended consequence of development strategies in other sectors of society, such as the economy. Vulnerability may also be the intended consequence of aggression and war. Certain groups are especially vulnerable and, in addition to the frail elderly, they include women, children and non-economically productive persons in a society.

4.3.1   Women

Women are disproportionately vulnerable to disease. In comparison with men they fare less well in terms of disease prevalence, utilization of services and allocation of resources within the family. Such gender differences are found throughout the world from birth onward.[8,9]

Türmen[10] notes that women's health status is too often characterized by neglect, abuse and victimization. Some conditions either affect only women or hit women the hardest, as in the case of female infanticide, genital mutilation, malnutrition and anaemia, early marriage, high fertility, abortion, sexually transmitted diseases, maternal mortality and morbidity, violence, rape and incest. Türmen goes on to propose for priority action three indicators which reflect the unequal health status of women—nutrition, fertility and maternal mortality.

Every year half a million women die of causes related to pregnancy and childbirth. Their deaths leave a million children motherless. Even though more women are reaching childbearing years in good health, maternal mortality and morbidity figures will continue to rise unless there is improved coverage and quality of care. A considerable proportion of maternal deaths are the result of unsafe abortion,[6] and the associated mortality and morbidity will rise unless safe preventive measures are made widely available. The disparity between maternal mortality in developing countries and that in developed countries is greater than for any other major health indicator. Maternal mortality in 1988 varied from about 737 per 100 000 live births in the least developed countries to about 34 per 100 000 in developed countries. For example, a woman in sub-Saharan Africa who becomes pregnant is 75 times more likely to die as a result than a woman in western Europe.[4] Despite improvements in coverage, in some developing countries less than 20% of deliveries are attended by trained personnel, many of whom are trained not as physicians, nurses or midwives but as birth attendants able to address only the most basic needs. In the developed world highly trained personnel and sophisticated equipment are available at levels in excess of that required for the majority of births, but in the developing world the needed facilities may not always exist and, even if they do, they are frequently too few and too inaccessible for most people.

4.3.2 Children

Despite gains in life expectancy, children living in poverty continue to experience disproportionately the effects of avoidable mortality and morbidity. One-third of the developing world's children suffer from malnutrition. The diarrhoeal diseases together kill approximately 4 million young children each year and they are also a major cause of child malnutrition.[5] Every year, vitamin A deficiency results in a third of a million children going blind, and 60% of these children die within a short time of losing their sight. Iodine deficiency is a major health risk for one-fifth of the world's population, resulting in stunted growth, mental retardation and defective speech, hearing and movement.[5] The problems of malnutrition may arise from the consequences of poverty, but the cause may also lie in children's exposure to frequent infections and a lack of knowledge about the special feeding needs of the young child.

Children are frequently the group worst affected by local wars, conflict and disaster. UNICEF reports that unknown numbers of children have been killed, wounded, abandoned, orphaned or taken as hostages. Millions will never see their families again. Even in times of peace there is child exploitation in factories, sweatshops, agriculture or domestic service. An estimated 30 million children live on the streets of the world's expanding cities. They have run away, have been abandoned or are orphaned. Most of these children are deprived of health care and education; almost all face the difficult choice of either resisting or falling in with violence, crime, prostitution and drug abuse.[5]

If nursing is to contribute effectively in the next century to the achievement of a level of health that permits all citizens to lead socially and economically productive lives, nurses and midwives must address the nature of their role with respect to the health needs of vulnerable groups.

5. Access to Health Care Personnel and Services

In view of the global diversity in health needs and the extremes of the range of gross national product (GNP) between different countries—in 1991, GNP ranged between US$ 80 and US$ 33 610 per capita[6]—it is not surprising that people's opportunities for access to medical, nursing and midwifery care are also strikingly unequal. In 1990, world spending on health totalled about US$ 1700 billion, or 8% of global income. Spending within countries ranged from less than US$ 10 per person in several African and Asian countries to more than US$ 2700 in the United States.

Yet health spending alone does not explain all the variation in health among countries. At any level of income and education, higher health spending should yield better health, all else being equal. But there is no evidence of such a relationship. The *World development report* gives the following average ratios of nurses to population in 1984[11] and physicians to population in 1990[6] and ranges for the proportion of births attended by health staff in 1985 and for infant mortality rates in 1991[6]:

1. Low-income economies
   —1 nurse to 2180 population
   —1 physician to 6760 population
   —3 to 87% health personnel attendance at birth
   —infant mortality rate of 18 to 161 per 1000 live births.
   —(If China and India are excluded from the above data, the average ratio of nurses and physicians to population in low-income economies is reduced to 1 nurse per 3670 and 1 physician to 11 730.)
2. Middle-income economies
   —1 nurse to 980 population
   —1 physician to 2060 population
   —19 to 100% attendance at birth
   —infant mortality rate of 11 to 115 per 1000 live births.
3. High-income economies
   —1 nurse to 140 population
   —1 physician to 420 population
   —98 to 100% attendance at birth
   —infant mortality rate of 5 to 9 per 1000 live births.

The search for better indicators continues. For example, the *World development report 1993*[6] presents a range of health data relating to demographic regions and economies. These include nurse to doctor ratios ranging from 0.3 to 16.4, with a world average of 1.4. The report suggests that, although doctors are needed for supervising essential clinical care and handling complications, most of the services in the minimum package of health services can be delivered by nurses and midwives. The World Bank suggests that a ratio of fully qualified nurses to physicians of between 2:1 and 4:1, and of one or two physicians per 10 000 population is adequate. However, achieving an optimal skill mix of physicians, nurses, midwives and less qualified personnel is a major challenge.

6. Trends in Nursing and Midwifery

6.1 The Role of Nurses and Midwives

In most countries nursing and midwifery personnel make up the largest single group of human resources for health in both hospital and community. In almost all countries there is imbalance in the supply of nurses, midwives, physicians and other health professionals. For nurses and midwives, the most frequent problem is shortage of personnel. Of course, shortage of personnel can reflect a wide variety of situations. For instance, a personnel shortage can be defined in terms of perceived health care needs, or in terms of demand from the health services sector. It may indicate maldistribution of the health workforce or imbalance among different categories of health workers. In many countries the number of different kinds of health personnel reflects the willingness or ability of governments to fund positions. In a recent (unpublished) opinion survey of nursing personnel resources worldwide,* respondents from 70% of developing countries reported a shortage of nurses in the public sector, especially in rural areas. Reluctance to practise in rural areas exacerbates the shortage of health care personnel.

Some responses to the survey reported that many nurses leave the public sector for the private sector in search of better working conditions and pay, producing acute personnel shortages in the public sector. Yet many replies also indicated unemployment of nurses because positions had been cut in health services. While half the responses from industrialized countries reported a shortage of nurses, several also mentioned

---

*Hirschfeld MJ, Henry B, Griffith H. *Nursing personnel resources: results of a survey of perceptions in ministries of health on nursing shortage, nursing education and quality of care.* Geneva, World Health Organization, 1993 (unpublished document WHO/HRH/NUR/93.4; available on request from Nursing, Division of Development of Human Resources for Health, World Health Organization, 1211 Geneva 27, Switzerland).

nurse unemployment caused by a cut in positions as a result of economic retrenchment or by over-supply of nurses as a result of inaccurate projections of need.

The cost-effectiveness of nursing and midwifery care across settings has been demonstrated in research reviews,[12] but many countries still do not devote adequate resources to planning the effective employment and deployment of nursing and midwifery staff. The objective of human resource planning is to balance supply with demand—to ensure that sufficient (but not excessive) numbers of appropriately qualified personnel are available, in the right place and at the right time, to match the demand for their services. Demand for nursing and midwifery services is but one aspect of demand for health services in general, and must be measured in this wider context. Planning of human resources for nursing and midwifery cannot be properly conducted in isolation from planning for other health care workers or from planning of the service as a whole.

Three closely linked elements appear to influence the development of nursing: power, gender and the medicalization of health care. Nurses face these issues to varying degrees, depending on the stage of development of the country.[13]

Nurses play a full part in policy-making and decision-making at all levels of the health care system in very few countries. Even in countries whose health ministries have large nursing departments, nurses must continually fight to ensure that their voice is heard. This lack of formal power at the top is reflected elsewhere, as in the lack of democratic decision-making among members of health care teams in hospital and community.

One means of addressing this problem would be for countries to create a multisectoral forum of relevant partners (e.g. health, education and finance sectors, as well as professional associations, regulatory bodies and consumers) involved in practice, research, education, management and policy development for nursing and midwifery services. This forum should meet regularly to develop, and monitor implementation of, a national plan to ensure that nursing and midwifery, as integral parts of the health service, can meet current and projected health care needs with available resources. The plan should specifically ensure nursing and midwifery participation in policy-making and decision-making at all levels. It should also address the changing needs of nursing and midwifery personnel, the preparation of personnel for their tasks, and the development of educational systems that enable personnel to move to new career levels.

In nearly every country women are the vast majority of the nursing and midwifery workforce. Nursing everywhere is women's work and shares the characteristics of other female-dominated occupations—low pay, low status, poor working conditions, few prospects for promotion and poor education. For example, nurses' salaries in a third of the world's countries are lower than those of other occupations that require a similar level of education, and in some of the least developed countries salaries are actually decreasing. Pizurki et al.[14] contend that, of all the professions subject to sex-role stereotyping, nursing is the most severely handicapped in that "nurses are doubly conditioned into playing a subservient role: first by society generally, and secondly by the medical establishment."

The prestige associated with the practice of medicine in high technology environments compounds this situation. In spite of the rhetoric of the community care approach, acute curative interventions receive the lion's share of prestige and resources in many countries. Nurses are sometimes seen as medical assistants whose job is to carry out physicians' orders, and nursing in high technology settings is more prestigious and brings better pay than, for example, community nursing. This situation may be one of the reasons for the enormous shortage of community nurses, especially in rural communities. In the recent opinion survey of nursing personnel resources, 95% of respondents from the least developed countries and 83% from developing countries reported shortages of nurses in rural communities. In many of these countries, however, nurses and midwives do not work in rural areas because there are no positions for them there.

These issues provide the backdrop for the evolution of nursing and midwifery in the twenty-first century. The problems they pose must be considered along with the global trends in health needs and resources described in sections 4 and 5 above. As the Director-General of WHO has noted, "Until society values caring work and women's work more highly, and rewards them accordingly, measures taken to attract new recruits will not succeed; well educated, motivated women will continue to seek careers in occupations that have a higher social standing and higher remuneration. The social consequences of this for the health and well-being of populations will be disastrous."[15]

In discussing nursing and midwifery we must consider the changing approach to health care worldwide arising from new technology, growing demands and the pressure of lack of resources. Health care is becoming the province of all. Consumers of health care are demanding safe, affordable, comprehensive and acceptable service. At the same time, there is a growing movement towards self-care. In the next century individuals, families and communities will play a larger role both in determining and in meeting their own health needs. The roles of nurses and other health care providers will change as individual behaviour and lifestyle choices are seen as more important for health. With increasing numbers of elderly and children, a range of informal care-givers will be needed. Everyone may need to be taught the basic skills and knowledge of caring, and everyone will be involved in matters relating to health. Traditional labels such as qualified/unqualified care-givers or formal/informal care will cease to be as important as they are today. Providers of care must seek partnerships with communities to help them plan and implement health services so as to ensure an equitable distribution of health care. Nurses and midwives must become enablers and facilitators by, for example, providing information and guidance to adolescents on safe sexual practices and educating communities on the consequences of early marriage, early pregnancy and unsafe abortion. Nurses will help people to help themselves and will do for people what they cannot do for themselves. The aim will be to make the best use of all available resources in order to provide the best possible health care for all.

This new approach will require great change both on the part of individuals who need care and on the part of those who provide care. This has major implications for the development of nursing and midwifery practice, education and research.

6.2   Implications for Practice

The most effective use of health care personnel involves the appropriate mix of direct care-givers (nurses, doctors, etc.) with support staff, plus a suitable balance of staff of different disciplines. However, planning of the workforce, and more specifically planning for nursing and midwifery services, is impossible until answers are found to the basic questions of what the identified health needs are, what services should be provided and with what objectives, and what human, financial and material resources are available to support them. The answers to these questions may vary widely according to the socioeconomic, political and cultural context and in light of the health needs that are to be given highest priority. Thus a range of scenarios of nursing and midwifery practice may be needed so that countries can choose the approaches to practice and education that are most appropriate to changing conditions.

One extreme yet possible future scenario is that the very notion of nursing and medicine as separate occupations may disappear. Nurses, physicians and other health care professionals might be replaced by a generic health care workforce made up of workers trained to carry out a range of specific tasks for specific care groups. For example, a person who comes into hospital with a fractured femur could be cared for by one or two workers who handle the range of tasks from X-ray to discharge. In another future scenario, well educated nurses with broad general preparation and additional specialization may provide, directly or indirectly, a range of promotive, curative and rehabilitative services— including the management of other workers under their supervision. Between these two extremes, there may be health care professionals with clusters of skills and with job titles we may not recognize today. Each of these scenarios raises questions about how best to ensure an appropriate cost-effective level of clinical or public health skills together with professional accountability.

In many countries government spending may be concentrated on selected groups of interventions (bigger or smaller in content according to available resources) provided chiefly through public facilities and focusing on primary care and prevention. At the same time, the trend towards private health care is increasing. It seems very likely that private health care will play a major role in both developed and developing countries in the future. There will thus be a growing need to monitor the quality of care of private medical, nursing and midwifery services. A recent study of 100 private physicians identified 80 treatment regimens for tuberculosis, of which only four followed WHO treatment recommendations.[16]

In future it is likely that some tertiary care, specialist care and other services outside a country's basic health care package will rely to a great extent on private or insurance-based financing. Nurses with highly specialized training (whether they are called nurses or not) will be involved in this high technology tertiary care. At the same time, nurses with broad education will play an essential role in directing the range of public services. For example, the work of a community midwife might involve education about safe delivery, as well as development of women's health care programmes that would include prevention of unwanted early pregnancy and sexually transmitted diseases, family planning, nutrition and healthy childbirth.

Nurses and midwives in poor or remote districts often face a lack of basic services such as clean water, sanitation, immunization or basic drugs. Some lack syringes or needles to give an injection. Some lack facilities to maintain the cold chain with the result that vaccines become ineffective. On the other hand, nurses and midwives who work in highly technical environments may face problems related to the use of technology. They may have to make difficult ethical decisions about when not to use, or to stop using, technological intervention. At the same time the development and routine use of technology (e.g. dentures, joint replacements) may significantly improve life for the elderly and disabled. Thus health care personnel will increasingly need to consider whether particular technologies are effective, culturally acceptable and politically supportable. In addition, because of the problem of iatrogenic illness, nurses working in hospitals—both public and private—will need to monitor the quality of care and develop alternative approaches to improving outcomes for patients.

In the future, health care professionals such as nurses and midwives will be expected to provide increased coverage of health care to groups of patients who are poor, socially marginal or culturally different from the mainstream of society. If this challenge is to be met, the many reasons why nurses, midwives and other health personnel have difficulty working in remote areas or with the disadvantaged (refugees, AIDS patients, the chronically mentally ill, the homeless) will have to be addressed. One reason is the desire for the higher status and higher pay associated with complex medical technology, but social and physical conditions are also factors. Nurses who are not in urban hospitals not only earn less but often live and work in situations where facilities are inadequate, without electricity, water or postal service. They may be concerned about substandard schooling and living conditions for their children in remote communities. In addition, nurses' security and safety in the workplace must be ensured. Awareness of these factors should help future governments create conditions conducive to equitable delivery of care.

Countries must consider developing regulatory systems for nursing and midwifery in order to:

- define the scope of nursing and midwifery and the categories of personnel;

- establish educational standards;
- take measures to check and maintain practitioners' competence;
- set up and maintain administrative mechanisms for dealing with such problems as disability and for taking disciplinary action in cases of misconduct and malpractice[13];
- address ethical concerns.

In some countries, nursing and midwifery practice is constrained by inflexible and out-of-date public service requirements which regulate employment and career pathways. Regulatory systems must be flexible so as to enable nurses and midwives to redirect their practice to meet changing health care needs (for instance, certified midwives should be able legally to undertake essential life-saving emergency measures when necessary).

6.3   Implications for Education

Changing nursing practice to meet the health care needs of the twenty-first century calls for fundamental change in nursing education. The shape of nursing and midwifery education for the future will in part depend on a country's policy and planning regarding the health workforce. For instance, education of nurses will vary widely according to whether the nurse will be a highly specialized manager in a tertiary care setting, a direct care-giver under the direction of a manager, or a community nurse who not only provides care in the community but assists and enables people to meet their own health needs, fostering the maintenance and promotion of health and providing health education.

In many countries today, nurses and midwives are now educated at university level. Indeed, in some countries, the current trend is towards university education for all nurses. In others, however, the trend is towards the use of a small core of highly educated nurses and a large number of auxiliary personnel, which means there is an overall lowering of skill levels. Systematic planning of a country's health workforce may lead to nursing programmes being developed at various educational levels in order to reflect the nursing contributions needed in a changing health care system. In some countries the variety of educational levels now represented in nursing is considered a weakness of the profession. In fact, it is a weakness if there is little differentiation in the role of the nurse in different practice settings. It is a strength when nurses are used in a wide variety of ways in a broad range of settings.

Discussion about levels of nursing education inevitably raises questions about the intellectual development of women and career mobility of nurses and midwives. There are related questions about the role of education generally and the role of training that is narrowly focused on teaching very specific tasks. Nursing education has for generations been one of the few avenues of education open to women. As such, it has provided employment opportunities and social and career mobility. On the other hand, developing countries need low-cost provision of care, and enhanced career mobility of nursing personnel through formal education may limit countries' ability to provide such services. If the differences in grade between qualified and other categories of nursing personnel are to become more distinct, then questions about the role of education in providing or obstructing mobility between grades must be addressed. Decisions about the numbers and levels of nurses and their education therefore involve far-reaching decisions about women's role in the social structure.

Placing basic nursing education in the university may improve the status of nursing, enhance recruitment of able students and ensure that all practitioners are broadly educated, become equal members of health care teams and are mobile. On the other hand, it may encourage elitism among nurses, prompt countries to increase the proportion of unqualified personnel and reduce the overall cost-effectiveness of the workforce. Thus, in deciding about basic nursing education, national authorities and the nursing profession may need to consider the overall need for nursing personnel, the level of general education in the country, the extent of opportunities for higher education and the training of other similar professions.

The issue goes beyond questions of professional competence to the question of women's entitlement to participate in all the benefits that only higher education offers them. The demand for nurses trained by cheaper, alternative educational programmes may therefore have to be set against the wider benefits of further education for women.

Crucial issues in planning nursing education include:

- an understanding of the nature of nursing, which has consequences for the value placed on different subjects in the curriculum and how they are taught and assessed;

- what constitutes nursing knowledge (whether it comes from a unique discipline, via the nursing process and models of nursing, or whether it is an amalgam of knowledge from several disciplines);
- an understanding of how best to foster the development of the nurse.[13]

For instance, if nursing is viewed as derived from the humanities and the physical, social, medical and biological sciences[13] yet requiring understanding and application of knowledge and skills specific to one discipline, educational requirements will differ from those that would come from a definition of nursing as a purely technical skill.

The question of how best to foster the development of nurses raises other issues. When students are taken out of rural communities to be educated in a central, specialized location, many do not return to the rural community to practise. Even if they do return, their education and their exposure to outside influence often result in nurses being alienated from the community. On the other hand, multiple, widely dispersed, small schools of nursing operating without adequate resources are ill-equipped to provide good nursing education.

In planning nursing education, both the content and method should be considered.[17] Countries may need to consider a variety of approaches—including problem-based learning, distance learning, self-directed learning, community-based education, continuing education credits and professional experience—in order to expand educational opportunities and career mobility for nursing and midwifery personnel.

6.4   Implications for Research

In terms of research, the challenge to nursing and midwifery in the future is to show the link between inputs (by an appropriate mix of nurses, physicians and other health care professionals) and health outcomes. This calls for the inclusion of nursing and midwifery issues in health systems research to a far greater extent than before.

The lack of involvement by nurses and midwives in multidisciplinary research and the problems in developing appropriate research (in addition to costs and complexity) are related to traditional structures of power and status. In the past there has been considerable investment of professional power and status in particular forms of research focused on only one discipline. As a result, much research on nursing which has been highly developed in terms of methodological rigour has been too narrowly focused, in terms of both the health problems addressed and the wider issues of cost-effective care delivery. Some of the most highly developed research of this kind has been conducted in the United States of America, to which many nurses in developing countries look for research education and inspiration.

Unfortunately there is little research that documents the efficacy of nursing care activities, especially in relation to activities of other health care providers. In part that is a consequence of the complexity of health services research, for a multiplicity of inputs may affect the outcome for the client. The context of health care, the type of health care provider and the processes used by providers must all be defined in relation to the outcome for the client. In addition, health systems research must recognize the complexity and breadth of clients' problems, the resources they possess to deal with the problems, and the processes they may use in addition to health care as they move towards health and healing. A special problem for multidisciplinary health services research is the lack of adequate consensual language to describe care delivery in relation to client outcomes.

Usually research on client outcomes focuses on a change in the health status of the patient/client that is attributed to an intervention by a health care provider or by the health care system. Client outcomes may include indicators of functional status, measures of quality of life, length of stay in hospital, utilization of resources, satisfaction with care delivery and so on. In the search for global indicators of health outcomes, the World Bank, in conjunction with WHO, has developed the concept of the global burden of disease (GBD). This concept combines losses through premature death with loss of healthy life resulting from disability. The GBD is measured in units of disability-adjusted life years, or DALYs.[6] In future it seems highly probable that health care providers, including nurses and midwives, will be increasingly called upon to show the efficacy of their interventions in terms of such global outcome indicators.

As consumer satisfaction becomes an important variable in determining the beneficial outcomes of health care services, it will be important to determine whether health services are delivered in a manner acceptable to community norms and at costs that can be borne by the recipient. Improved health outcomes may be due not to delivery of health care but to an interaction of personal, socioeconomic and cultural resources in addition to the care. Among this mix of inputs, distinguishing the contribution of nursing care to health outcomes for the client will be a significant challenge in the future.

Meeting this challenge will require major reorientation of programmes for nursing and midwifery education. All nurses and midwives will need to be aware of and be able to appreciate research findings in order to see the relevance of research to nursing practice. They should be able to understand the benefits of research both to nurses and to the groups of clients they care for. A sizeable number of nurses and midwives will need to be enabled to develop research skills in order to participate as equal members in multidisciplinary research teams which address the health problems discussed in this report. In giving priority to research related to nursing and midwifery services, the aim will be to seek solutions to problems in health care situations where nurses and midwives are the principal care providers or make a major contribution. Consequently nurses and midwives at all levels of practice will need to be involved in developing research questions and in conducting the research itself. A major question for health care researchers everywhere is how to develop locally appropriate methodologies in which local health care providers and communities can be involved.

A further challenge is to disseminate research results so that they can be used both in health care delivery and in policy formulation for nursing and midwifery care. Even in countries where research in nursing is encouraged and research results are regularly published in journals, much of what is currently written is over-technical and difficult to decipher and lacks clear discussion of the implications for practice. In some countries the problems of dissemination are more severe. There may be few channels for the communication of research results to those in practice and few practitioners who are prepared to read and critically evaluate research. In many countries the problem of disseminating research findings is compounded by the fact that the dominant scientific language is English, making published research inaccessible to large numbers of practitioners. In addition, the research journals never reach some countries or may never get to communities or hospitals where the research might be used.

The use of research to change practice and policy will require not only major efforts to disseminate research results widely in language that is easily understood by practitioners and policy-makers but also ongoing administrative support for change. Ideally, local and countrywide data sets will include nursing and midwifery input and output variables so that monitoring of the effects of changes in practice and management can be evaluated.

7. Conclusions

As the twentieth century closes, there is increasing inequity in income distribution and access to health care. The vulnerable are becoming more vulnerable, and the divisions between the technical and human aspects of health care are widening. The deterioration of national economies in many parts of the world, particularly in least developed countries, is reflected in rising infant mortality rates and falling standards of infant nutrition as well as a worsening of other indicators of health. Earlier gains in health and health care are being lost as costs escalate, resources shrink, currencies are devalued and the debt burden continues. While health has been declared a fundamental human right, many governments are unable to provide basic health care to their citizens.

Meeting the health care needs of the future calls for careful use of resources and the targeting of health care interventions at those population groups where they will have most effect. It will also require less hierarchical, more flexible health care systems that are multidisciplinary and indeed multisectoral in scope. Health care personnel must be prepared quickly to reorient education and practice to meet changing needs, working with central governments, local authorities and communities in order to set priorities. All levels of health care personnel, including auxiliary personnel and informal care-givers, will need to collaborate in practice, education and research.

In the future, health care needs and the factors that affect health care delivery are likely to be complex, multifaceted and constantly changing. Health care systems will be radically different from those we now know. It is thus critical that WHO, Member States and all partners with an interest in the future of nursing and midwifery should anticipate these developments and begin the process of change without delay. This process also applies to the individual responsibility of nurses and midwives to be full partners in a caring and competent health workforce. It is essential to recognize the need for continuing review and evaluation in order to facilitate rapid response to change.

8. Recommendations

The recommendations of the Study Group on Nursing beyond the Year 2000 should be understood to include the need for continuing assessment and change. The recommendations have three strategic aims:

- a new multisectoral systems approach to health care delivery and full collaboration of health care personnel at all levels;
- a shift in the focus of workforce development in nursing and midwifery to reflect country health needs, with particular emphasis on vulnerable groups;
- revitalization and reorientation of nursing and midwifery education and practice to meet the challenges of the future.

8.1 Recommendations to WHO and Member States

1. WHO should encourage Member States to review their current strategies for providing basic health care, especially for vulnerable populations, to identify gaps in services, and to plan an appropriate mix of skills and responsibilities (including those of nurses and midwives) in order to provide the care needed in the future.

2. WHO should encourage governments to obtain the input of nurses and midwives in formulating health care policy at country, district and subdistrict levels. In order to ensure the appropriate involvement of these personnel in policy formulation, WHO and Member States should prepare nurses and midwives to deal with policy issues through leadership development and participation in policy forums.

3. WHO and Member States should explore the gap between approval of recommendations about nursing and midwifery at previous WHO forums and their implementation. For those recommendations that have not been implemented, the reasons should be analysed, alternative strategies developed and a continuous monitoring system created, with indicators of progress.

4. WHO and Member States should continue to support the development of innovative, cost-effective programmes for nursing and midwifery education which focus on the development of critical thinking and a caring attitude. In particular, WHO should

support management training and the development and use of relevant learning materials.

8.2   Recommendations to WHO

1. WHO, the WHO collaborating centres and other institutions should develop collaborative research, facilitate the exchange of relevant research findings, develop strategies to utilize the findings of research in practice and policy, collect and evaluate models of nursing development, and share successful models across countries.
2. WHO should encourage development of an international multi-disciplinary project that:
   —identifies the core competencies in health and social sciences that are common to all health professions (e.g. ethics, communication, research, consultation skills, teaching skills);
   —identifies the unique competencies for each profession;
   —examines the implications of these findings for the education of the different health professions.
3. WHO should make a commitment to include nursing and midwifery care in special initiatives (e.g. safe motherhood, the sick child, urban health, sustainable development) and should monitor progress towards this goal.
4. WHO should act as a catalyst by working with Member States and donors to include nursing and midwifery issues in relevant health systems research and to seek needed funds for such research.

8.3   Recommendations to Member States

1. Member States should create a multisectoral forum of relevant partners (e.g. health, education and finance sectors, as well as professional associations, regulatory bodies and consumers) involved in practice, research, education, management and policy development for nursing and midwifery services in order to address the changing needs of nursing and midwifery personnel, their preparation and the development of educational systems that allow personnel to move from one career level to another.

2. Member States should continually assess their needs for health care personnel to provide community-based health care interventions, especially to vulnerable groups. The data obtained should be shared with health professionals, including nurses and midwives, so that they can redirect their practice and prepare personnel to meet future needs.

3. In view of the growing need for informal care-giving, Member States should be encouraged to include self-care and basic care-giving skills at appropriate points in school curricula.

4. Member States should ensure that students entering nursing and midwifery programmes have a good basic education and have reached a level of maturity consistent with the responsibilities of their work.

5. In deciding on the appropriateness of basic and postbasic education in nursing at university level, Member States should consider:
    —future health care needs and the roles of nurses and midwives;
    —the level of general education in the country;
    —the educational patterns of other professions in the health care field.
    When appropriate, Member States should move basic nursing education to the university.

6. Member States should ensure that basic and continuing nursing and midwifery education focuses on knowledge and skills that are relevant to, and attitudes that are respectful of, the needs and values of local communities, and that innovations which are introduced through continuing education become part of basic professional education.

7. Member States should develop multidisciplinary programmes for management development within universities and colleges and in agencies at country, district and subdistrict levels.

8. Through flexible and enabling legislation and regulation, Member States should support the development of nursing and midwifery practice to meet changing health care needs. Member States should consider regulatory controls for nursing and midwifery auxiliary personnel.

9. Member States should review their public service regulations to ensure that a variety of educational pathways to nursing and

midwifery are recognized, and that requirements are flexible in regard to changing functions, professional practice and career structures.

10. In their health systems research, Member States should include questions related to nursing and midwifery education and care, and should consider these a priority for funding. Member States should also encourage local communities to collaborate in developing research questions and in raising funds to support such research, in order to ensure its relevance to local needs.

11. Member States should develop information systems for the management of nursing and midwifery personnel as an integral part of countrywide health information systems.

Acknowledgements

The Study Group acknowledges the important assistance given to its work by Professor E. Abou Youssef, Regional Nursing Adviser, WHO Regional Office for the Eastern Mediterranean, Alexandria, Egypt, and Dr S.A. Bisch, Regional Nursing Adviser, WHO Regional Office for South-East Asia, New Delhi, India, and the considerable and essential input of the temporary advisers (Professor P. Archbold, Professor J. Robinson and Ms E. Tornquist). Professor Robinson's theoretical overview of the global health situation and policy provided the conceptual framework for the Study Group's discussions.

The contribution of the following persons in preparing background documentation for the Study Group is gratefully acknowledged:

James Buchan, Senior Policy and Research Analyst, Royal College of Nursing, England (*World nursing "shortages" and human resource planning*);

Anne J. Davis, Professor, School of Nursing, University of California, USA, and Ruth Stark, Suva, Fiji (*Health care ethics and international nursing*);

Nelly Garzon, Professor Emeritus, School of Nursing, The National University of Colombia, Colombia (*World view of nursing education*);

William Holzemer, Professor and Associate Dean for Research, School of Nursing, University of California, USA (*The impact of nursing care: a focus on outcomes*);

Margretta Madden Styles, Livingston Professor of Nursing, University of California, USA (*Laws and regulations*);

R. Margaret Truax, Nurse Scientist, Division of Development of Human Resources for Health, WHO, Geneva, Switzerland (*Management information systems for nursing/midwifery personnel*).

REFERENCES

1. *Global Advisory Group on Nursing and Midwifery. Report of the first meeting, Geneva, 30 November to 2 December, 1992.* Geneva, World Health Organization, 1993 (unpublished document WHO/HRH/NUR/93.1; available on request from Division of Development of Human Resources for Health, World Health Organization, 1211 Geneva 27, Switzerland).

2. *Handbook of resolutions and decisions of the World Health Assembly and the Executive Board*, Vol. III, 3rd ed. (1985–1992). Geneva, World Health Organization, 1993:45–46.

3. *Health dimensions of economic reform.* Geneva, World Health Organization, 1992.

4. *Implementation of the Global Strategy for Health for All by the Year 2000, second evaluation. Eighth report on the world health situation. Volume 1: Global review.* Geneva, World Health Organization, 1993.

5. **UNICEF.** *The state of the world's children 1991.* Oxford, Oxford University Press, 1992.

6. **The World Bank.** *World development report 1993: investing in health.* Oxford, Oxford University Press, 1993.

7. **Cooper Weil DE et al.** *The impact of development policies on health: a review of the literature.* Geneva, World Health Organization, 1990.

8. **Cook RJ.** *Women's health and human rights: the promotion and protection of women's health through international human rights law.* Geneva, World Health Organization (in press).

9. *Women's health: across age and frontier.* Geneva, World Health Organization, 1992.

10. **Türmen T.** *Priority health issues affecting women: address by Tomris Türmen to the Global Commission for Women's Health, Geneva, 8 March 1993.* Geneva, World Health Organization, 1993 (unpublished document WHO/FHE/WHD/93.1; available on request from Women, Health and Development, World Health Organization, 1211 Geneva 27, Switzerland).

11. **The World Bank.** *World development report 1991: the challenge of development.* Oxford, Oxford University Press, 1991.

12. **Buchan J, Ball J.** *Caring costs: nursing costs and benefits.* Brighton, Institute of Manpower Studies, 1991.

13. **Salvage J, ed.** *Nursing in action: strengthening nursing and midwifery to support health for all.* Copenhagen, World Health Organization, 1993 (WHO Regional Publications, European Series, No. 48).

14. **Pizurki H et al.** *Women as providers of health care.* Geneva, World Health Organization, 1987.

15. **World Health Organization.** More than ever we need nurses [editorial]. *World health*, September–October 1992.
16. Urban slums and primary health care: the private doctor's role [editorial]. *British medical journal*, 1993, **306**:667–668.
17. **Hammond, M, Mazibuko R.** Nurse education: in need of radical change for PHC? *Tropical doctor*, 1991,**21**:5–8.

Members

Mrs G. Betts, President, Sierra Leone Association for Maternal and Infant Health, Freetown, Sierra Leone

Ms G. Miscoe, Chief Executive, Australian Capital Territory Department of Health, Canberra, Australia (*Rapporteur*)

Dr M. Jato, Senior Lecturer, Faculty of Medicine, Yaoundé, Cameroon

Dr H. Lapsley, Health Economist, School for Health Service Management, University of New South Wales, Kensington, New South Wales, Australia

Dr W. May, Principal, Institute of Nursing, Ministry of Health, Yangon, Myanmar

Dr H. Minami, President and Professor, College of Nursing Art and Science, Hyogo, Japan

Mrs B. Misconiova, Chief Nurse, Ministry of Health, Prague, Czech Republic

Dr S. Mokabel, Head and Professor, Nursing Department, College of Applied Medical Sciences, King Saud University, Riyadh, Saudi Arabia

Dr R. Ndlovu, Senior Lecturer, Department of Nursing Science, University of Zimbabwe, Avondale, Harare, Zimbabwe (*Chairman*)

Mr H. Rouis, Director, School of Public Health, Ministry of Public Health, Sousse, Tunisia

Dr A. de Almeida Souza, Associate Professor, Department of Public Health, University of Brasilia, Brasilia Federal District, Brazil

Representatives of Other Organizations

International Confederation of Midwives
Sister A. Thompson, Treasurer, International Confederation of Midwives, London, England

International Council of Nurses
Ms F. Affara, Nurse Consultant, International Council of Nurses, Geneva, Switzerland
International Federation of Red Cross and Red Crescent Societies
Ms E. Ortin, Technical Adviser, Nursing, International Federation of Red Cross and Red Crescent Societies, Geneva, Switzerland

Secretariat

Dr P. Archbold, Professor, School of Nursing, Oregon Health Sciences University, Portland, OR, USA (*Temporary Adviser*)

Dr E. Goon, Director, Division of Development of Human Resources for Health, WHO, Geneva, Switzerland

Dr M.J. Hirschfeld, Chief Scientist for Nursing, Division of Development of Human Resources for Health, WHO, Geneva, Switzerland (*Secretary*)

Dr J. Robinson, Head and Professor, Department of Nursing and Midwifery Studies, University of Nottingham, Queen's Medical Centre, Nottingham, England (*Temporary Adviser*)

Ms E. Tornquist, Lecturer, University of North Carolina at Chapel Hill, Chapel Hill, NC, USA (*Temporary Adviser*)

APPENDIX A

A Model Assessment Guide for Nursing in Industry

Components	Questions to Ask
The Company	
Historical development	How, why, and by whom was the company founded?
Organizational chart	What is the formal order of the system, and to whom are the health providers responsible?
Company Policies	Is there a policy manual? Are the workers aware of existence of the manual?
Length of the work week	How many days a week does the industry operate?
Length of the work time	Are there several shifts? How many breaks? Is there paid vacation?
Sick leave	Is there a clear policy, and do the workers know it?
Safety and fire provisions	Is management aware of situations or substances in the plant that represent a potential danger? Are there organized fire drills? (The *Federal Register* is the source of information for federal standards and serves as a helpful guide.)
Support services (benefits)	Is there a system for health insurance and life insurance, and is it compulsory?
Insurance programs	Does the company pay all or part? Who fills out the necessary forms?
Retirement program	Are the benefits realistic?
Educational support	Can the workers further their education? Will the company help financially?
Safety committee	If there is no committee, do certain people routinely handle emergencies? The Red Cross First Aid Course through programmed instruction is excellent (for information consult your local Red Cross).
Recreation committee	Do the workers have any communication with or interest in each other outside the work setting?
Employee relations	Are there problems in employee relations? (This is difficult information to get, but it is important to get a sense of how employees feel generally about management and vice versa.)
The Plant	
General physical setting	What is the overall appearance?
The construction	What is the size and general condition of buildings and grounds?
Parking facilities and public transportation stops	How far does the worker have to walk to get inside?
Entrances and exits	How many people must use them? How accessible are they?
Physical environment	What conditions exist in the physical environment? (Comment on heating, air-conditioning, lighting, glare, drafts, and so forth)
Communication facilities	Are there bulletin boards and newsletters?
Housekeeping	Is the physical setting maintained adequately?
Interior decoration	Are the surroundings conducive to work? Are they pleasing?

Components	Questions to Ask

The Plant
Work areas
  Space — Are workers isolated or crowded?
  Heights: workplace and supply areas — Is there a chance of workers falling or being injured by falling objects? (Falls and falling objects are dangerous and costly to industry.)
  Stimulation — Is the worker too bored to pay attention?
  Safety signs and markings — Are dangerous areas well marked?
  Standing and sitting facilities — Are chairs safe and comfortable? Are there platforms to stand on, especially for wet processes?
  Safety equipment — Do the workers make use of hard hats, safety glasses, face masks, radiation badges, and so forth? Do they know the safety devices that the OSHA regulations require?

Nonwork areas
  Lockers — If the work is dirty, workers should be able to change clothes. Are they accidentally carrying toxic substances home on their clothes?
  Hand-washing facilities — If facilities and supplies are available, do workers know how and when to wash their hands?
  Rest rooms — How accessible are they, and what condition are they in?
  Drinking water — Can workers leave their jobs long enough to get a drink of water when they want to?
  Recreation and rest facilities — Can a worker who is not feeling well lie down? Do workers feel free to use the facilities?
  Telephones — Can a worker receive or make a call? Does a working mother have to stay home for a call because she can't be reached at work?
  Ashtrays — Are people allowed to smoke in designated areas? Are they safe areas?

The Working Population: Include worker and management, but separate data for comparison.
General characteristics — (Be as accurate as possible, but estimate when necessary.)
  Total number of employees — (Usually, if an industry has 500 or more employees, full-time nursing services are necessary.)
  General appearance — Are there records of heights, weights, cleanliness, and so forth? Ask to see them.
  Age and sex distribution — What are the proportions of the different groups? (Certain screening programs are specific for young adults, whereas others are more for the elderly. Some programs are more for women; others are more for men.) Is there any difference between day and evening shift populations? Are the problems of the minority sex unattended?
  Race distribution — Does one race predominate? How does this compare with the general community?
  Socioeconomic distribution — Are there great differences in worker salaries? (This can sometimes cause problems.)
  Religious distribution — Does one religion predominate? Are religious holidays observed?
  Ethnic distribution — Is there a language barrier?
  Marital status — What proportion of the workers are widowed, singles, or divorced? (These groups often have different needs.)
  Educational backgrounds — Can all teaching be done at approximately the same level?
  Lifestyles practiced — Is there disapproval of certain lifestyles?
Types of employment offered
  Background necessary — What educational level is required? Skilled versus unskilled?
  Work demands on physical condition — What level of strength is needed? Is the work sedentary or active?
  Work status — How many employees work full-time? Part-time? Is there overtime?

(continued)

Components	Questions to Ask

The Working Population: Include worker and management, but separate data for comparison.

Absenteeism	Is there a record kept? By whom? Why?
Causes	What are the five most common reasons for absence?
Length	What are the patterns of absences? (Absenteeism is costly to the employer. There is some difference between one 10-day absence and 10 one-day absences by the same person.)
Physically handicapped	Does the company have a policy about hiring the handicapped?
Number employed	Where do they work? What do they do?
Extent of handicaps	Are they specially trained? Are they in a special program? Do they use prosthetic devices?
Personnel on medication	What medication does each of these employees take? Where does each person work?
Personnel with chronic illness	At what stage of illness is the employee? Where does the employee work? Will he or she be able to continue at this job?

The Industrial Process: What does the company produce and how?

Equipment used	Is the equipment portable or fixed? light or heavy?
General description of placement	Ask to have each piece of large equipment marked on a scale map.
Type of equipment	Fans, blowers, fast moving, wet, or dry?
Nature of the operation	Ask for a brief description of each stage of the process so that you can compare the needs and abilities of the worker with the needs of the job.
Raw materials used	What are they and how dangerous are they? Are they properly stored? Check the *Federal Register* for guidelines on storage.
Nature of the final product	Can the workers take pride in the final product or do they make parts?
Description of the jobs	Who does what? Where? (Label the map.)
Waste products produced	What is the system for waste disposal? Are the pollution-control devices in place and functioning?
Exposure to toxic substances	To which toxins are the workers exposed? What is the extent of exposure? (Include physical and emotional hazards. Remember that chronic effects of industrial exposure are subtle; a person often gets used to having mild symptoms and won't report them. The *Federal Register* contains specifications for exposure to toxins, and some states issue state standards.)

The Health Program: Outline what is actually in existence as well as what employees perceive to be in existence.

Existing Policies	Are there informal, unwritten policies?
Objectives of the program	Are they clear?
Preemployment physicals	Are they required? Are they paid for by the company? Is the information used to select?
First aid facilities	What is available? What is not available?
Standing orders	Is there a company physician who is responsible for first aid or emergency policy? (If so, work closely with him or her in planning nursing services.)
Job descriptions for health personnel	Are they in writing? (If there are no guidelines to be followed, write some.)
Existing Facilities and Resources:	Sometimes an industry that denies having a health program has more of a system than it realizes.
Trained personnel	Who responds in an emergency?
Space	Where is the sick worker taken? Where is the emergency equipment kept?
Supplies	What are they? Where are they kept? (Make a list and describe the condition of each item.)

Components	Questions to Ask
The Health Program: Outline what is actually in existence as well as what employees perceive to be in existence.	
Records and reports	What exists? (The OSHA requires that employers keep three types of records: a log of occupational injuries and illnesses, a supplemental record of certain illnesses or injuries, and an annual summary [forms 100, 101, and 102 are provided under the act]. Good records provide data for good planning.)
Services rendered in the past year:	Describe as specifically as possible.
Care needed	Chronic or acute? Why?
Screening done	Where? By whom? Why?
Referrals made	By whom? To whom? Why?
Counseling done	Formal or informal? (Often informal counseling goes unnoticed.)
Health education	What individual or group education was offered by the company?
Accidents in the past year	During working hours? After hours? (Include those that occur after work hours; some may be directly or indirectly work related.)
Reasons why employees sought health care	What are the five major reasons?
Stressors	
As identified by employees	What pressures are felt on the job?
As identified by health providers	What problems do they perceive?

(Adapted from Serafini, P. (1976). Nursing assessment in industry: A model. American Journal of Public Health, 66(8),755–760.)

APPENDIX B

Assessment of an Industry

Components	Description
The Company	

	The AAB Chemical Company
	   Hampton Industrial Complex
	   Located west of State Highway 519 and Loop 177

Historical development	The AAB Chemical Company separated from the AAB Refinery in 1957, and the present plant was completed in 1961. The parent company is a major oil company with headquarters in Chicago. The plant is today the most complex and versatile in the AAB system.
Organizational chart	A formal organizational chart was not available. However, by observation and interview, a structure consisting of a plant manager, with a supervisor in charge of each production area, safety, and maintenance was noted. There are overseers for each area of operation for each shift. The medical staff, which consists of one doctor and one nurse, are not hired by the plant personnel department but by the parent company in Chicago.
Company policies	The plant operations are never shut down. There are shifts around the clock for operators and craftspeople. Employees such as clerical, administrative, and medical staff work 8-hour days, 40-hour weeks. Breaks are provided during the work period. Employees are eligible for 2 weeks of paid vacation per year after working 1 year. This increases in 5-year increments. A 20-year employee is eligible for 5 weeks of vacation. Employees are eligible for sick leave after 6 months of service. Benefits vary with length of service. All benefits are published in an employee handbook, distributed to all employees.
	Management is well aware of situations and substances that pose danger to the workers. The safety program, run by a safety supervisor and a safety engineer, is extensive. Organized fire drills are held frequently. Procedures for dealing with spills and other hazards are also well organized. Fire-fighting equipment and an ambulance are available on the plant site at all times. Certain employees are trained as firefighters. There are EMTs available inside the plant in addition to the nurse. Fire extinguishers are placed throughout the plant in strategic locations.
Support services	A comprehensive medical expense plan is compulsory for all employees. In addition, disability up to 40 weeks owing to occupational illness or injury is provided to all employees regardless of length of service. Term life insurance under a group plan is available at a low rate. A long-term disability plan is available to employees covered under the basic life insurance plan. A retirement plan is provided at complete cost to the company. A savings plan in which employees may invest in company stock and U.S. Savings Bonds is also available.
	Employees are offered an educational assistance program and are encouraged to advance their careers. On-the-job training is provided to help employees advance.

Components	Description
Employee relations	The workers are affiliated with the Oil, Chemical and Atomic Workers International Union, a part of the AFL-CIO. It was difficult to perceive how management and labor relate to each other. However, several workers mentioned the familylike atmosphere among employees, and hopefully, this bridges the gap between labor and management. The last strike occurred approximately two years ago.
The Plant General physical setting	The appearance of the plant is best described as an intimidating maze of pipes, towers, and vessels. The main building, in which the clinic is located, is modern and attractive, with well-tended grounds. Ample parking is available, with areas provided for the handicapped. The building is air conditioned, spacious, and clean, with a pleasing interior. The grounds and buildings inside the plant are also neat and well maintained. Scattered through the plant in strategic locations are eye-bubbling devices for flushing the eyes and showers for removing irritants from the skin. Danger areas are clearly marked with yellow paint and warning signs. Employees working in areas where hydrofluoric acid is used are provided with complete protective covering, and they shower immediately upon leaving the area. Ear plugs and ear muffs are required in high-noise areas. Compliance in use of safety devices is good, and workers are aware of Occupational Safety and Health Administration (OSHA) regulations.
Work areas	Some work areas, especially where craftspeople are involved, are cramped and close, owing to the physical structure of the myriad pipes and lines. Some areas are also elevated in height. One problem noted by the plant nurse is occasional heat stress during summer months when employees are working in these areas on equipment that reflects heat. Another problem noted was the stress, manifested in muscle and joint discomfort, of working in cramped quarters, especially when employees work a lot of overtime. Occasionally employees are injured by falling objects such as heavy wrenches. Burns are the most common type of injuries. Operators who work in the processing units and monitor the gauges and flow rates are in stressful jobs because a mistake could be costly and dangerous.
Nonwork areas	Each work area has a kitchen area, restrooms, and water fountains that are easily accessible. Lockers and showers are also available. Communication by phone is possible in all areas of the plant. Facilities are available in the clinic so that workers who are ill may lie down. However, in some areas, repeated visits to the clinic are discouraged. Employees are instructed regarding handwashing and prompt attention to small wounds by the nurse as part of new employee orientation. Smoking is permitted only in specifically designated parts of the fenced area of the plant, the docks, and warehouses.
The Working Population General characteristics	AAB Chemicals employs approximately 500 people. Age and sex distribution data were not available. However, the plant nurse stated that employees range in age from age 18 to retirement at age 65, and that male employees outnumber female employees. The nurse also stated that some women were moving into previously male-dominated jobs. Race distribution data were not available. By observation, the distribution appeared to be predominantly white, followed by black and then hispanic employees, which is in line with the population

(continued)

Components	Description

The Working Population

General characteristics

distribution in the community. Data regarding religious and marital status were not available. Wages and salaries are commensurate with education, qualifications, and years of service. Educational backgrounds range from high school graduates to advanced degrees in engineering and the sciences. Therefore, health teaching must be geared to match the educational level of the group being instructed.

Type of employment offered

Types of employment include skilled craftspeople, operators, lab analysts, chemists, engineers, clerical and administrative personnel, and a nurse and a physician. The background required for each area varies with the complexity and nature of the job. Most employees are full-time and work overtime as required.

Absenteeism

Records of absences are kept in the employee's work unit. The nurse keeps records on illness- or injury-related absences. An employee who has been absent owing to an extended or serious illness, an injury, or surgery must report to the medical department before returning to work and must supply a statement from a doctor regarding the nature of his or her disability and the limitations, if any, on permissible work. The medical department then determines the physical condition of the employee and notifies his or her supervisor regarding the employee's return to work. Strict record keeping also is done for OSHA requirements. According to the nurse, the most common reasons for absence are not occupationally related. They are most often for upper-respiratory infections and other common health problems or for accidents that occurred away from the plant.

Physically handicapped

The AAB Company is an equal opportunity employer. Information regarding handicapped employees, the nature of their handicaps, and the jobs they fill was not available.

Personnel on medication
Personnel with chronic illness

The nurse keeps records of employees on medication. This information is confidential. The confidentiality of employees' medical records is strictly enforced.

The Industrial Process

Equipment used
Nature of the plant operation

The basic job of the plant is to produce specialty chemicals and petrochemical intermediates for manufacture of products that range from boats and surfboards to carpets and furniture. Production of these chemicals involves moving raw materials (called "feedstock") from AAB's Hampton Refinery and another chemical plant and mixing them with xylenes and benzenes. Some of the chemicals produced are propylene, styrene, paraxylene, metazylene, aromatic solvents, oil-recovering chemicals, oil-producing chemicals, and polybutenes. The equipment used involves miles of pipes and many towers and vessels. Process units are designed to be energy efficient, and in many instances energy-producing hydrocarbons are a by-product of a process. These are then recovered and used as fuel in other operations.

Flammability and danger of explosion are major concerns when dealing with the above-named chemicals. Proper storage is essential and is carried out with care in this plant.

The final product of the production process is barrels of chemicals. Workers take pride in turning out a certain number of barrels in a time period and in keeping the plant operating efficiently.

The treatment of wastewater is through an effluent water-control system that is one of the most sophisticated in the industry. The facility handles wastewater not only from AAB Chemicals but also from the AAB Refinery and another chemical

Components	Description
The Industrial Process	plant in the area. Air-pollution control is done in two steps, first by eliminating potential contaminants whenever possible and then through the use of devices such as scrubbers, filters, cyclone separators, and a flare system to burn up the waste hydrocarbons.
Exposure to toxic substances	The major substances of concern are benzene and xylene. Benzene is a colorless, flammable, volatile liquid. The major hazard with this chemical is chronic poisoning by inhalation of small amounts over a long time. It is one of the most dangerous organic solvents in common use. Benzene acts primarily on the blood-forming organs. Skin contact also is to be avoided. Benzene is suspected of being carcinogenic. Xylene resembles benzene in many chemical and physical properties but is not involved in causing chronic blood diseases. It has a narcotic effect and can cause dermatitis with repeated contact. Benzene screening is done on all employees on a yearly basis.
The Health Program Existing policies	The objectives of the program are to monitor the status of each employee's health in order to pinpoint problems at an early stage and to provide prompt attention to accidents or emergencies as they occur at the worksite. The employees perceive the second objective more readily than the first. Many of them perceive the yearly physicals as a low priority. Preemployment physicals are done by the nurse and company doctor at no charge to the client and are used as a baseline for future reference. The ambulance kept at the plant is equipped for all emergencies. Injured or ill employees requiring more than initial first aid are taken immediately to Jefferson Memorial Hospital. There is a set of comprehensive standing orders, written through collaborative effort by the nurse and doctor. Yearly physicals include chest roentgenogram, blood work that includes benzene screening, urinalysis, vision and hearing assessments, and physical exams by the physician. Pregnant women are seen each month by the doctor in addition to their own private doctors. No screening programs alone are done, but they are incorporated into the yearly physical. Health teaching and informal counseling are done on an individual basis by the nurse and doctor. CPR is taught to selected personnel through the plant by the nurse.
Existing facilities and resources	The medical department consists of one full-time nurse and a physician who cover this plant and AAB's larger plant near Avina, as well as a part-time secretary. The facilities include the nurse's office, where all medical records are kept and where employees check in when visiting the clinic; a treatment room; a small lab and dispensary; a roentgenogram room; an exam room, and the physician's office. Fist aid facilities are extensive and well supplied. EKG equipment also is available. The nurse sees between 12 and 15 clients per day in the clinic. The major reasons employees seek health care are nonoccupationally related sicknesses or accidents, stress-related complaints, and minor accidents on the job.
Stressors Employees	Job pressure, as with operators who control the process units Overtime hours, when worked frequently Knowledge of potential fire or explosion

(continued)

Components	Description
Stressors	
Employees	Shift work that may not be in sync with normal body rhythms
	Strikes or layoffs
Health care providers	Problems with role definition. Nurse wishes to do more health teaching but feels Safety Department has taken over many of her functions. Feels powerless to change the situation. Feels that physician also perceives her role as limited to specific, traditional areas.

Index

Page numbers followed by *f* indicate figures; those followed by *t* indicate tabular material.